HEALTH, SAFETY, AND NUTRITION FOR THE YOUNG CHILD

Lynn R. Marotz, MEd, BSN, RN
Jeanettia M. Rush, MA, BS, RD
Marie Z. Cross, PhD, MS, BS

Department of Human Development and Family Life
University of Kansas
Lawrence, Kansas

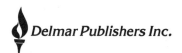

Delmar Publishers Inc.

This book is dedicated to our husbands and children for their love, encouragement and continued support of our efforts.

Cover photo: Joseph Schuyler Photography

Delmar staff
  Administrative editor: Adele O'Connell
  Production editor: Ruth Saur

For information, address Delmar Publishers Inc.
2 Computer Drive West, Box 15-015
Albany, New York 12212

Printed in the United States of America
Published simultaneously in Canada
by Nelson Canada,
A division of International Thomson Limited

10 9 8 7 6 5 4 3 2

Library of Congress Cataloging in Publication Data

Marotz, Lynn R.
  Health, safety, and nutrition for the young child.

  Includes index.
    1. Children—Care and hygiene. 2. Children—Nutrition. 3. Children's accidents—Prevention. I. Rush, Jeanettia M. II. Cross, Marie Z. III. Title.
  [DNLM: 1. Child Care. 2. Child Nutrition. 3. Accident Prevention—in infancy & childhood. WS 113 M355h]
  RJ101.M347 1985   649'.1   84-23845
  ISBN 0-8273-2052-3

CONTENTS

PREFACE

A child's health status, a safe but challenging learning environment, and proper nutrition affect the care, nurturance and optimal physical and cognitive development of the young child. A decade ago, each of these subject areas was viewed as a separate entity, but research has shown that the correlation among them is so intertwined that they cannot be completely separated. Philosophies concerning health care have also undergone notable change. Today, there is a great deal of attention being focused on the concept of preventive health care—care that recognizes the relationship between health status, safety, and nutrition, as well as the need for individuals to become involved and responsible for their own well-being.

Health, Safety, and Nutrition for the Young Child is intended for students working in an educational setting, for child care providers, and for adults and parents who desire additional information about current concepts in the fields of health, safety, and nutrition and their relationship to the young child. The text is also intended to help adults assist young children to develop good habits and attitudes, and to assume lifelong responsibility for their own well-being.

Each unit of this book begins with learning objectives. Key words are noted and italicized in the text and defined in the glossary. Those who are using the book as a text will find the summaries, learning activities, and unit review material of special interest. The Instructor's Guide includes answers to review questions, additional test items, audiovisual resources, and discussion topics that can be used to focus attention on particular subject areas.

The material included in this book is based on professional and popular information that is both current and accurate at the time of writing. The authors realize, however, that new developments and research may alter some current philosophies and techniques. Therefore, the reader is encouraged to keep abreast of current literature from sources similar to those cited in the text, and to keep informed of recent developments and research cited or conducted by professional early childhood organizations.

ABOUT THE AUTHORS

Lynn R. Marotz received her M.Ed. from the University of Illinois and a B.S. in Nursing from the University of Wisconsin. Currently she is the health and safety coordinator for the Edna A. Hill Child Development Laboratories at the University of Kansas. She teaches several courses in health and safety and works closely with graduate and undergraduate students in the early childhood program. She has made many professional presentations to academic, professional and community groups on health and safety issues and has written several items on these topics.

Jeanettia Rush, R.D., received her M.A. and is currently pursuing a doctorate in human development from the University of Kansas. A graduate of the dietetics and institutional management program at Kansas State University and the dietetic internship program of the University of California, she worked as a hospital dietitian for five years. She has experience as a nutrition consultant for Meals On Wheels and Educare Laboratory Child Care Center. She is currently involved in teaching basic nutrition courses at the University of Kansas, Lawrence, Kansas.

Marie Cross received her B.S., M.S. and Ph.D. degrees from the University of Wisconsin and is currently an associate professor in the Department of Human Development at the University of Kansas. Her teaching experience includes undergraduate courses in basic and applied nutrition and graduate courses related to nutrition and child development. Current research involves the development of appropriate materials for nutrition education programs at levels ranging from preschool to college.

AN ACKNOWLEDGMENT TO THOSE WHO HELPED

The authors wish to express their appreciation to a number of special people whose encouragement and technical assistance helped to bring this book to fruition. They wish to thank K. Eileen Allen, Professor of Human Development and Family Life, University of Kansas, for her recommendations and support of their interest and work in the area of child health, safety and nutrition. They also wish to thank Gary Mason, Associate Professor of the School of Journalism, University of Kansas, for his unique ability to photograph young children. They are very grateful to their typists Jennifer Lamb, Andy Knickerbocker, Peggy Baker, and Alberta Wright for their extraordinary assistance. Also, they wish to thank the editorial and production staff at Delmar Publishers for their encouragement and guidance in preparing this book.

The authors also wish to express appreciation to the following reviewers for their comments and recommendations:

Jan Smith, MEd, BS
Coordinator, Child Development Program
College of the Mainland
8001 Palmer Highway
Texas City, TX

Sue Creech, MAEd, MAHE, BSEd
Chair, Childhood Education Programs
Pitt Community College
Greenville, NC

Margaret Dotson, MS, BS
Associate Professor, Early Childhood Education
Sinclair Community College
Dayton, OH

Florence Munuz, MA
Associate Professor, Early Childhood Development
Oakton Community College
Des Plaines, IL

Jeanne M. Machado, MA
Department Chairperson, ECE
San Jose City College
San Jose, CA

Bess-Gene Holt, PhD
Early Childhood Consultant
Ames, IA

Tom Gordon, MS, BA
Chair, Department of Human Services
Montgomery Technical College
PO Drawer 487
Troy, NC

L.M.
J.R.
M.C.

Section

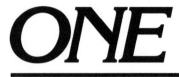

ONE

HEALTH, SAFETY,
AND NUTRITION:
AN INTRODUCTION

INTERRELATIONSHIP OF HEALTH, SAFETY, AND NUTRITION

Terms to Know

sedentary	*nutrient*
heredity	*malnutrition*
health	*overnutrition*
obese	*undernutrition*
preventive	*resistance*
habit	

Objectives

After studying this unit, you will be able to:
- *Describe the interrelationship of health, safety and nutrition.*
- *List five environmental factors that have a negative effect on health.*
- *List five environmental factors that have a positive effect on health.*
- *State how nutrition affects children.*
- *Differentiate between overnutrition and undernutrition.*
- *Define preventive health care.*
- *Identify three factors that affect children's safety.*
- *State three ways through which early childhood care providers can protect the health, safety, and nutrition of their young children.*

Many positive changes have taken place over the last several years in attitudes and practices relative to personal *health*. The concept of *preventive* health care has grown in response to costly medical care and realization that the medical profession is not always able to cure every health problem. New research data have provided conclusive evidence that changes in basic life-style can lead to improved health status (Saward 1978; Iverson 1983).

The basic philosophy of preventive health care is based on the principle that individuals can exercise control over many of the factors that affect their health. Every child and adult can learn to accept greater responsibility for developing and maintaining attitudes, *habits* and practices that will promote good health (Gephart 1984). This responsibility includes the need to establish good dietary habits and safety practices such as eating balanced meals and wearing seat belts in addition to regular physical exercise and early treatment of occasional illness and injury. Personal and professional medical approaches work together to help ensure a state of long-term well-being.

HEALTH

Definitions of health are as numerous as the factors which affect it. In the past, the term referred only to an individual's physical status and emphasis was placed on the treatment of apparent disorders. Today, the concept of health is much broader and encompasses more than the absence of illness and disease. International professional groups such as the World Health Organization describe health in terms of a state or quality of total physical, mental and social well-being; each element is assumed to make an equally important contribution to health. Furthermore, factors affecting the quality of one element are known to have an effect on the others. For example, a stressful home environment may lead to frequent illness, such as stomachaches, headaches, or asthma in children. Also, the presence of a chronically ill child in the home can have profound effects on the state of the parents' mental health.

This broader concept of health also recognizes that children and adults do not exist in isolated settings. Rather, they are important members of a variety of social groups, including families, peers, community and society. The quality of their social interactions and contributions to these groups often affects, and is affected by, their state of health, Figure 1-1.

Factors Influencing Health

Health status is determined, in part, by specific biological materials that are inherited at conception and influenced by numerous factors in the environment. Thus, health status is a dynamic quality that can change from setting to setting, moment to moment, day to day and year to year.

Heredity. Characteristics transmitted from parents to their children at the time of conception determine all of the genetic traits of a new, unique individual. *Heredity* sets the limits for growth, development and health potential, Figure 1-2. It partly explains why children in one family are short while those from another family are tall. Heredity helps to explain why some individuals have allergies or need glasses to see while others do not.

The heredity factor can be useful for predicting those children who are likely to inherit certain health problems such as heart disease, cancer or diabetes. Early

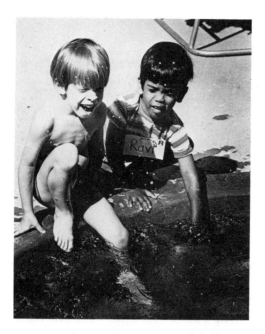

FIGURE 1-1   The quality of children's social interactions affects, and is affected by, their state of health.

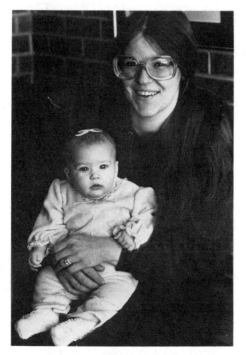

FIGURE 1-2   Heredity sets the limits for growth, development and health potential.

recognition of these conditions is very important for minimizing their long-term effect on a child's health.

Environment. Heredity provides the basic building materials for health status but the environment also plays an important role. In a simplified way, an environment is made up of physical, social and cultural factors that influence the way people perceive and react to their surroundings. Environmental factors affect physical, mental and behavioral patterns, and ultimately influence the way in which an individual's inherited potentials will be realized (Mullin 1983). Some environmental factors are positive and promote good health:

- good dietary habits
- physical exercise and adequate rest
- quality medical and dental care
- a safe and sanitary environment
- limited stress
- good interpersonal relationships with others

On the other hand, exposure to chemicals and pollution, abuse, illness, obesity, *sedentary* life-styles, stress, poor diet and inadequate medical and dental care are negative influences and interfere with the achievement of optimal growth and development.

Early childhood is a prime time to introduce good health habits and attitudes. Many behavior patterns that affect the long-term quality of health, such as personal cleanliness, exercise, and methods for expressing one's emotions, are learned through early and repeated experiences, Figure 1–3. They often become well established during the early years and are frequently carried over into adulthood (Mahoney 1982). For these reasons, it is very important that parents and care givers provide young children with accurate information and help them develop attitudes and practices that will promote good health. Learning positive behaviors from the very beginning is much easier than having to reverse poor habits later in life.

SAFETY

Safety refers to the behaviors and practices that protect children and adults from risk or injury. Safety is of special concern with young children because their well-being is directly affected by a safe environment. Accidents account for the greatest single cause of death among children 1 to 14 years of age. Consequently, effective prevention of accidental injury and death is a primary task of the adult care provider (Lubchenco 1982).

Accidents resulting in even minor injuries have an immediate effect on children's health. Learning and participation in activities are temporarily interrupted, and if an injury is serious, a child may be absent from the classroom for a prolonged period of time. Serious injuries also result in added medical expenses and increased stress for both the child and family.

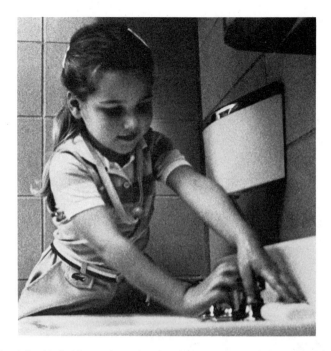

FIGURE 1-3   Good health habits such as handwashing are learned through early and repeated experiences.

Factors Affecting Children's Safety

An awareness of children's developmental abilities at various stages is a critical factor that affects their safety (Smolensky 1977; Cataldo 1982). Adults can use this information to identify sources of potential danger in the child's environment. Knowing that an infant enjoys hand-to-mouth activities should alert adult care givers to continuously check the environment for small objects or poisonous substances that could be accidentally ingested. Recognizing the toddler's curiosity and desire to explore the unknown should make adults concerned about such things as children wandering away, pedestrian safety, unsupervised pools and availability of unsafe materials, Figure 1-4.

Limits or rules set by concerned adults are another important factor affecting children's safety. Rules must be expressed in simple terms that children can understand, yet not be so overly restrictive that they create fear. Rules should be taught and consistently enforced. However, care providers must be cautious not to become overly trusting of a child who has supposedly ''learned the rules'' because spontaneity frequently overcomes learned behaviors.

The Importance of Safety Education

During the early years, it is the care provider's responsibility to protect young children from injury. However, as children grow older, safety education also be-

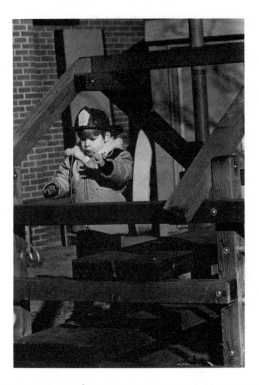

FIGURE 1–4 In order to provide a safe environment, care providers must be aware of children's desire to explore.

comes an important factor in accident prevention. Eventually, explanations must be included in rules so as to instill the importance of these behaviors, such as, "I don't want you to run out into the street. A car might not see you in time and you could get hurt." Educational experiences related to safety instruction must gradually go beyond teaching children only simple facts and rules. They should interest and excite children in participating in their own protection.

The fact that children often learn more from what they see than what they are told cannot be overlooked in safety education. Setting good examples of positive safety practices, such as wearing seat belts, obeying pedestrian signs, and keeping stairways clear of objects, is one of the most important responsibilities that care providers and parents share. Such good examples help to create safe environments where young children begin to learn, understand and assume responsibility for their own safe behaviors.

NUTRITION

Nutrition can be defined as "all the processes used by the adult or child to take in food and to digest, absorb, transport, utilize and excrete food substances"

(Endres 1980). The components or substances found in foods are called *nutrients*.

Food is essential for life; what children and adults eat affects their nutritional status as well as their health. Food supplies essential nutrients that the body requires for:

- energy
- growth and development
- normal behavior
- resistance to illness and infection
- tissue repair

A daily intake of essential nutrients depends on eating a variety of foods in adequate amounts. However, the availability of food is often determined by one's environment—the availability of money, geographic location, cultural preferences and consumer knowledge of good nutrition. The majority of children in the United States live in a time and place where food is abundant. Yet, there is growing concern for the number of children who may not be getting enough or the right types of food to eat.

Effects of Nutrition on Children

Nutritional status affects children's behavior. Well-nourished children are more alert and attentive and are better able to benefit from physical activity and learning experiences. Poorly-nourished children may be quiet and withdrawn, or hyperactive and disruptive during class activities. *Obese* children also face many problems. They are often slow and less able to participate in physical activity. They may suffer from added ridicule and emotional stress by being excluded from peer groups (Brownell 1984).

Children's *resistance* to infection and illness is also definitely influenced by their nutritional status (Weisel 1982). Children who are well nourished are less likely to become ill; they also recover more quickly when they are sick. Poorly-nourished children are more susceptible to infections and illness. Illness increases the need for some nutrients. Thus, poor nutrition creates a cycle of illness, poorer nutritional status, and lowered resistance to illness.

Malnutrition. *Malnutrition* is a serious problem for many children but it is not always associated with poverty or a deprived environment. Children of middle and upper income families may also be malnourished because of unwise food selections (Pliner 1983). Frequent fast food meals, snacking habits, and skipped meals can seriously limit the variety of food choices which, in turn, limit the nutrients ingested.

Malnutrition occurs when there is a prolonged imbalance between the nutrients that are required and the nutrients that are actually eaten. Malnutrition may be the result of:

- *undernutrition*—an inadequate intake of one or more nutrients
- *overnutrition*—overconsumption of one or more nutrients

It is important that both of these conditions be avoided in the infant and young child. An adequate intake of all required nutrients is most critical during periods of active growth and development. Also, the effects of nutritional deficiency on physical development during certain stages of infancy and early childhood cannot always be reversed with improved dietary intake (Alford and Bogle 1982; Hurley 1979).

Nutrition Education

Children do not always know how to make correct food choices based on nutritional needs. Proper eating habits are a learned behavior and children must be trained to select and consume foods that contain essential nutrients and energy. Food habits developed during early childhood often last into adulthood.

Children gather much of their information and food preferences from adults who serve as important role models. Therefore, it is critical that parents, teachers and care providers work together to provide children with sound nutritional information and training. Food experiences that help children develop good attitudes toward food must be an integral part of early childhood education.

HEALTH, SAFETY, AND NUTRITION: AN INTERDEPENDENT RELATIONSHIP

Health, safety and nutrition are closely related because the quality of one affects the quality of the others. A healthy child is more likely to accept and eat a nutritious meal than a child who is ill. Pain, injury and infection decrease a child's appetite. At the same time, they place additional stress on the child's body and increase the need for certain nutrients, e.g. protein, carbohydrates, vitamins and minerals. Recovery from illness and injuries occurs more rapidly if these nutrients are supplied in adequate amounts. In other words, health affects nutritional requirements, while at the same time essential nutrients are necessary to restore and maintain health.

Good nutrition also plays an important role in safety and accident prevention. The child or adult who arrives at school having eaten little or no breakfast may experience low blood sugar. This results in decreased alertness and slowed reaction time which causes the individual to be more accident-prone and less able to avoid serious injury. Children and adults who are overweight are also more likely to have accidents. Excess weight impedes physical activity. Children who are overweight tire more quickly and may be slower to react in accident situations.

IMPLICATIONS FOR EARLY CHILDHOOD CARE PROVIDERS

Today, increasing numbers of children are being cared for outside of the home. Preschools, child care centers and day-care homes serve more children now than at any other time in the history of the United States. Because these children spend many hours away from their home environment, early childhood programs must direct greater attention to children's health, safety and nutritional needs. Activities, environments, meal planning and supervision should reflect a commitment to promoting the optimal growth and development of each infant and child served. Programs can fulfill this commitment by providing:

- protection
- services
- education

Protection

Early childhood programs have a moral and legal obligation to protect the children they serve. The physical arrangement of all spaces occupied by children should receive special attention. Both indoor and outdoor areas must be planned carefully to provide environments that are safe and designed to meet the developmental needs of young children. Daily inspections and prompt removal of hazardous materials, equipment and activities help to prevent accidents. Careful teacher supervision and the establishment of rules also reduce the chance for accidental injury.

Policies that address the health, safety and nutritional needs of children are important for early childhood programs to establish. These policies should reflect the goals and philosophy of an individual program. Examples of some general policy areas might include:

- who is responsible for providing first aid
- what types of emergency information should be obtained from parents

State licensing requirements make it necessary for child care facilities to adopt additional health policies, such as:

- the way sanitary conditions in the classrooms and food preparation areas are to be monitored
- the types of children that will be accepted into the program

For legal protection centers may also need to establish policies such as:

- the types of activities that require special parental permission
- when information concerning a child can be released

To be most useful, policies must be written in clear, concise terms which can be easily understood. Policies should describe the expectations and actions the program considers important and the penalty for noncompliance. New poli-cies should be fully explained and copies of the policies made available to those persons who are directly affected.

Measures taken to protect infants and young children from unnecessary ill-ness and disease are also an important responsibility of child care providers. Adherence to good sanitary standards and personal health practices such as disinfecting tables after each diaper change and careful handwashing help to control the spread of infectious disease in group settings. Education of both chil-dren and adult care providers also helps to ensure success.

Services

As a result of changes in society and family structure, responsibility for children's total health care is often shared by parents and care providers (Christi-ano 1982). However, primary responsibility for a child's health care still belongs to the parents. Parental consent must always be obtained before arrangements are made for any special testing, screening procedures, or treatment. To function effectively in this new role, teachers and care providers must have up-to-date information, a sound understanding of health, safety and nutrition issues that affect young children, and a cooperative relationship with parents.

Early identification of health impairments is critical to optimal realization of a child's growth and development. Care providers occupy an ideal position for

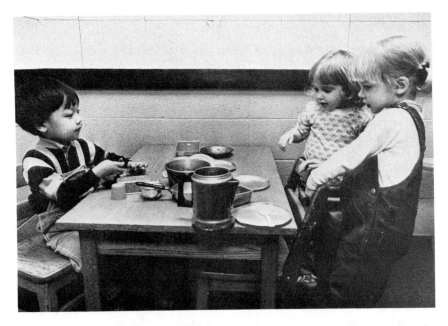

FIGURE 1-5   Daily experiences provide ideal opportunities for learning about health, safety and nutrition.

observing children's health and identifying children who require additional evaluation by health professionals. Various screening tests, such as vision, hearing and speech, should be made available to children. Families can be referred to appropriate sources in the community that provide these screenings.

Education

Caring for young children involves more than providing healthful, safe environments and serving nutritious meals. If children are to assume responsibility for their own well-being, they must be knowledgeable about health, safety and nutrition (Hindson 1979; Knobel 1983).

As part of early learning experiences, early childhood programs have an obligation to provide children with accurate information and to help them develop good attitudes and habits. Health, safety and nutrition concepts can be woven into daily experiences, making them more meaningful for the young child, Figure 1–5. For example, exercise can accompany musical activities, good nutrition can be stressed during snack time, and the importance of handwashing can be combined with cooking activities. In this way, young children can begin to see that health, safety and nutrition have important implications; they can then begin to integrate these concepts naturally into their everyday lives.

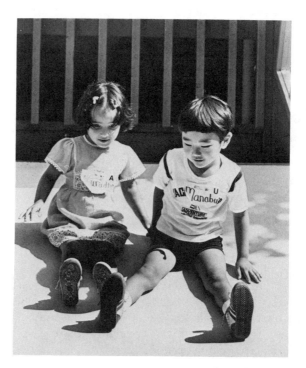

FIGURE 1–6 Good health allows children to function effectively with their peers.

SUMMARY

Preventive health care is a relatively new concept. It recognizes that health attitudes and practices are learned behaviors. It encourages individuals to take an active role in developing and maintaining practices that promote good health. Early childhood is perhaps the most critical time for establishing these habits.

Health is a dynamic state of physical, mental and social well-being. It allows children to realize their inherited potentials. It also permits children to function effectively as members of peer groups, families and society, Figure 1–6.

Genetic characteristics and environmental factors together shape the quality of an individual's health. Environments that are clean and safe, quality medical and dental care, and good nutrition all contribute to children's optimal growth and development.

A strong commitment to health, safety and nutrition is essential for early childhood programs. It encourages children's maximum growth and development by providing protection, services, and educational experiences to the children.

LEARNING ACTIVITIES

1. Find out what preventive health care programs are available to children in your community. Make a list of the various services each provides.

2. Observe a child eating lunch or dinner. What foods does the child eat? What foods are refused? Based on your observation, do you think the child is developing healthy eating habits? If there is an adult present, observe the adult's eating practices. Do you think the adult exhibits healthy eating habits? Do the adult's food likes and dislikes have any influence on what the children eat?

3. Review a menu from a child care center. Are a variety of foods served to children? Are meals and snacks offered at times when children are likely to be hungry? Does the staff encourage children to try different foods?

4. Contact your local public health department. Make arrangements to observe a routine well-child visit.

5. Compile a list of child care services available in your community. Note the variety of programs and services offered. Select five programs at random; check to see if they have waiting lists. If there is a waiting list, how long can parents expect to wait for placement of their child? How many of these programs accept children with special needs, e.g., physical disabilities, behavior problems, giftedness, learning disabilities?

UNIT REVIEW

A. Define the following terms:

 1. preventive health care

 2. nutrient

 3. heredity

 4. undernutrition

 5. overnutrition

B. Multiple Choice. Select the best answer.

 1. Current definitions of health include
    a. physical status
    b. emotional status
    c. social interactions
    d. all of these

 2. Health care is *primarily* the responsibility of
    a. teachers
    b. parents
    c. the extended family
    d. each child

 3. Environmental factors which may influence health include
    a. physical activity
    b. difficulty making friendships
    c. adequate nutrition
    d. all of these

 4. All essential nutrients can be obtained daily by
    a. eating the same foods every day
    b. eating fruits and vegetables in season
    c. eating a wide variety of foods daily
    d. none of these

 5. Factors that affect children's safety include
    a. careful supervision
    b. awareness of developmental skills
    c. set limits and rules
    d. all of these

 6. Undernourished children may exhibit the following behavior(s)
    a. withdrawal
    b. disruptive behavior
    c. hyperactivity
    d. all of these

7. The *limits* of growth and development are set by
   a. heredity
   b. good nutrition
   c. adequate medical supervision
   d. all of these

8. Health, safety, and nutrition education should be
   a. taught as a separate subject
   b. woven into daily experiences
   c. the responsibility of the parents only
   d. treated lightly in the preschool environment

C. Briefly answer each of the following:

1. List five environmental factors that have a negative effect on health.

2. List five environmental factors that have a positive effect on health.

3. Explain how heredity contributes to health.

4. Explain why an abundant food supply does not assure good nutrition for everyone.

5. List three bodily processes that are sustained through the consumption of food.

6. Explain how illness affects a child's nutritional needs.

7. Name three ways through which a preschool or child care center can fulfill its obligations to protect the health, safety, and nutrition of the children enrolled.

REFERENCES

Alford, B.B., and Bogle, M.L. *Nutrition During the Life Cycle.* Englewood Cliffs, NJ: Prentice-Hall, 1982.

Brownell, K.D. "The Psychology and Physiology of Obesity: Implications for Screening and Treatment." *Journal of American Dietetic Association,* April 1982.

Capitol Publications, Inc. "Dramatic Changes in Families Make Child Care Necessary." In *Report on Preschool Programs,* May 1, 1984.

Capitol Publications, Inc. "National Center for Educational Statistics." In *Report on Preschool Programs,* May 18, 1982.

Cataldo, C. *Infant and Toddler Programs: A Guide to Very Early Education.* Menlo Park, CA: Addison-Wesley Publishing Co., 1982.

Christiano, M.M. "Health Care of Children: A Continuing Struggle." *Early Childhood Development and Care* 8(1):45–53, 1982.

Gephart, J.; Egan, M.; and Hutchins, V. "Perspectives on Health of School-age Children: Expectations for the Future." *Journal of School Health* 54(1):11–17, January 1984.

Hindson, Paul. "Preschool Potential: A Health Educator's Perspective." *Australian Journal of Early Childhood* 4(3):7–12, September 1979.

Hurley, L.S. *Developmental Nutrition.* Englewood Cliffs, NJ: Prentice-Hall, 1982.

Iverson, Donald C., and Kolbe, L.T. "Evolution of the National Disease Prevention and Health Promotion Strategy: Establishing a Role for the Schools." *Journal of School Health* 53(5):294–302, May 1983.

Knobel, R.J. "Health Promotion and Disease Prevention: Improving Health While Conserving Resources." *Family/Community Health* 5(4):16–27, February 1983.

Lubchenco, A. "Good Measure of Safety: Safety in the Home Day Care Program." *Day Care and Early Education* 10:19–23, Winter 1982.

Mahoney, M.E. "Attitudes Affecting Child Health Care: A Perspective on the 1980s." *Advances in Pediatrics* 29:247–57, 1982.

Mullin, P.D. "Promoting Child Health." *Family and Community Health* 5(4):52–68, February 1983.

Pliner, P. "Family Resemblance in Food Preferences." *Journal of Nutrition Education,* December 1983.

Saward, E., and Sorenson, A. "The Current Emphasis on Preventive Medicine." *Science* 200:889–94, May 26, 1978.

Smolensky, J. *A Guide to Child Growth and Development.* 2nd ed. Dubuque, IA: Kendall/Hunt Publishing Co., 1977.

Weisel, W.R. "Single Nutrients and Immunity." *American Journal of Clinical Nutrition,* February supplement, 1982.

Additional Reading

"Better Health for Our Children: A National Strategy, Vol. III and Vol. IV." Report of the Select Panel for Promotion of Child Health, 1980.

"Healthy People." *The Surgeon General's Report on Health Promotion and Disease Prevention.* Washington, DC: U.S. Department of Health, Education and Welfare, 1979.

School Health in America, A Survey of State School Health Programs, 3d ed. Kent, OH: American School Health Association, December 1981.

Section

TWO

HEALTH OF THE YOUNG CHILD: MAXIMIZING THE CHILD'S POTENTIAL

PROMOTING
GOOD HEALTH

Terms to Know

autonomy	normal
characteristics	head circumference
growth	parallel play
development	deciduous teeth
developmental norms	bonding

Objectives

After studying this unit, you will be able to:

- *Identify growth and developmental characteristics of the infant and preschool child.*
- *List three areas of special concern regarding children's health.*
- *Describe how teachers can provide for the safety of preschool children.*
- *Explain how care providers influence children's mental health.*
- *State the relationship between good dental health and learning.*

The period of infancy is truly a marvel when one considers the dramatic changes in *growth* and *development* that occur. The infant progresses from a stage of complete helplessness and passiveness to one that enables the child to explore the environment and interact with others. The spectacular changes in growth and development that occur during this first year will never again be repeated throughout the entire lifespan.

The toddler years are characterized by an explosive combination of improved locomotion, seemingly unending energy, delightful curiosity, and an eagerness to become independent. Driven by the desire for *autonomy* or personal identity, toddlers display an intense determination to do things for themselves. As a result, special attention to safety and accident prevention must be a prime concern for care providers.

The preschool years are a time of great excitement and tremendous accomplishments. As children pass through this stage of life they continue to explore the enchanted world around them, but with an added dimension of understanding. The preschool child's efforts and skills become increasingly sophisticated, while concentration on basic needs such as eating, sleeping, mobility and communication grows less intense. Moving toward a sense of independence becomes a major task. Unlimited amounts of energy are united with a spirit of curiosity, imagination and adventurous instincts to create a dynamic child who continues to need careful adult supervision and guidance.

GROWTH AND DEVELOPMENT

Early childhood programs encompass education and care for infants through preschool; in some areas programs include after-school services. For this reason, it is important that teachers and care providers be familiar with the normal changes in growth and development that take place during each of these ages. A basic understanding allows adults to work more effectively with young children (Hendrick 1984). They are better prepared to help children master the critical skills and behaviors that are necessary during each stage by providing activities that are both appropriate and interesting and by setting performance standards that are realistic. This is also important information to have when setting up educational programs and environments that will protect and promote the health, safety and nutrition of young children. Knowledge of growth and development aids in the recognition of health impairments and deviations in children's skill levels and behaviors. Through such an understanding, adults can maximize the child's good health and zest for life.

Discussions of normal growth and development often make reference to the "average" child; such a child probably does not exist. Every child is a unique individual—a product of different experiences, environments, interactions and heredity, Figure 2–1. As a result, each child differs in some way from all other children (Tudor 1981).

This fact also leads to considerable variation in the rate at which children grow and acquire skills and behaviors (Department of Health, Education and Welfare 1979). Growth and *developmental norms* have been established to serve as a useful frame of reference. These norms represent the average or approximate age when the majority of children demonstrate a particular behavior or skill. Therefore, the term *normal* implies that while many children can perform a particular skill, some will be more advanced, and others may be somewhat slower, yet they are still considered to be within the normal range.

Growth

The term *growth* refers to the many physical changes that occur as a child matures. Although the process of growth takes place without much conscious

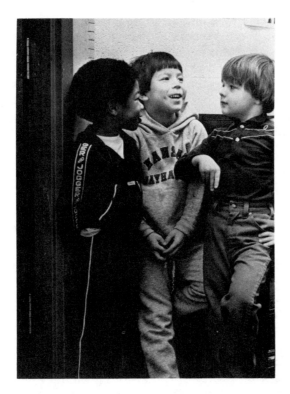

FIGURE 2-1 Each child is a unique individual—a product of different experiences, environments, interactions and heredity.

control, there are many factors that affect both the quality and quantity of growth:

- genetic potential
- cultural influences
- adequate nutrition
- health status
- level of emotional stimulation
- socioeconomic factors

Infants. The average newborn weighs approximately 7–8 pounds at birth and is approximately 20 inches in length. Growth is rapid during the first year; an infant's birth weight nearly doubles by the fifth month and triples by the end of the first year (Leach 1982). An infant weighing 8 pounds at birth should weigh 16 pounds at 5 months and approximately 24 pounds at 12 months.

Increases in length during the first year represent approximately 50 percent of the infant's original birth length. An infant measuring 21 inches at birth should reach a length of approximately 31.5 inches at 12 months of age. A larger percentage of this gain takes place during the first six months when an infant may grow as much as one inch per month.

Rapid growth of the brain causes the infant's head to appear very large in proportion to the rest of the body. Measurements of *head circumference* are important indicators of normal growth. Measurements should increase steadily and equal the chest circumference by the end of the first year.

Other physical changes that occur during the first year include the growth of hair and the eruption of teeth (four upper and four lower). The eyes begin to focus and move together by the third month and hearing becomes more acute. Areas of special concern with regard to infant health include:

- nutritional requirements
- adequate provisions for sleep
- *bonding* or maternal attachment
- early stimulation—emotional, sensory, motor
- safety and accident prevention
- identification of birth defects and health impairments

Toddlers. The toddler continues to make steady gains in height and weight, but at a much slower rate than during infancy. A weight increase of 6–7 pounds per year is considered normal and reflects a total gain of nearly four times the child's birth weight by the age of two. The toddler grows approximately 3–5 inches in height per year. Body proportions change resulting in a more erect and adultlike appearance.

Eruption of "baby" or *deciduous teeth* is completed by the end of the toddler period. (Deciduous teeth consist of a set of 20 temporary teeth.) Toddlers should be taught how to brush and care for their new teeth as an important aspect of preventive health care. Although appetite may decrease during the toddler period, special attention should be given to providing foods that contain all of the essential nutrients and that promote good dental health. These foods include fruits and vegetables, cheese, meats, milk and milk products.

High activity levels require that the toddler get at least 10–12 hours of rest and sleep daily. Also, the need for safety and accident prevention continue to be a top priority for care providers of toddlers.

Preschoolers. During the preschool years a child's appearance becomes more streamlined and adultlike in form. Head size remains approximately the same, while the child's trunk (body) and extremities (arms and legs) continue to grow. Gradually, the head appears to separate from the trunk as the neck lengthens. Legs grow longer and at a faster rate than the arms, adding extra inches to the child's height. The characteristic chubby shape of the toddler is gradually lost as muscle tone and strength increase. These changes are also responsible for the flattening of the abdomen or stomach and straighter posture.

Gains in weight and height are relatively slow but steady throughout the preschool years. At 3 years of age, children weigh approximately five times their weight at birth. An ideal weight gain for a preschool child is approximately 4–5 pounds per year. However, a greater proportion of the preschool child's growth is the result of increases in height rather than weight. The typical preschool child grows an average of 2 to 2½ inches per year. By the time children reach 6 years of age, they have nearly doubled their original birth length (from approximately 20 inches to 40 inches). This combination of growth changes causes the preschool child to take on a longer, thinner appearance.

Adequate nutrition must continue to receive high priority during the preschool years (Endres 1980). High activity levels replace the rapid growth of earlier years as the primary demand for calories. However, this period is often marked by lessened appetite and poor eating habits. As a result, parents and care providers must pay very careful attention to children's actual food intake as well as their development of good nutritional habits.

Sleep is also an important requirement for optimum growth. When days are long and tiring or unusually stressful, the young child's need for sleep may be even greater. However, bedtime and afternoon naps are often a source of conflict between children and care providers. Preschool children tend to be so intensely busy and involved in play activities that they are reluctant to take time out for sleep. Nevertheless, young children benefit from a rest or break in their normal daytime activities. Planned quiet times with books, puzzles or a small toy may be sufficient for many children. Eight to twelve hours of uninterrupted sleep at night, in addition to daytime rest periods, are needed by the preschool child.

Development

In the time span of one year, the infant progresses from a stage of complete helplessness to a stage that is marked by locomotion, deliberate motor skills and the beginning of language. Infants become more social and outgoing near the end of the first year and seemingly enjoy and imitate the adults around them (Le francois 1980).

The toddler and preschool periods see a continued refinement of language, motor, cognitive and social abilities. Improved motor and verbal skills enable the toddler to explore, test and interact with the environment for the purpose of determining personal identity or autonomy.

Development of the preschool-aged child includes increased ability to perform self-care skills and improved strength, speed, accuracy and ease of performing tasks that require fine motor control. The beginning of a conscience slowly emerges. This is an important step in the process of socialization as it allows children to exercise control over some of their own emotions. Friendships with peers become increasingly important as preschool children begin to extend their sphere of acquaintances beyond the limit of family members.

A summary of major developmental achievements is presented in Table 2-1. It should be remembered that such a list represents the accomplishments that the majority of children can perform at a given age. It should also be noted that not every child achieves all of these tasks. Many factors, some of which are beyond the control of the individual child, influence the acquisition of such skills.

TABLE 2-1   Developmental Characteristics

2 months	Lifts head up when placed on stomach. Holds head erect when supported in a sitting position. Follows moving person or object with eyes. Imitates or responds to smiling person with occasional smiles. Rolls over from side to back. Turns toward source of sound. Begins to make simple sounds and noises.
4 months	Has good control of head. Reaches for and grasps objects with both hands. Laughs out loud; vocalizes with coos and giggles. Waves arms about. Rolls from side to side.
6 months	Grasps objects with entire hand; transfers object from one hand to the other and from hand to mouth. Sits alone with minimal support. Deliberately reaches for, grasps and holds objects. Rolls over; can turn self completely over. Babbles using different sounds. Raises up and supports weight of upper body on arms.
9 months	Sits alone; able to maintain balance while changing positions. Picks up objects with pincer grasp (first finger and thumb). Begins to crawl. Attempts words such as "mama" and "dada." Hesitant toward strangers. Explores new objects by chewing or placing them in mouth.
12 months	Pulls up to a standing position. May "walk" by holding on to objects. Stacks several objects one on top of the other. Responds to simple commands. Talks using 2–3 word sentences. Uses hands and eyes to investigate new objects. Can hold own eating utensils.
18 months	Climbs up and down stairs one at a time. Walks and runs with confidence. Enjoys being read to; likes toys for pushing and pulling. Vocabulary consists of approximately 5–12 words. Helps feed self, manages spoon and cup.
2 years	Runs, walks with ease; can kick and throw a ball; jumps in place. Speaks in 2–3 word sentences; asks simple questions; knows about 200 words. Displays parallel play. Daytime toilet trained. Voices displeasure.

3 years	Climbs stairs using alternate feet.
	Can hop and balance on one foot.
	Feeds self.
	Can help dress and undress self; washes own hands and brushes teeth with help.
	Is usually toilet trained.
	Curious; asks and answers questions.
	Enjoys drawing, cutting with scissors, painting, clay and make-believe.
	Can throw and bounce a ball.
	States name; recognizes self in pictures.
4 years	Dresses and undresses self; helps with bathing and manages own toothbrushing.
	Enjoys creative activities: paints, draws with detail, models with clay, builds imaginative structures with blocks.
	Rides a bike with confidence, turns corners, maintains balance.
	Climbs, runs and hops with skill and vigor.
	Enjoys friendships and playing with small groups of children.
	Enjoys and seeks adult approval.
5 years	Expresses ideas and questions clearly and with fluency.
	Vocabulary consists of approximately 2500–3000 words.
	Substitutes verbal for physical expressions of displeasure.
	Dresses without supervision.
	Seeks reassurance and recognition for achievements.
	Play is active and energetic, especially outdoors.
	Can throw and catch a ball with relative accuracy.
	Can cut with a scissors along a straight line.
	Draws with attention to detail.
6 years	Plays with enthusiasm and vigor.
	Develops increasing interest in books and reading.
	Displays greater independence from adults; fewer requests for help.
	Forms close friendships with several peers.
	Improved motor skills; can jump rope, hop and skip, ride a bicycle.
	Enjoys conversation.

PROMOTION OF GOOD HEALTH

Today, concern for children's health and welfare is shared by a variety of people. Changes in current life-styles, trends and expectations have resulted in a shifting of some of the responsibilities for children's health to the cooperative efforts of parents, teachers, child care providers and health professionals.

How are parents, care providers and teachers to determine whether or not children are healthy? What are the qualities of a "well" child? *Characteristics* of normal growth and development can be helpful in evaluating children's overall health status and developmental progress. However, they must be used cautiously, as there is much variation within the so-called normal range. Table 2–2

TABLE 2-2 Characteristics of the "Well" Preschool Child

A. Physical Characteristics		
1. alert and enthusiastic	X	
2. enjoys vigorous, active play	X	
3. appears rested when child arrives		
4. firm musculature		
5. growth—slow, steady increases in height and weight		
6. not easily fatigued		
7. inoffensive breath		
8. legs and back straight		
9. teeth well formed—even, clean, free from cavities		
10. lips and gums pink and firm		
11. skin clear (color is important) and eyes bright		
12. assumes straight posture		
13. large motor control well developed		
14. beginning to develop fine motor control		
15. good hand–eye coordination		
B. Social Behaviors		
1. enthusiastic		
2. curious—interested in surroundings		
3. enters willingly into a wide range of activities		
4. happy and friendly; cheerful most of the time		
5. developing self-confidence; anticipates success, copes with failure		
6. shares in group responsibilities		
7. works and plays cooperatively with peers		
8. respects other's property		
9. appreciates and understands other's feelings		
10. adapts to new situations		
11. enjoys friends and friendships		
12. participates in cooperative play		
13. understands language; can express thoughts and feelings to adults and peers		
14. demonstrates courage in meeting difficulties; recovers quickly from upsets		
15. begins to exercise self-control		
C. Characteristic Work Behaviors		
1. attentive		
2. begins to carry tasks through to completion		
3. increasing attention span		
4. is persistent in activities; is not easily frustrated		
5. can work independently at times		
6. demonstrates an interest in learning; curiosity		
7. shows originality, creativity, imagination		
8. accepts responsibility		
9. responds quickly and appropriately to directions and instructions		
10. works and shares responsibilities with others		
11. accepts new challenges		
12. adaptable		

identifies some of the physical and behavioral qualities based on these norms which can be observed in the "well" preschool child. Similar lists can be generated for infants and toddlers based on characteristics of growth and development.

SPECIAL CONSIDERATIONS

Preschool and child care programs have a substantial influence on the well-being of children. Many opportunities exist within these programs to promote good health and strengthen the concepts of preventive health care.

Teachers, parents, and care providers should give special consideration to important aspects of health, safety, and nutrition based on a child's age and stage of development. Three of these areas will be discussed: accident prevention, dental health, and mental health.

Accident Prevention

Accidental injuries are one of the greatest threats to the lives of young children (Arena 1978). They are also responsible for more than one-third of all deaths among children under 4 years of age. Accidental deaths result from motor vehicles, drownings, burns, falls and poisonings and are also responsible for thousands of additional injuries to children each year. For these reasons, safety awareness and accident prevention must be given prime consideration in schools, child care centers and the child's own home.

An understanding of normal growth and development is particularly useful when planning for the safety of young children. Many of the characteristics which make children exciting and a joy to work with are the same characteristics which make them likely victims of accidents. Children's skills are seldom as well developed as their determination, and in their zealous approach to life they often fail to recognize inherent dangers. Their limited experiences make it difficult for them to always anticipate the consequences of their actions.

Accidents are more likely to occur when certain conditions exist. Teachers and care providers must keep in mind that extra precautions should be taken whenever:

- they are not feeling well or are tired
- there are new staff members or visitors who are unfamiliar with the children
- they are upset or faced with a difficult experience, e.g. an uncooperative child, an unpleasant experience with a parent, a strained relationship with another staff member or a personal problem
- there is a shortage of staff members
- children are not able to play outdoors because of bad weather, e.g. snow, rain, extreme cold
- conditions are rushed
- there are new children in the classroom
- rules have not been carefully explained

Teachers and parents have a tremendous responsibility to protect the safety of young children (Olson 1980). This task requires adults to be continuously alert to situations or activities that involve any element of danger, Figure 2–2. Also, special precautions may need to be taken when children with physical disabilities are present. Basic measures which help to ensure children's safety include:

- advanced planning
- careful organization
- the establishment of rules
- close adult supervision

Taking these precautions will not necessarily eliminate all risks of accident. However, the chances of serious accidents or injuries can be lessened. Children should gradually learn how to avoid injury and protect themselves by developing good safety behaviors.

Dental Health

An area of health that is commonly overlooked in the young child is that of good dental care. The U.S. Department of Public Health estimates that as many as one-half of the children in this country under 15 years of age have never been

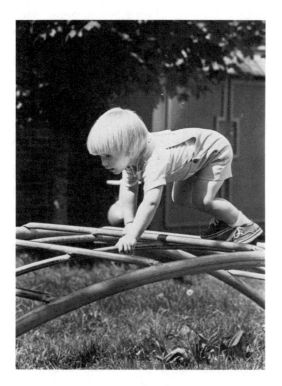

FIGURE 2–2 Adults must be continuously aware of hazards in children's environments.

seen by a dentist (National Center for Health Statistics 1972). This figure may actually be higher in poverty areas. Many parents hold the mistaken belief that "baby" or deciduous teeth are relatively unimportant because they eventually fall out. This belief is incorrect because these temporary teeth are necessary for:

- chewing
- the spacing of permanent teeth
- shaping of the jaw bone
- development of speech

The condition of children's teeth can also have a direct effect on their behavior and ability to learn. Neglected dental care can result in painful cavities and infected teeth making it difficult for children to concentrate and maintain interest in tasks and activities. Proper dental care must be practiced from birth, with special attention given to:

- diet
- hygienic practices—e.g. toothbrushing, flossing
- regular dental examinations
- prompt treatment of dental problems

A child's first visit to the dentist should be scheduled when the child is between 2 and 2½ years of age. These initial visits should be a pleasant experience. They should give the child an opportunity to become acquainted with the dentist and routine examinations without the discomfort of painful dental work. Hopefully, such positive dental experiences will discourage children from anticipating future dental examinations with fear and anxiety. Routine checkups at six to twelve month intervals are generally recommended as part of a preventive dentistry program.

Diet has an unquestionable effect on children's dental health (Newbrun 1982). Proper tooth formation depends on an adequate intake of protein and minerals, particularly calcium. One of the most devastating influences on diet, however, is the consumption of large amounts of highly refined carbohydrates, such as those found in cakes, cookies, candies, gum, soft drinks, and sweetened dry cereals. Obviously, a great deal of education of adults as well as children is necessary in this area (Hart 1980; Houle 1982). Care providers can help young children begin to adopt good dietary habits by limiting the frequency and amounts of sweets they are served and by substituting nutritious foods for those that are highly sweetened.

A daily routine of good oral hygiene is also essential for the promotion of good dental health. Children can begin brushing their teeth around 15 months of age. Several steps care providers can take to increase children's interest in learning to brush their own teeth include:

- purchasing a small, soft toothbrush in the child's favorite color
- storing the toothbrush where the child can reach it
- providing a footstool or chair so the child can reach the sink. **Caution:** Supervise the child closely to prevent slipping or falling.

- demonstrate the toothbrushing procedure so the child has an idea of what to expect
- encourage the child to brush teeth at least twice daily—once in the morning and again before going to bed
- construct a simple chart where children can place a check each time they brush their teeth; this provides a good method for reinforcing regular tooth-brushing habits.

Toddlers can be taught to brush their teeth with an adult's help. Preschool children are usually able to brush with minimal adult supervision. When a child is first learning toothbrushing skills, it is a good idea for an adult to brush over the teeth at least after one of the brushings each day to be sure all areas are clean. Children can also be taught alternative methods for cleaning teeth between brushings. These methods include rinsing out the mouth with water after eating and eating raw foods such as apples, pears, carrots, and celery that provide a natural cleansing action on the teeth.

Although their technique may not always be perfect, preschool children are, hopefully, establishing a life-long habit of good toothbrushing. In addition to proper technique, the use of a toothpaste containing fluoride has proven to be very beneficial in reducing dental cavities.

The question of whether or not young children should learn to floss their teeth is best answered by the individual child's dentist. Although the practice is regarded as beneficial, much depends on the child's maturity and fine motor skills. Parents can floss the teeth of children who are too young to floss their own teeth.

Regular dental supervision also contributes to good dental health. However, it cannot replace daily attention to good nutrition and hygiene. During routine examinations, dentists look for signs of any dental problems. They also review the child's toothbrushing technique and diet and personal habits that may have an effect on their teeth such as thumbsucking or grinding the teeth. Many dentists also include cleaning and an application of fluoride with their routine examinations. Fluoride added to city water supplies also has proven to significantly reduce tooth decay. X-ray examinations at every visit remains a controversial issue.

Mental Health

The preventive approach to health care recognizes the close relationship which exists between mental and physical health. Therefore, the promotion of children's well-being must also include a concern for their emotional health. Early childhood educators have long practiced preventive mental health concepts. They help young children learn to communicate with others, control their impulsive and aggressive behaviors, express their emotions, develop independence, handle success and failure, respond with ease to new situations and feel good about themselves. Teaching preschool children preventive concepts such as these improves their chances for enjoying good mental health.

The quality of children's mental health is determined by their ability to cope with their environment and adjust to change. The way children feel about themselves and others is also important (Crosby 1982). However, to be emotionally healthy, children must first experience satisfaction of their basic needs for food, water, sleep, shelter, safety, love, security, and achievement. These basic needs must be met before children can move on to develop a sense of autonomy, form good relationships with others and function effectively in group settings.

Teachers and care providers play a major role in fostering positive mental health among young children. They can best achieve this goal by:

- promoting good mental health practices
- preventing emotional problems
- identifying children with possible emotional disturbances.

The teacher's and care provider's own state of emotional or mental health is very important if they are to be successful in helping young children achieve good mental health. Teachers and care providers must have a sense of self-worth; they should feel confident that what they are doing is worthwhile. At the same time, they should be aware of their capabilities as well as their limitations. Teachers must also be able to exercise control over their emotions if they expect children to do the same. Teachers and care providers need to be honest and understanding. They should be able to accept success and failure, set realistic goals for themselves and the children they work with, and communicate effectively with others.

The emotional climate of a classroom or child care setting has a significant impact on children's mental health. Consider the following situations and decide which classroom is most inviting:

Kate enters the classroom excited and eager to tell her teacher about the tooth she lost last night and the quarter she found under her pillow from the "tooth fairy." Without any greeting, the teacher hurries to check Kate in and informs her that she is too busy to talk right now, "but maybe later." When they are finished, the teacher instructs Kate to find something to do without getting into trouble. Kate quietly walks away to her locker.

Ted arrives at the child care center and is reluctant to leave his mother. The care provider greets Ted and his mother. "Ted, I am so glad that you came to school today. We are going to build with the wooden blocks, and I know that is one of your favorite activities. Perhaps you would like to build something for your mother before it is time for her to go home." Ted eagerly builds a barn with several "animals" in the yard around it and proudly looks to his mother for approval. When Ted's mother is ready to leave, he waves good-bye.

Clearly, the classroom atmosphere or mood is influenced by the teacher's actions and responses, which in turn have a direct effect on children's behavior,

Figure 2–3. Young children are more receptive and likely to respond enthusiasti-cally to care providers who are warm, loving and sensitive to their special needs. Using ridicule, sarcasm, threats or unfair treatment is inappropriate and will have a negative impact on children's emotional development. When children are forced to cope with unpleasant situations of this type, they often develop and respond with undesirable behaviors. However, an emotional climate that encour-ages and supports mutual cooperation, respect, trust, acceptance, and indepen-dence allows children to build a strong foundation of positive mental health atti-tudes.

Understanding the developmental characteristics of young children facilitates the care provider's efforts to promote good mental health. Respect must be shown for a child's individuality for each child has qualities that are worthy of recognition. All children like to be praised for their efforts. However, they should also be accepted for what they are and not for what they can do. Teachers and care providers should be impartial; favoritism cannot be tolerated.

Teachers and care providers can promote children's mental health in other, more subtle ways. For example, activity or curriculum planning should take into account the developmental levels and abilities of children. By providing tasks and activities which are appropriate for their skill levels, it is possible for children to attain success more often than failure and frustration. Children need to experi-ence the rewards of achievement for continued motivation and interest in learn-ing. Schedules should also be planned carefully to allow for alternating periods of activity and rest, work and play, and indoor and outdoor times.

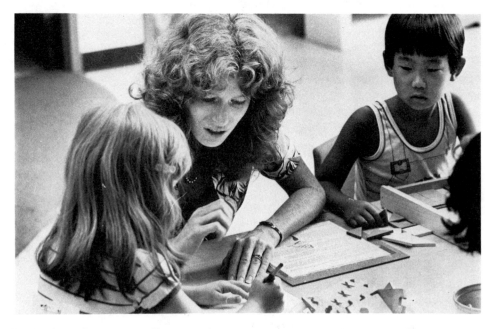

FIGURE 2–3 The teacher affects the classroom atmosphere which, in turn, affects children's behavior.

Stress in children's lives has a definite effect on the state of their mental health (Chandler 1982). It may be evident in children's behaviors in the form of unusual aggressiveness, withdrawal, hostility and nervousness, or it may present itself in symptoms of physical illness such as ulcers, headaches, vomiting, diarrhea, or difficulty breathing. Many experiences adults take in stride provoke feelings of anxiety, tension and stress in the young child:

- separation from parents
- new experiences—e.g. moving, placement in a day care center, mother going to work, the birth of a sibling, a new teacher, being left with a baby sitter
- illness and hospitalization
- divorce of parents
- death of a pet, family member or close friend
- conflict of ideas and confrontations with parents, friends or teachers
- overstimulation—hectic schedules, participation in numerous extracurricular activities.

Inexperience and immature development of children's coping mechanisms make it more difficult for the young child to handle stressful experiences in a healthy fashion (Mental Health 1973). Techniques of stress management can be implemented by teachers and care providers to help children learn effective means for dealing with stress (Cherry, 1981). Some of these methods include:

- the use of music for relaxation
- progressive relaxation techniques—the process of contracting and relaxing various body parts, beginning at one end of the body and moving toward the other
- relaxation activities—the use of imagery and visualization, make-believe, let's pretend, books and stories, movement activities
- short periods of vigorous physical activity followed by rest.

The topic of stress and children is receiving increased attention in current literature and research projects. As mental health problems and deaths from suicide continue to escalate among children, stress management should be an area of utmost concern to parents and care providers.

Care providers also have an important responsibility to help identify children with existing emotional problems. Early identification is extremely important to the success of treatment. Signs of behavior disturbances can range from those that are less serious, such as nailbiting, hair twisting, body rocking, or shyness, to more serious problems, such as repeated aggressiveness, destructiveness, withdrawal, extreme nervousness, depression, psychosomatic illnesses or poor performance in school.

Teachers should always be alert to sudden changes in children's behavior. Abnormal behaviors often result from stress, anxiety, or inner turmoil a child is experiencing (Honig 1984). However, all children undergo occasional periods of emotional instability or undesirable behavior. Short-term or onetime incidences of such reactions are usually not cause for concern. However, when a child consistently demonstrates abnormal behaviors, some form of intervention or treatment program may be necessary.

In many instances, it may be difficult for parents to recognize abnormal behaviors in their own children. Some emotional problems develop slowly and over a long period of time, and are hard to differentiate from normal behaviors. Some parents may find it hard to talk about or admit that their child has an emotional disturbance. For these reasons, it may be the teacher or child care provider who first recognizes abnormal behaviors. Teachers are in an ideal position to identify children's mental health problems and to help parents understand and accept them. Teachers can use their expertise to counsel parents in appropriate methods for managing certain undesirable behaviors. For more serious problems, teachers may need to advise parents to seek professional mental health care for their child.

SUMMARY

Growth during infancy is rapid while the preschool years are marked by a relatively slow rate of growth. Children grow taller and more adultlike in the process. As their gross motor skills improve, more time and effort is spent acquiring fine motor skills. Although children are able to manage much of their own personal care by the end of the preschool period, adults should continue to make certain that children's need for nutrition, sleep, love, security, and protection are adequately met.

Perhaps one of the most dramatic transformations that occur from infancy through the preschool period relates to socialization. Whereas the infant is initially a nonsocial being, friendships and group interaction become important to the preschool child. However, the process of separation from parents sometimes is very difficult.

Today, many persons are concerned with children's health. Growth and development norms are one effective means for evaluating children's health status and developmental progress. An evaluation of children's physical and social characteristics, as well as their work habits can also provide additional clues. Teachers and care providers must remember that there are many differences in the so-called "normal" range.

Because of the influential position early childhood teachers and child care providers occupy, they must demonstrate a commitment to the health and safety of young children. This obligation can be met by providing adequate health services, health education programs and healthy, safe settings. Three areas of special concern for the preschool child are accident prevention, dental health, and mental health.

LEARNING ACTIVITIES

1. Observe a group of preschool-aged children during free-choice or outdoor times for two 15-minute intervals. For each observation, select a different child and record the number of times that child engages in a cooperative play situation. If possible, repeat this observation procedure with a group of toddlers. Note any differences.

2. Read the book *Think of Something Quiet* by Clare Cherry. Discuss your reactions to the book. Do you see this information as having any value in your own life? In small groups, practice some of the techniques suggested.

3. Write to the American Dental Association and request information on children's dental care. Decide how you could implement this knowledge in a preschool classroom that meets daily for a 2½ hour session.

4. Invite a child mental health specialist to speak to your class. Find out what types of problems are treated most often and how care providers can help prevent these problems in young children.

UNIT REVIEW

A. Multiple Choice. Select the best answer.

1. The leading cause of death among preschool children is
   a. birth defects
   b. accidents
   c. communicable illnesses
   d. hereditary diseases

2. Dental care of deciduous or "baby" teeth is
   a. controversial
   b. unnecessary
   c. very important
   d. only needed by some children

3. Good dental hygiene for preschool children should include all of the following *except*
   a. regular dental examinations
   b. use of toothpaste containing fluoride
   c. proper brushing technique
   d. elimination of all sweets and carbohydrates from the diet

4. Growth during the preschool years
   a. is slow but steady
   b. occurs only in height, not weight
   c. increases rapidly
   d. is insignificant

5. Norms for growth and development
   a. state definite ages when children should be able to perform specific skills
   b. give an average age when most children are able to perform a behavior or skill
   c. have little relevance for most children
   d. list characteristics of the "well" child

6. At one year of age, a boy who weighed 7 pounds 9 ounces at birth can be expected to weigh
   a. 22 pounds 11 ounces
   b. 18 pounds
   c. 30 pounds 4 ounces
   d. 15 pounds 2 ounces

B. Answer the following questions by filling in the blanks. Then, take the first letter of each answer and place it in the appropriate square that follows question 6 to form an important word.

1. Major gains in the preschool child's growth are due to increases in
   _____.

2. A comprehensive health program should include services, _____ and provisions for a healthy environment.

3. The leading cause of death among children under 4 years of age is the result of _____.

4. Teachers can promote children's mental health by planning activities that are appropriate for their _____ of skill.

5. _____ and care providers have a tremendous responsibility to protect the safety of young children they care for.

6. Good dental care depends on a nutritious diet, good oral _____ and routine dental examinations.

C. Briefly answer each of the following questions.

1. How many hours of sleep are recommended for the toddler each day?

2. An infant is expected to grow what percent in length during the first year?

3. What is another term used to describe "baby" teeth?

4. How does environment affect children's mental health?

5. Explain the relationship between good dental health and learning.

6. Would it be realistic to expect an 11-month-old infant to be toilet trained? Explain. Should parents be concerned if their 9-month-old infant cannot sit up without support?

7. List the purposes served by deciduous teeth.

REFERENCES

Arena, J.M., and Bachar, M. *Childhood Safety Is No Accident: A Parent's Handbook of Emergencies.* Durham, NC: Duke University Press, 1978.

Chandler, L.A. *Children Under Stress: Understanding Emotional Adjustment Reactions.* Springfield, IL: Charles C. Thomas Publisher, 1982.

Cherry, C. *Think of Something Quiet.* Belmont, CA: Pitman Learning, Inc., 1981.

Crosby, R. "Self-Concept Development." *Journal of School Health* 52(7):432–36, September 1982.

Endres, J., and Rockwell, R. *Food, Nutrition and the Young Child.* St. Louis, MO: C.V. Mosby Co., 1980.

Hart, E.J., and Behr, M.T. "The Effects of Educational Intervention and Parental Support on Dental Health." *Journal of School Health* 50(10):572–76, October 1980.

Haynes, U. *A Developmental Approach to Casefinding.* Washington, DC: U.S. Department of Health, Education and Welfare, Public Health Service, Government Printing Office (DHEW No. 79–5210).

Hendrick, J. *The Whole Child: Early Education For The Eighties.* 3d ed. St. Louis, MO: Times Mirror/Mosby College Publishing, 1984.

Honig, A. "Risk Factors In Infants and Young Children." *Young Children* 39(4):60–73, May 1984.

Houle, B. "The Impact of Long-term Dental Health Education on Oral Hygiene Behavior." *Journal of School Health* 52(4):256–61, April 1982.

Joint Commission on the Mental Health of Children. *Mental Health: From Infancy Through Adolescence: Reports of Task Forces I, II, and III.* New York: Harper and Row Publishers, Inc., 1973.

Leach, P. *Your Baby and Child: From Birth to Age Five.* New York: Alfred A. Knopf, 1982.

Le francois, G. *Of Children.* 3d ed. Belmont, CA: Wadsworth Publishing Co., 1980.

National Center for Health Statistics. *Periodontal Disease and Oral Hygiene Among Children.* Series 11, No. 117. Washington, DC: U.S. Government Printing Office, 1972. (DHEW No. 72–1060)

Newbrun, E. "Sugar and Dental Caries: A Review of Human Studies." *Science* 217(30):418–23, July 1982.

Olson, N. *Personal and Family Safety and Crime Prevention.* New York: Holt, Rinehart and Winston, 1980.

Tudor, M. *Child Development.* New York: McGraw-Hill Book Company, 1981.

Additional Reading

Curtis, S. *The Joy of Movement In Early Childhood.* New York: Teachers College Press, 1982.

Gonzalez-Mena, J. "What Is A Good Beginning?" *Young Children* 34(3):47–53, 1979.

Jalongo, M.R. "Using Crisis-Oriented Books With Young Children." *Young Children* 38(5):29–36, July 1983.

Lee, A.J. "Daily Dry Toothbrushing in Kindergarten." *Journal of School Health* 50(9):506–9, September 1980.

Smardo, F., and Willis, T.B. "Looking Critically at Dental Health Books for Children." *Journal of School Health* 53(10):626–29, December 1983.

Sapon-Shevin, M. "Teaching Children About Differences: Resources for Teaching." *Young Children* 38(2):24–32, January 1983.

Unit 3
HEALTH
APPRAISALS

Terms to Know

appraisal
impairment
chronic
observations

anecdotal
atypical
symptom
diagnosis

Objectives

After studying this unit, you will be able to:

• State why it is important for teachers and care providers to make health observations.
• Explain the relationship between health and learning.
• List four sources for gathering information about a child's health.
• Identify five health specialists who may be called upon to evaluate children's health.
• State how to perform a health inspection.
• Discuss the value of parent contacts.

A major goal of early childhood programs is to encourage and enhance the growth and development potential of each child. However, in order to achieve these goals, a child must enjoy good health. Even the most sophisticated teaching methods and learning theories are likely to fail if a child is troubled by illness or health *impairments.* A hearing defect, for example, can distort what the child actually hears, the child's perception of letter and word sounds, pronunciation and voice tone. Consider the long-term effects such misperceptions can have on a child's future learning skills.

Health problems do not necessarily have to be obvious or complex to have a negative effect on a child's ability to learn. Even a simple cold, toothache, temporary hearing loss or bothersome sprained ankle interfere with a child's energy level, cooperation, attention span, interest, and enjoyment of learning. It is imperative that early childhood educators and care providers be continuously aware of the health status of young children. They must learn to recognize the early signs of potential health problems before any lasting effect on learning occurs (Allen 1971).

CONCERN FOR CHILDRENS' HEALTH

Child care programs and schools make a significant contribution to the well-being of young children through health services, educational programs, and provisions for a healthy learning environment. A successful health program depends on health *appraisals* to identify, supply information about, and adequately meet the needs of children with health impairments. The term health appraisal, refers to an evaluation or assessment of an individual's state of health. Because health is not a static quality, the process of appraising health must be carried on continuously. A child's state of health can change dramatically in a relatively short time span as illustrated in the following example.

> *Erin appeared to be feeling perfectly healthy when he was checked upon arrival at the center that morning. By 10:00 AM, however, he became restless and was not interested in any of the classroom activities offered to him. The teacher noticed that Erin was constantly rubbing his right ear. By 11:30 AM Erin was crying and complaining of an earache.*

Thus, it is important for teachers and care providers to be observant and alert to changes in a child's appearance or behavior at all times, Figure 3–1. Such changes can be the first indication of an illness or *chronic* health impairment.

Information Gathering

Information necessary for evaluating children's health can be gathered from a variety of sources, including:

- health histories
- results of medical examinations
- teacher health inspections
- dental examinations
- vision and hearing screenings
- speech evaluations
- psychological testing
- developmental evaluations.

Several of these procedures can be administered by early childhood educators while others require the services of specially trained health professionals. Often, the process of identifying the child's specific health impairment requires the cooperative efforts of specialists from several different fields:

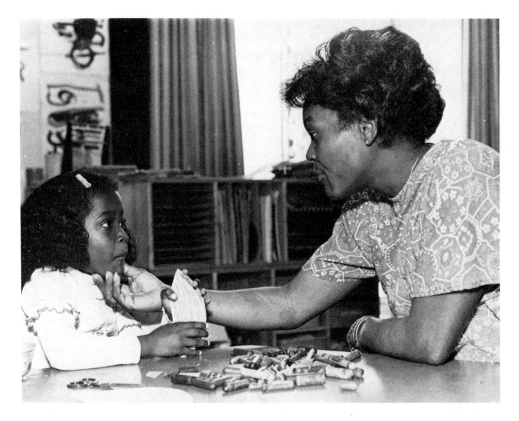

FIGURE 3-1   Care providers should be alert to changes in children's appearance and behavior.

- pediatric medicine
- nursing
- speech
- dietetics
- dentistry

- psychology
- education
- opthamology
- social work
- audiology

Health information should be collected from a variety of appropriate sources before any final conclusions are reached about a child's condition. The results of one health appraisal method alone are often too limited and may present a biased picture of the problem. A child faced with strange surroundings or an unfamiliar adult examiner may behave in *atypical* ways, thereby making screening evaluation difficult. The anxiety of new experiences may also cause the young child to behave in abnormal ways. Gathering pertinent information about the child from several sources helps to eliminate some of these problems. Such an approach also presents the most accurate picture of an illness or impairment and its effect on the child's daily life. For example, a combination of care provider and parent observations coupled with the results of a hearing test may confirm the need for referral of a child to a hearing specialist.

OBSERVATION AS A SCREENING TOOL

Teachers and care providers are important members of the health team who watch over the orderly growth and development of young children. It is not necessary for them to have extensive training in health and medicine. Rather, they make their most valuable contributions through skilled *observations*. Watching children work and play provides the teacher with many clues about potential health problems, Figure 3–2.

Health observations are one of the simplest, least costly, and most useful screening techniques available to child care providers. They already have many of the tools necessary for making objective health observations at their disposal. Sight is perhaps the most important of these natural gifts. Much can be learned about children's health by merely watching them in action. A simple touch can detect a fever or enlarged lymph glands; odors may indicate lack of cleanliness or an infection. Careful listening may reveal breathing difficulties or changes in voice quality. Conversations may reveal poor peer relationships or children who

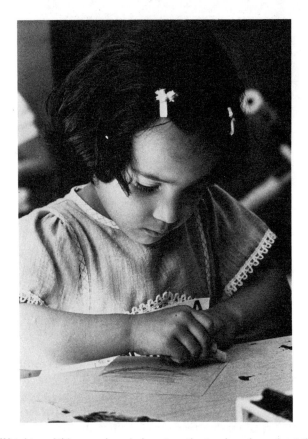

FIGURE 3–2   Watching children work and play gives the teacher clues about the child's health.

voice frequent complaints. Developing the use of the senses to their fullest—
seeing children as they really are, hearing what they really have to say, and
responding to their true needs—requires time, patience, and practice to perfect.

Teachers and child care providers occupy an excellent position for observing
the health of young children (Looking For Health 1969). They see children functioning in a variety of settings and activities for extended periods of time, Figure
3–3. Observation skills coupled with a knowledge of normal growth and development permit careful assessment of a child's skills and abilities. A baseline of what
constitutes the usual behavior and appearance for each child can be established
through continuous observation; changes or deviations can then be quickly
noted.

Assessment of children's growth and development must be done cautiously.
Teachers and care providers must remember that a wide range of normal behaviors and skill attainment exists within each developmental stage. Norms merely
represent the average age at which most children are able to perform certain
skills. For example, many three year olds can reproduce the shape of a circle, cut
with a scissors and walk across a balance beam. There will be some three year
olds, however, who will not be able to perform these tasks. This does not imply
that these children are not "normal." Some children simply take longer than
others to master certain skills. Teachers can use developmental norms to alert

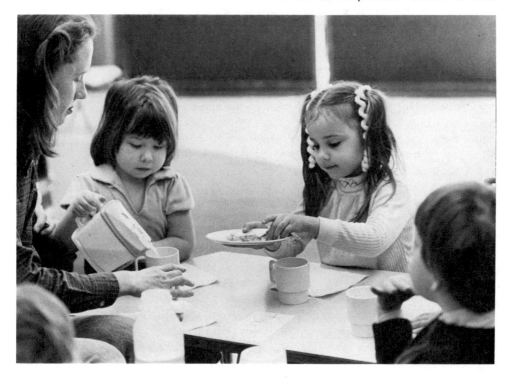

FIGURE 3–3   Teachers and care providers see children functioning in various settings. This gives
them an excellent opportunity to observe the children for potential health problems.

themselves to the child with potential health impairments, as well as those who may require extra help acquiring certain skills.

HEALTH INSPECTIONS

The daily inspection or checking of each child requires only a minute or two of the care provider's time, and should be carried out in addition to continuous observations. Checking children in this manner enhances the care provider's ability to detect early signs and symptoms of illness and health impairments (Powell 1981).

Method

A quiet area set aside in the classroom is ideal for conducting health inspections. The observer may choose simply to sit on the floor with the children or provide a more structured setting with a table and chairs. By designating the same area each day for health inspections, young children will know where they are expected to check in.

A systematic approach is the surest and most efficient method for conducting health inspections. By establishing a routine, the care provider can be assured that health inspections will be consistent and thorough each time. Table 3–1 gives a sample checklist that can serve as a guideline for observations. It is organized so that inspections are made from top to bottom of the child and then front to back. This list is by no means exhaustive or the only method available. Care providers may wish to adapt the procedure to their own setting and particular needs of children with whom they work.

A teacher should begin health inspections by observing children as they enter the room and approach the teacher. Many clues about their well-being, e.g. personal cleanliness, weight changes, signs of illness, facial expressions, posture, skin color, and coordination can be noted quite easily. A teacher or care provider can also utilize this opportunity to gain important insight into the quality of relationship between parent and child by observing as they arrive and interact together. These observations can help to explain why some children exhibit certain behaviors. For example, does the parent have a tendency to do everything for the child—take off boots, hang up coats, pick up items the child has dropped—or does the parent encourage the child to try to do these things? Is the child allowed to answer question or does the parent provide all of the answers?

Following these initial observations, the teacher can begin checking individual children. First, a flashlight is used to inspect the mouth and throat, Figure 3–4. A quick look inside the mouth can alert the care provider to the child with an unusually red throat, swollen or infected tonsils, dental caries or any other apparent disorder. Additional observations of the hair and face, including the eyes, ears, and nose, can also be made at this time.

TABLE 3-1   Health Observation Checklist

1. *General appearance*—weight change (gain or loss), fatigue, excitability, skin color, size for age group

2. *Scalp*—observe for itching, sores, cleanliness

3. *Face*—general appearance, expression (e.g., fear, anxious, happy), color

4. *Eyes*—look for redness, tearing, puffiness, coordinated eye movements, sensitivity to light, squinting, frequent rubbing, styes or other sores

5. *Ears*—check for drainage, frequent earaches, bewildered looks or inappropriate responses

6. *Nose*—runny, sneezing, deformity, frequent rubbing, congestion

7. *Mouth*—inspection of teeth for cavities or malformations; inside of mouth for redness, spots or sores, or malformations; mouth breathing

8. *Throat*—look for enlarged, red or infected tonsils or red throat with or without white spots

9. *Neck*—check for enlarged glands if you question any of the other findings

10. *Chest*—watch child's breathing for wheezing, rattles, labored breathing (shortness of breath), frequent coughing with or without other symptoms

11. *Skin*—observe the child's front and back for color, rashes, scratches, bumps, bruises, unusual scars or injuries

12. *Speech*—clarity, substitution of letter sounds, stuttering, monotone voice, nasality, appropriate for age

13. *Extremities*—equal length, straight, check posture, coordination, pigeon-toed, bowed legs

14. *Behavior*—observe level of activity, alertness, degree of cooperativeness appropriate for age, appetite, sleep habits, irritable or excitable, motor skills

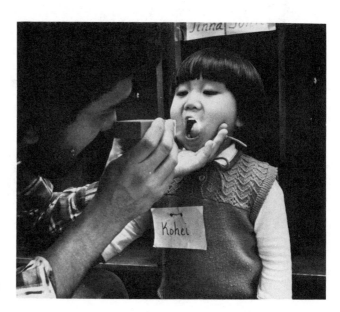

FIGURE 3-4   A flashlight is used to inspect the inside of the mouth and throat.

Next, the front of the body, including the chest, abdomen and arms, is inspected for signs of rashes, skin color, or unusual scratches, bumps or bruises. Because many of the rashes associated with communicable disease begin on the warmer areas of the body, e.g. chest, back, neck and forearms, these areas should be looked at carefully, Figure 3–5. The child's back should then be inspected for the same conditions.

When the more formal aspects of the health inspection process are completed, the teacher should continue to make observations. Qualities of balance, coordination, posture and size can be easily noted as the child walks away to join in group activities. Information gathered from both formal health inspections and teacher observations contribute to an awareness of a child's total state of health—physical, mental, emotional and social well-being.

With time, observers become more skillful in conducting health inspections and making significant observations. Experience enables the teacher or care provider to gain the sensitivity and skills necessary to distinguish between signs and *symptoms* which are normal and those that are abnormal. Gradually, it becomes easier for the observer to recognize not only very obvious changes, but also the more subtle differences that may be cause for concern.

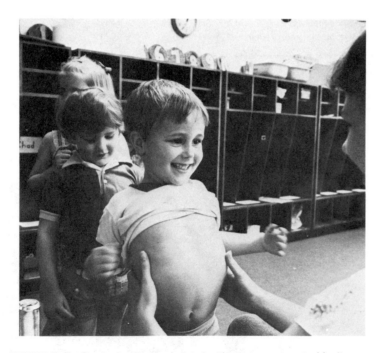

FIGURE 3–5 Because rashes associated with many communicable diseases begin on the chest and back, these areas should be checked carefully.

Recording

Care providers are indispensable as observers and recorders of children's health information. Their frequent and close contact with children permits them to play an important role in the promotion of health. Written notes should be made following the inspection of each child. Space provided on daily attendance records is one very good method for recording important *anecdotal* information. Simple checklists are also useful for systematically observing and recording children's health status.

Recorded observations must be precise and specific. To say that a child "looks sick" is much too vague and can be interpreted differently by everyone reading it. To state that a child is flushed, has a fever of 101°F, and is covered with a fine red rash is much more meaningful.

Carefully recorded observations can be useful for the early detection of illness and health impairments. Such information is often very beneficial to health professionals when making a *diagnosis.* Recorded observations can be useful for determining whether a child is too ill to remain in group care. Patterns of illness or behavior changes can also be traced from the daily notes kept by the care provider. Children known to have had close contact with an identified case of head lice, for example, can be watched closely for the next several weeks.

Whatever recording method is used, the important thing to remember is that the information should be available and meaningful to other personnel working with the child. Notes scribbled on scratch paper and tucked in the back of a notebook are often lost and useless to others. Also, it must be remembered that information about a child's health status is confidential and should only be shared with other care providers or teachers who are working directly with the child.

Interpretations

Observations are an essential component of the overall health appraisal process. Teachers and care providers, however, must be careful not to try to diagnose the specific nature of children's health problems. Skillful questioning, careful listening, watching, and keen interest in the problems of children make the observer's contribution invaluable. The teacher can provide much of the information necessary for evaluating a child's health status and reaching a final diagnosis. By recording one's findings, information is accurate and can be shared with other involved professionals. Final interpretation of the various signs and symptoms, however, should be left to qualified health professionals.

Managing Health Risks

In addition to assessing the progress and needs of individual children, the teacher or care provider also has an obligation to protect the health of other children in the classroom; observations provide an effective means for accomplishing this task. Communicable illnesses, and the risks associated with each, pose one of the most frequent threats to the well-being of young children in group settings. The task of identifying sick infants and preschool children is made easier because they usually look and act as though they are ill. Changes in their appearance and behavior are often the first sign of an impending illness. It is during the early stages of an illness that a child is most contagious and most likely to infect other children. Removing a sick child from the classroom helps to reduce the chances of exposing other children.

Other Benefits

Teacher health observations are conducted primarily to aid in the early identification of health problems (Hansom 1980). The sooner health impairments are discovered and treatment is begun, the less damaging they may be to a child's future learning experiences.

While early identification is probably the most important consideration, there are other benefits which can be gained from the opportunity. Time can be spent talking with children on an individual basis, which busy schedules too often discourage. Young children especially enjoy these private conversations. They often are more spontaneous in their expressions, sharing the joy of a new pet, the pain of a scrapped knee, the fear of harsh discipline at home or the excitement of having captured a fuzzy caterpillar.

INVOLVING PARENTS

Daily health inspections provide an excellent opportunity for actively involving parents in children's preventive health care. Frequent parent contacts help to build a relationship of understanding and confidence between staff and parents, Figure 3–6. Some parents may be hesitant, at first, to initiate contacts with the teacher or care provider regarding their child's health needs. Through repeated encouragement, interest and personal contacts, however, effective lines of communication can quickly be established.

Parents should remain with their child until the health inspection process is completed. Parents should be encouraged to ask questions or voice concerns they may have about their child's behavior, physical condition, habits, or feelings while they wait. Another distinct advantage of having parents wait is that often they can offer simple explanations for the problems a teacher or care provider observes. For example, a child's fatigue or aggressiveness may be the result of a new puppy, a grandmother's visit, a new baby in the home or a seizure the night before. Allergies or a red vitamin taken at breakfast may be the cause of a questionable red throat. Without this direct sharing of information, such symptoms might otherwise be cause for concern.

Contacts made with parents during health inspections are also a good time to alert them to outbreaks of communicable illnesses. They can be told of specific signs and symptoms to watch for. When parents are informed ahead of

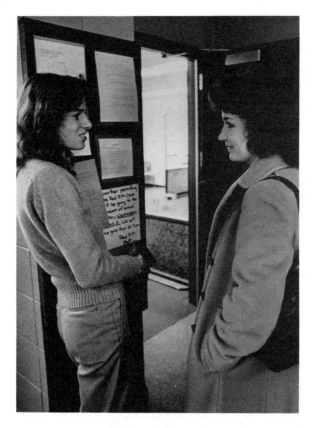

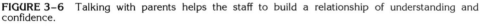

FIGURE 3-6 Talking with parents helps the staff to build a relationship of understanding and confidence.

time, they are more likely to keep sick children at home, avoiding exposing other children in the group.

Parent's Responsibility

Primary responsibility for a child's health care belongs to the parents. Parents are ultimately responsible for maintaining their child's health, following through with recommendations and obtaining any necessary evaluations and treatments.

In most instances, parents are often the first to sense that something is wrong with their child. Some parents delay seeking professional advice, either denying that the problem is real or else hoping that the child will outgrow it. They may not realize the serious consequences health problems can have on a child's ability to learn successfully. Also, it is often difficult for parents to determine the exact nature or cause of a child's health impairment and where to turn for appropriate health care or treatment.

Occasionally, parents fail to take the initiative to provide for any type of routine health care. Some parents find it hard to understand the need for medical care when a child does not appear to be sick, while others cannot afford preventive health care. With today's rising medical care costs, it is fairly easy to see why this might occur. Cost, however, should not discourage parents from obtaining necessary health care because most communities offer a variety of free or low-cost health services for young children, including:

- Head Start Programs
- Child Find Clinics
- Medicaid Assistance
- Well Child Clinics
- Crippled Children's Services
- University Training Centers and Clinics
- Public Health Immunization Centers

Teachers and care providers can be very instrumental in helping parents understand the importance of and need for regularly scheduled health care for their child. Familiarity with community health resources facilitates knowledgeable referrals and helps parents secure the type of health care needed for each child (Mennie 1984).

HEALTH EDUCATION

Daily health inspections also provide an opportunity for informal health education. Care providers can help young children begin to develop an awareness of their own health. Simple questions about many topics, such as hygiene, nutrition, exercise, and sleep, can be discussed with even very young children. For example:

- "Sandy, did you brush your teeth this morning? Brushing helps to keep teeth healthy and prevents cavities."
- "Alexander, what did you eat for breakfast this morning before coming to school?"
- "Marion, have you had a drink of water yet today? Our bodies need water in order to grow and stay healthy."

Spontaneous conversations such as these help young children assume some interest in their own health care. Even the young child can begin to recognize and establish preventive health practices which promote good health. Also, the cooperation and trust that is gained through daily health inspections is important for future contacts a child may have with health professionals.

Parent Education

Health inspections provide an effective means for educating parents. Many aspects of children's care and health education lend themselves to informal discussions with both parents and children during the health inspection process:

- toy safety
- the importance of eating breakfast
- nutritious snack ideas
- the benefits of exercise
- cleanliness
- children dressing appropriately for the weather
- dental hygiene.

Including parents in health education programs brings about an improved understanding of the health principles and goals stressed with the children. It also helps to encourage a greater degree of consistency in the health practices and attitudes between school and the child's home.

SUMMARY

Teachers and child care providers play a valuable role in the promotion of children's health. Good health is essential for effective learning. Illness and health impairments interfere with this process. Because a child's health status can change very quickly, it is necessary to make continuous health observations.

Health observations are a valuable tool for evaluating all aspects of a child's state of health—physical, mental, social and emotional. It is one of the simplest and most inexpensive screening techniques available. The information gathered from health observations may be useful to health specialists for diagnosing or ruling out many health problems.

Caution should be exercised when using developmental norms to determine whether a child is "normal." Conditions which threaten the well-being of an individual child or others in a classroom can be quickly identified and referred for treatment.

There are many benefits to be gained from health observations and inspections. One of the most important is the early identification of children's health impairments. They also provide an excellent opportunity for personal or one-to-one conversations with young children. Health appraisals provide an opportunity for involving parents in children's health care and health education.

The responsibility of the parents must not be overlooked as teachers become more involved in children's health care. Rather, the efforts of the care provider should compliment those of the parents. Teachers can help parents accept the need to provide care for their child and assist them in locating appropriate health services in the community.

LEARNING ACTIVITIES

1. With another student, role play health inspections. Record your findings.

2. Invite a public health nurse from a well-child clinic or a local pediatrician to speak to the class about routine health care for children under 6 years of age.

3. Visit several preschools and child care centers in your community. Note whether any type of health inspection is performed as children arrive. Describe the method used at each center.

UNIT REVIEW

A. Match the term in column II with the correct definition in column I.

Column I	Column II
1. the process of writing down health data	a. health
2. a problem which interferes with one's ability to function	b. impairment
3. evaluation or assessment of an individual's health	c. observations
4. to gather information by looking and listening	d. symptom
5. physical maturation	e. appraisal
6. a bodily change noticed by the affected individual	f. recording
7. to examine or look at carefully	g. diagnosis
8. formal or informal meetings	h. parent contacts
9. a state of complete physical, mental and social well-being	i. development
10. development toward maturity	j. inspection
11. the act of determining an illness or disorder from signs and symptoms	k. growth

B. Read the following case study and answer the questions that follow.

> Lynette's teacher has recently become concerned about her ability to see. He has noticed that when stories are read to the children, Lynette frequently leaves her place in the circle and crawls closer to him in order to see the pictures he holds up. The teacher has also observed that Lynette looks very closely at puzzles and pictures she is coloring. Lynette's parents have expressed some concern about her clumsiness at home. An initial vision screening test, administered by the school nurse, reveals that Lynette's vision is not within normal limits. She was referred to an eye specialist for further evaluation.

1. What behaviors did Lynette exhibit that made her teacher suspect some type of vision disorder?

2. Identify the various sources from which information concerning Lynette's vision problem was obtained before she was referred to an eye specialist.

3. If the teacher suspected a vision problem, why didn't he just go ahead and recommend that Lynette get glasses?

4. What responsibilities do teachers and care providers have when they believe that a child has a health impairment?

C. Briefly answer the following questions.

1. List four sources for gathering information that can be useful in evaluating children's health.

2. Name five professionals that can be asked to identify specific health impairments of children.

3. What is the relationship between health and learning?

4. Name six areas to observe during a health inspection.

5. How can teacher observations benefit the health of a child?

6. How can daily health inspections involve parents in the preventive health care of their children?

REFERENCES

Allen, K.E.; Rieke, J.; Dmitriev, V.; and Hayden, A. "Early Warning: Observation As A Tool For Recognizing Potential Handicaps In Young Children." *Educational Horizons* 50(2):43–55, Winter 1971–72.

Hansom, M.A., and Levine, M.D. "Early School Health: An Analysis of Its Impact on Primary Care." *Journal of School Health* 50(10):577–80, December 1980.

Looking For Health. New York: Metropolitan Life Insurance Company, 1969.

Mennie, J., and Klinger, M.J. "Health Department Services for Preschools and Day Care Centers." *Journal of School Health* 54(4):160–61, April 1984.

Powell, M. *Assessment and Management of Developmental Changes and Problems In Children.* 2d ed. St. Louis, MO: C.V. Mosby Co., 1981.

Additional Reading

Brink, S., and Nader, P.R. "Comprehensive Health Screening In Elementary Schools: An Outcome Evaluation." *Journal of School Health* 54(2):75–78, February 1984.

Maddox, M., and Edgar, E. "Implementing EPSDT Screening in the Public School: Resolving Some Issues." *Journal of School Health* 53(9):536, November 1983.

Willis, W.O. "The Health of Preschoolers In Child Care Settings: Some Possibilities For Nursing Intervention." *Child Care Quarterly* 6(3):189–95, 1977.

Unit 4
HEALTH
ASSESSMENT TOOLS

Terms to Know

intervention	hyperopia
skeletal	misarticulation
neurological	speech
amblyopia	language
strabismus	referral
myopia	

Objectives

After studying this unit, you will be able to:
- List seven screening procedures that can be used to assess a child's health status.
- List three uses for children's health records.
- Name three vision defects which can be detected through vision screening.
- Match the recommended screening test to the condition or behavior that indicates its need.

It is essential that teachers and care providers familiarize themselves with some of the preventive methods for assessing children's health. A variety of screening tools are available for collecting objective data; several common ones are described in this unit. The purpose of all such methods is the promotion of good health and the identification of potentially disabling or handicapping conditions that may have an effect on children's growth and intellectual development.

Health observations and appraisals are the most valuable health assessment tools. Another valuable assessment tool is the information and explanations parents contribute about conditions affecting their child's well-being or academic performance. Screening test results, "well-child" assessments, and health records also contribute a wealth of information about a child's state of health. Data assembled from a combination of these sources are most desirable for health promotion, the early detection of health problems, and the adjustment of programs to meet the needs of individual children.

HEALTH RECORDS

Information contained in children's permanent health records can help promote well-being, if the data are current and sufficiently detailed. Unfortunately, the types of records maintained by early childhood programs vary considerably in quality and quantity from one center to another. State licensing regulations often specify the kinds of records a center must keep on file. Because licensing requirements generally reflect only minimal standards, child care centers may want to consider additional forms of documentation. Selection of appropriate health-related records and forms should be consistent with the program's goals and philosophy. Records should provide comprehensive information about individual children and afford adequate legal protection for the children, staff, and center.

A permanent health record should be kept on file for each child enrolled in a program. It should contain the following essential information:

- child/family health history
- copy of a recent medical assessment (physical examination)
- immunization records
- emergency contact information
- record of dental examinations
- attendance data
- school-related accidents or injuries
- parent conferences related to the child's health
- results of special testing, e.g., vision, hearing, speech
- medications administered while the child is at school

Information found in children's health records can be used for many purposes:

- determining health status
- identifying possible problem areas
- developing *intervention* programs
- evaluating the success of treatments
- coordinating services
- making *referrals*
- following a child's progress
- research

Health records contain much private information about children and their families. Teachers and care providers must respect the confidential nature of these records. Only information which will improve effectiveness and interaction should be shared with those who are working directly with a child. Personal facts about a child or family must not be made public or serve as topics of casual conversation among teachers, staff members, or with other parents. No portion of a child's health record should ever be released to another agency, school, health professional or clinician until written permission is obtained from the child's parent or guardian. A special release form such as the one shown in Figure 4–1 can be used for this purpose. The form should clearly designate the nature of information that is to be released and the agency or person to whom it is to be sent. It must be dated and signed by the parent.

Recordkeeping is most efficient when one person is responsible for the maintenance of all health records. However, meaningful contributions regarding concerns, findings, or conversations related to a child's health should be added by any teacher or staff member working with the child. This makes records more

---

INFORMATION RELEASE FORM

I understand the confidentiality of any personally identifiable information on my child shall be maintained in accordance with PL 93–380, federal and state regulations and used only for the educational benefit of my child. Personally identifiable information about my child will be released only with my consent. With this information, I hereby grant the

_____
(Name of program, agency or person)

permission to release the following types of information:

Medical information   _____
Assessment reports   _____
Child histories   _____
Progress reports   _____
Clinical reports   _____
(Other) _____

to: _____
(Name of agency or person to whom information is to be sent)

regarding _____ _____ ____
              Name   Birthdate   Sex

_____
Signature of Parent or Guardian

_____
Relationship of Representative

_____
Date

FIGURE 4–1 A sample information release form

complete and useful. Health records can serve as legal documentation and should be kept on file by the center for approximately five years.

Child Health Histories

Health histories contain important background and current information about a child. Questions about family members are usually included in order to provide a more comprehensive picture of the child. Parents should be asked to complete a child health history form when their child is accepted into a preschool or child care program.

Much variation can be found in the type of background information which is requested. Unless a center is required to use a standard form, it can adapt or develop a format which best suits its own specific needs. Sample forms can be obtained from other centers and reviewed to determine the types of questions a program wants to include. A child health history form should request certain basic information:

- facts related to the child's birth
- family circumstances, e.g., numbers and ages of family members, predominant languages spoken
- developmental milestones
- previous injuries, illnesses or surgery
- personal habits, e.g., toileting, food preferences, napping
- parent concerns, e.g., behavior problems, social development, language skills
- special health conditions, e.g., allergies, asthma, epilepsy, diabetes, blindness, hearing loss

Information found in children's health histories contributes to a better understanding of individual children, including the factors which make each one unique. This knowledge is also extremely useful for assessing a child's general state of health and enables care providers to set reasonable goals and expectations for individual children. Programs can be adjusted to meet children's special needs, such as a hearing loss, the use of crutches and braces for locomotion or a mild language delay. However, caution must be exercised not to set expectation levels for children unnecessarily low based on this information alone (Haslam 1975). A child's ability to learn must never be discounted unless an impairment is definitely known to interfere with the educational process or performance. Lowering goals and expectations may limit what a child is willing to try, for often children will achieve only what is expected and may not be encouraged to progress or strive to develop their true potential.

Child health histories also provide the teacher with insight into the kind of routine medical supervision a child has received in the past. This knowledge may be very useful when making referrals, because it often reflects the value parents place on preventive health care.

Medical and Dental Examinations

In many states, children are required to have a thorough health examination before entering preschool or child care programs. It is generally recommended that well children, who are less than one year of age, have a routine checkup every 2–3 months. Children two to three years of age should be examined every 6 months and children four and older should be seen by their doctor annually. More frequent medical supervision may be necessary when health problems exist.

Current health information is obtained from the parent and child during the course of the examination. Questions related to physical, mental and social development are asked to help the examiner assess the child's total state of health. Body parts and systems, such as the heart, lungs, eyes, ears, *skeletal* and *neurological* development, and gastrointestinal function (stomach and intestines) are carefully examined. Measurements of height and weight are taken and compared with past records to determine if a child's growth is satisfactory. Lack of growth may be an indication of other health problems. The child's blood pressure should also be checked at this time. Specialized tests, such as blood tests for anemia, sickle cell disease or lead poisoning, urinalysis or tuberculin testing, may be ordered as part of the medical examination. The child's immunization record should be reviewed and additional immunizations given as indicated.

SCREENING PROCEDURES

The stated objective of various screening procedures is traditionally described as the "identification of those children who require further study because of suspected handicaps" (Spodek 1984). This approach, however, reinforces the negative aspect of testing and supports the disease/illness approach to health care. The identification role is an important, but secondary function of screening procedures and should not overshadow the fact that the majority of children tested will perform satisfactorily. This is an era of transition; it is important to instill in young children positive attitudes toward health promotion and care.

Screening tests are essential to comprehensive health assessment of young children. Their purpose complements the preventive health concept by ensuring that a particular system is functioning as it should. Routine screening helps children become accustomed to evaluation procedures as a means of health maintenance and not as something that is done only when problems arise.

A variety of screening procedures are available for evaluating different aspects of children's health; they are not designed to diagnose the specific nature of problems. During routine screening, there may be some children identified who will need more extensive evaluation by a specialist. The results obtained from any screening procedure simply provide additional information and should be used to supplement the observations of parents and teachers. Some screening procedures can be administered by care providers, while others require the services of professional clinicians.

Measurements of Height and Weight

The first five years of life are an important period of growth. Changes are dramatic during infancy, while increases in the preschooler's height and weight continue steadily but at a much slower rate. Measurements of height are particularly important because they provide a rough indication of a child's long-term health and nutritional status (see Appendix for growth curves that show norms by age and sex of the child). Fluctuations in weight, on the other hand, usually reflect short-term variables, such as a recent illness, infection or temporary emotional stress. However, it must be remembered that a child's growth potential is ultimately governed by inherited characteristics.

The practice of measuring height and weight is one method care providers and teachers can use to assess children's health, Figure 4–2. It does not require any special skills or training and can be completed in a relatively short period of time. Whenever possible, these measurements should be conducted as a group activity. Children are fascinated to see how much they have grown or how big they are in comparison to their friends. Care providers can use this opportunity as a valuable learning experience to encourage the interests of young children in their own growth and health. Simple individual or group growth charts can be constructed with crayon and paper. By plotting measurements of height and

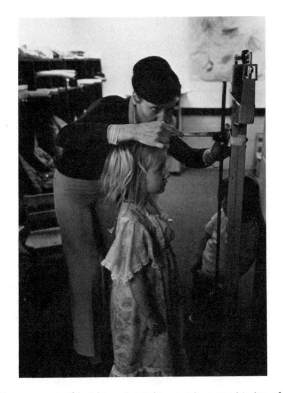

FIGURE 4–2   Measurement of height and weight provide a good index of children's health.

weight each time, children can visualize their growth from one measurement to the next.

Ideally, measurements of height and weight should be taken at 4–6 month intervals. A child's growth cannot be accurately evaluated from one measurement. Rather, what is most important are the changes in size which occur over a period of time. A single measurement is unlikely to identify the child who is experiencing a growth disturbance related to physical illness or emotional difficulties. Height and weight data should also be recorded in the child's permanent health file. Comparisons can then be made from previous measurements and standardized growth charts to determine if the child's growth is progressing normally. Growth charts are available from:

Mead Johnson Nutrition Division
2404 Pennsylvania Avenue
Evansville, IN 47721

Ross Laboratories
625 Cleveland Avenue
Columbus, OH 43116

Wyeth Laboratories
P. O. Box 8099
Philadelphia, PA 19101

Examples of growth charts are also included in the Appendix.

SENSORY DEVELOPMENT

The sensory system affects all parameters of a child's growth and development. Five special senses comprise the sensory system: vision, hearing, smell, touch, and taste. The young child receives, interprets, processes, and responds to external environmental cues and stimulation. Optimal functioning of the sensory system is, therefore, of critical importance, especially during the early stages of growth and development. Of the five senses, perhaps vision and hearing are two of the most critical to young children, since much of early learning is dependent on what the child hears and sees.

VISION SCREENING

Parents, teachers and care providers too often assume that because children are young and healthy they naturally have good vision. This assumption may not always be correct. Vision impairments affect approximately one out of every four children of school age (*Vision Screening in Schools*). They may be present at birth or develop as a child matures or experiences certain illnesses, infections or injuries. For this reason, all children should have their vision tested before the age of six to avoid the risk of permanent loss of sight. Early detection of vision impairments improves a child's chances for rapid and successful treatment.

Often, it is the teacher or care provider who first notices clues in the young child's behavior that indicate a vision disorder, Figure 4–3. One reason is that as greater demands are placed on a child to perform tasks accurately vision problems often become more apparent. Also, it is unlikely that young children will know when their vision is not normal, especially if they have never experienced good vision before. A careful comparison of screening results and observations provide the most accurate assessment of children with potential impairments of vision.

Special attention should be paid to children who have other known physical handicaps and to those who are repeatedly unsuccessful in achieving tasks that depend on visual cues. Delays in identifying vision problems can seriously affect the learning process and chances for successfully treating the condition. Children with vision impairments may also be inappropriately labelled. Many times visually impaired children are considered to be slow learners or mentally retarded when they simply cannot see well enough to learn (Allen 1972). The following case study illustrates the point:

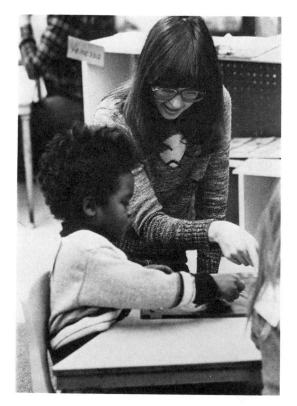

FIGURE 4–3 The teacher or care provider is often the first to notice signs of a child's vision problem.

The teachers were concerned about Tina. She was easily frustrated and unable to complete many preacademic tasks, such as puzzles, color identification, and simple object labelling. She appeared clumsy and often avoided participation in large motor activities during outdoor time. These problems were not typical of most children Tina's age (three years, eight months). Her teachers considered placing Tina in a special classroom for children with learning disabilities. However, during routine vision screening, Tina's vision was discovered to be 20/200. With corrective glasses and slight modifications in teaching techniques, immediate improvement was observed in Tina's performance.

Methods of Assessment

Early detection of visual defects requires observing young children carefully for signs of potential problems, Table 4–1. Some observable signs of visual impairments may include:

- rubs eyes frequently
- attempts to brush away blurs
- is irritable with close work
- is inattentive to distant tasks, e.g., a movie, catching a ball
- strains to see distant objects, squints or screws up face
- blinks often when reading; holds books too close or far away
- is inattentive with close work; quits after a short time
- closes or covers one eye to see better
- tilts head to one side
- appears cross-eyed at times
- reverses letters, words
- stumbles over objects; runs into things
- complains of repeated headaches or double vision

It is important that young children have their vision tested. The purpose of this routine vision screening is to be sure the child's vision is developing properly

TABLE 4–1 Detection of Visual Abnormalities in the Infant

Observe the infant closely for:
- roving eye movements that are suggestive of blindness
- one or both eyes continuously crossed
- eyes that wander in opposite directions
- inability to focus or follow a moving object (after three months of age)
- pupil of one eye larger than the other
- absence of a blink reflex
- eyelids not completely raised
- cloudiness on the eyeball

and to locate children with possible visual defects, Figure 4–4. Teachers, care providers, and parent volunteers can be trained by health professionals to administer most vision screening tests. Children of three and older are usually able to follow the instructions for vision testing after they have been carefully explained. It is very important that children understand the correct method of response before beginning any screening procedure.

Several standardized tests are available for use with young children. The Snellen E, or Illiterate E, is the method selected most often for testing the visual acuity of younger children (Brojkovich 1980). It does not require the child to know the letters of the alphabet and is considered to be fairly reliable. A child's eyes are first tested together, then separately. Standards for passing the Snellen E are age related. Generally, children 3 or 4 years of age should be able to correctly read the 20/40 or 20/30 lines. Five year olds should be able to read the 20/20 line. Any child who fails the initial screening should be rescreened at a later date. If the child does poorly on the second screening, parents should be encouraged to take the child for a professional examination. Also, children with more than one line difference between eyes should be referred to an eye specialist for additional evaluation. A home version of the Illiterate E test entitled, ''Home Test for Pre-schoolers,'' is available to parents from:

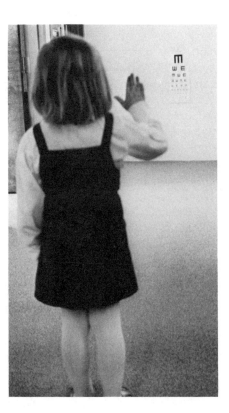

FIGURE 4–4 The purpose of routine screening is to be sure vision is developing properly.

National Society for the Prevention of Blindness
79 Madison Avenue
New York, NY 10016

Other vision tests which can be used with preschool children include the Children's Early Recognition Test, Michigan Junior Vision Screening Test, the Denver Eye Screening Test (DEST) and the Sjogren Hand Test. Information concerning symptoms of visual impairments, the various testing procedures and supplies can be obtained by writing to the National Society for the Prevention of Blindness or to the:

American Optometric Association
243 N. Lindbergh Boulevard
St. Louis, MO 63141

Common Disorders

Three vision defects which screening programs attempt to identify in young children include:

- amblyopia
- strabismus
- myopia

Amblyopia, or "lazy eye," is a condition that develops because of a distortion of the child's vision. This distortion is commonly thought to result from an imbalance of the eye muscles, although other causes have been suggested. A child with amblyopia shows no outward signs or symptoms of this visual impairment; it cannot be detected by merely looking at the child. Children with amblyopia often experience double vision because the images received from either eye cannot be focused together. In an effort to make sense out of the images it receives, the brain begins to ignore the vision from the weaker eye. Gradually, the vision in the weaker eye diminishes.

Prompt medical treatment can prevent the vision loss from becoming permanent. A significant amount of sight can usually be restored if amblyopia is discovered and treated before the child reaches the age of five or six. The results are even more favorable if therapy can be started sooner. Treatment for amblyopia consists of placing a patch over the child's stronger eye, forcing the weaker eye to work harder, Figure 4–5. When the muscles of the weak eye have been sufficiently strengthened, vision should be improved and the patch can be removed.

Strabismus, or cross-eye, also results from an imbalance of the eye muscles. Unlike most other defects of vision, however, strabismus can be recognized by observing the eyes as a child attempts to focus on objects. Generally, only one of the child's eyes is affected, causing it to turn either inward or outward. As in amblyopia, double vision occurs because the eyes are unable to focus together. Images from the weaker eye are blocked out by the brain to avoid confusion, and vision gradually deteriorates. Early recognition and treatment of strabismus is

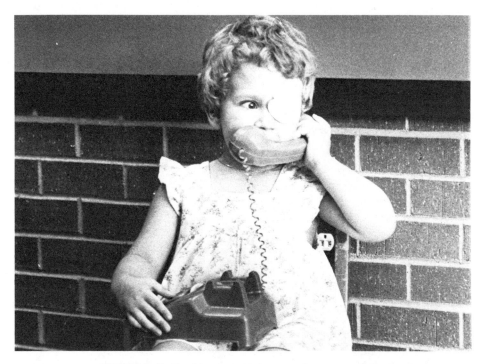

FIGURE 4-5 Patching is sometimes used to treat amblyopia.

essential to restore normal vision. Several methods are used for the treatment of strabismus, including surgical correction, patching of the unaffected eye, and eye exercises.

Myopia, or nearsightedness, is sometimes a problem for young children but is more common among school-aged children. A child who is nearsighted can see near objects, but has poor distant vision, Figure 4-6. Children with myopia appear clumsy and may stumble or run into things. Squinting is also typical behavior of these children as they attempt to bring distant objects into focus.

Farsightedness, or hyperopia, is considered by some authorities to be a natural tendency in very young children because of immature development of eye structures. However, as children grow older, this condition usually corrects itself. The older child who is farsighted will often complain of headaches, tired eyes, and blurred vision following periods of close work. Hyperopia cannot be detected with most routine screening procedures. Teacher and parent observations may provide the best clues to this disorder. Referral to a professional eye specialist is necessary.

Color blindness affects only a small percentage of children and is generally limited to males. Females may be carriers of this hereditary defect, but are rarely affected themselves. Children who are color blind usually cannot discriminate between red and green colors. It is very difficult to test young children for color blindness and is seldom done, since learning is not seriously affected and no treatment is available.

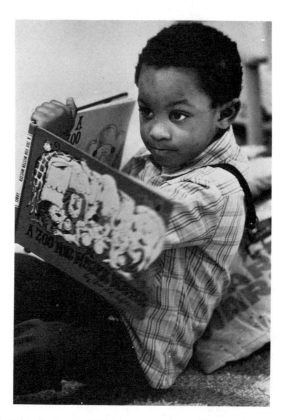

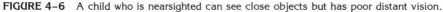

FIGURE 4-6   A child who is nearsighted can see close objects but has poor distant vision.

Management

Arrangements should be made for routine vision screening whenever there is documented concern that a child may be experiencing vision problems. Vision testing is available through a number of sources, including pediatricians, "well-child" clinics, public health departments, professional eye doctors, and public schools. Some local organizations also provide financial assistance for professional examinations and glasses.

Children who do not pass an initial vision screening should be retested. Failure to pass a second screening necessitates referral to a professional eye specialist for more extensive evaluation and diagnosis. However, results obtained from routine vision testing should be viewed with some caution because they are not necessarily a guarantee that a child does or does not have a problem. Most routine screening procedures are not designed to test for all types of vision impairments. Consequently, there will always be some over-referrals of children who do not have any problems, while other children with defects will be missed. It is for this reason that the observations of teachers and parents are so extremely important.

HEARING SCREENING

The development of speech patterns, *language,* and learning depend upon a child's ability to hear. Undetected hearing impairments may also affect a child's social interactions, emotional development and performance in school. The early diagnosis of any hearing loss is extremely critical. Unfortunately, children with hearing losses are sometimes inappropriately labelled as slow learners, retarded, or "behavior problems." Failure to hear properly often causes children to respond and behave in seemingly inappropriate ways.

Methods of Assessment

Inappropriate responses and behaviors may be the first indication that a child is not hearing properly (Gray 1984). Signs of hearing loss range from very obvious problems to those that are subtle and more difficult to identify. An observant parent or care provider may notice behaviors that indicate a hearing loss:

- frequent mouth breathing
- turns toward the direction of sound
- slowness in acquiring language; development of poor speech patterns
- difficulty understanding and following directions
- asks to have statements repeated
- rubs or pulls at ears
- mumbles, shouts or talks loudly
- appears quiet, withdrawn; rarely interacts with others
- uses gestures rather than words
- does well in activities that do not depend on hearing
- imitates others at play
- responds to questions inappropriately
- mispronounces many word sounds
- unusual voice quality—extremely high, low, hoarse or monotone

Hearing tests are most often conducted by either trained paraprofessionals or audiologists, Figure 4–7. An audiologist is a specially prepared clinician who uses nonmedical techniques to diagnose hearing impairments. Routine hearing screening procedures generally test for the range of tones normally used in speech. Children should have their hearing tested at least once during the preschool years. If a hearing problem is suspected, parents should make arrangements to have their child's hearing tested more often.

Most preschool children are able to complete routine hearing screening with little trouble. However, sometimes a strange situation involving new people, unfamiliar instruments and equipment, a novel task, or a lack of understanding or cooperation may interfere with the child's performance and cause unreliable results to be obtained from the test. These factors must be given special consideration when test results are analyzed.

Teachers and parents can be extremely helpful by preparing and training young children in advance for hearing screening (Brown 1982). In the classroom

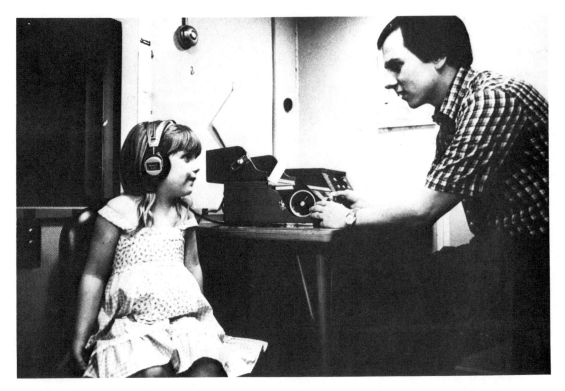

FIGURE 4-7 Hearing tests are conducted by audiologists or trained paraprofessionals.

and at home, children can practice concentrated listening for short periods of time. Also, activities which involve the use of headphones, e.g., telephone opera-tors, airplane pilots, radio announcers, will help children feel more comfortable when they are asked to put on headphones for screening purposes. Teachers should try to find out what response method, e.g., raising one hand, pressing a button, pointing to pictures or dropping a wooden block into an empty can, the children will be expected to use. This activity can also be practiced in the class-room. If a special room will be used for testing purposes, teachers should try to arrange for children to visit the facilities and look at the equipment beforehand. These special preparations will make hearing screening less frightening for young children and increase the reliability of test results.

Common Disorders

Many hearing impairments are present at birth (Haynes). Infectious illnesses, experienced by a mother during pregnancy and premature birth are two factors known to increase the risk of hearing loss in children. Hearing impairments are frequently present in children who have other physical handicaps. Permanent and temporary hearing impairments are often associated with other health conditions, including:

- allergies
- frequent colds
- repeated ear infections
- birth defects
- head injuries or trauma

Hearing defects should also be considered in children whose relatives have hearing losses. Parents who express concern about their children's hearing should be listened to carefully and encouraged to seek a professional evaluation.

The most common forms of hearing loss are classified as conductive and sensorineural.

- *conductive* affects the volume of word tones. (For example, a child usually hears loud, but not soft sounds. This type of hearing loss occurs because sound waves are transmitted improperly from the external ear to structures of the inner ear, as when fluid accumulates in the child's middle ear.)
- *sensorineural* affects the range of tones heard. (For example, a child usually hears high, but not low tones. This type of hearing loss occurs when the eighth cranial nerve or sensory cells of the inner ear have been damaged).

A less common form of hearing loss results when sound impulses cannot reach the brain because of previous damage to the auditory nerve. Also, there are some children who hear actual sounds and words but are unable to interpret what they hear because of previous brain damage.

Management

Many types of hearing impairments can be successfully treated if they are recognized in the early stages. Treatment of hearing impairments is based on the underlying cause and may range from drug therapy to surgery. In some cases, a hearing aid may be helpful or, in extreme cases, the child may need to learn sign language.

A child suspected of having a sudden or gradual hearing loss should be referred to a family physician for medical diagnosis or an audiologist for a hearing evaluation. Arrangements for testing can be made through the child's doctor, a speech and hearing clinic, public health department, public schools or an audiologist.

A teacher or care provider who understands how different impairments affect children's ability to hear can take appropriate steps to improve learning conditions. Such measures might include:

- giving individualized instructions
- facing or standing near the child when speaking
- bending down to the child's level to make it easier for the child to hear and understand what is being said
- speaking slowly and clearly
- using gestures to illustrate what is being said, e.g., pointing to the door when it is time to go outside

- demonstrating what the child is expected to do, e.g., picking up a bead and threading it on a shoestring

Additional information about various hearing impairments and testing procedures can be obtained from:

National Association of Speech and Hearing
919 18th Street, NW
Washington, DC 20006

or

American Speech and Hearing Association
9030 Old Georgetown Road
Washington, DC 20014

SPEECH AND LANGUAGE EVALUATION

Throughout the early years, impressive gains are evident in both the number of words children understand (receptive vocabulary) and use to express themselves (expressive vocabulary). Generally, children's receptive vocabulary is more extensive than their expressive vocabulary. For example, most young children can follow instructions and understand simple directions long before they can clearly express themselves.

Children's language becomes increasingly fluent with time. They can use it to express ideas in both past and present tenses, ask and answer questions in detail, voice satisfaction or dissatisfaction, and provide vivid descriptions of everyday events. Simple two and three word phrases are characteristic of most two year olds:

- Go bye bye?
- Me do it!
- My ball!

However, by the age of four a child generally speaks in more complex, adultlike sentences:

- When is Mommy coming home?
- I don't want to eat my green beans!
- Where did the firetruck go?

Many factors influence the development of *speech* and *language*. Young children acquire many of their early language skills by imitating speech heard in their homes (Bradley 1978). If parents speak with a particular accent or have an unusual voice tone, their children are likely to exhibit similar qualities. Cultural variations also have a strong influence on language usage and speech patterns. It would be easy to consider a child, for whom English is a second language, as having delayed language skills if a teacher were not aware of the child's background. For this reason, it is important that teachers become familiar with children and their families when evaluating speech and language development.

Methods of Assessment

Parents often realize that their child has a speech problem, but may not know what to do about it. Many people believe that children eventually outgrow such impairments. Indeed, some children have developmentally appropriate *misarticulations* which will improve as they grow older. Nevertheless, children who demonstrate speech or speech patterns that are not developmentally appropriate should be referred to a speech therapist for a thorough evaluation. A hearing test should also be included in this evaluation to rule out the possibility of a hearing loss which may be affecting the child's speech. Speech and hearing clinics are frequently associated with colleges and universities, medical centers, child development centers and public school systems. A listing of certified speech and hearing specialists can be obtained by writing to the American Speech and Hearing Association.

Common Disorders

The term speech impairment has many different meanings to persons working with children. For some, the term refers only to more obvious problems, such as stuttering, lisping, or unintelligent speech patterns. For others, a wide range of conditions are cause for concern, e.g., a monotone voice, nasality, improper pitch of the voice, a voice tone that is too high or too low, omissions of certain letter sounds or misarticulations of word sounds.

The range of speech and language disorders is as great as the variations in normal speech and language development (Haynes). Some deviant speech patterns include:

- no speech by two years of age
- stuttering
- substitution of word sounds
- rate of speech that is too fast or unusually slow
- monotone voice
- no improvement in speech development
- unintelligent speech by three years of age

Management

Parents, teachers and care providers must not overlook the important role they play as role models in child's speech and language development. Early language experiences and stimulation encourage the child's effective use of language. However, teachers and care providers should not hesitate to refer children for professional evaluation if their speech and language patterns interfere with or make communication difficult.

NUTRITION EVALUATION

There is no question that the quality of children's diets has a direct effect on their behavior and state of health. Problems related to over- and under-consumption of food and nutrients are of growing concern. Rising food costs and difficult economic conditions are forcing many families to sacrifice the quality and quantity of food they purchase and serve. Increased consumption of ''fast foods'' and the extensive use of prepackaged foods in meal preparation add to a further decline in the quality of many children's diets.

Common Disorders

Teachers and care providers need to be alert to several nutritional problems that may affect children's health. Poor dietary habits over a period of time can lead to malnutrition. Protein, vitamin C, and iron are nutrients most commonly missing from children's diets today. Long-term use of certain medications can also interfere with the absorption of some nutrients. Many children are undernourished simply because they do not get enough to eat. These children are often below average in height and weight, irritable, anemic, and listless. Their poor state of nutrition limits their ability to learn.

Not all malnourished children are thin and emaciated. Overweight children can also be malnourished. Because the bulk of their diet often consists of sugars and starches, they appear to be well fed, yet lack many of the nutrients essential for good health.

Another serious nutritional health problem is that of obesity (Wilson 1983). Approximately twelve to thirty percent of all children in the United States are considered overweight for their age (Haslam 1975; Little 1983). Suggested causes include metabolic disorders, emotional stress, heredity, lack of physical activity and, perhaps most significant, poor eating habits.

Children who are overweight or obese often face additional health problems. Excess weight limits their participation in much needed physical activity. Obese children tend to be less coordinated, experience shortness of breath with exertion and tire more quickly. Teasing, ridicule and rejection by others can also lead to maladjustment problems. Overweight children are more likely to remain overweight as adults and face an increased risk of medical complications, including heart disease, stroke and diabetes.

Management

Obesity in young children cannot be ignored. Prevention is always the most effective method. However, promising results can also be obtained by taking action while a child is young and still in the process of establishing lifelong eating habits (Lasky 1982). For maximum success, a treatment program for weight control must include the cooperation of the child, parents, teachers and health personnel.

The goal of any weight control program is to help young children and their parents develop a new awareness about:

- meal planning and nutritious eating habits.
- methods for increasing children's daily activity level, Figure 4–8. (For example, children can be asked to run errands, walk a pet or help with daily household chores.)
- acquainting children with new outside interests, hobbies or activities, such as swimming, dance, neighborhood baseball or learning to ride a bike. (Involvement in fun activities can divert children's attention away from food.)
- finding ways to help children experience success and develop a positive self-image. (For example, praise received for simple achievements can make children feel good about themselves—"Lonnie, you did a nice job of sweeping all the sand off the sidewalk." For many children, praise replaces food as an important source of satisfaction.)

Chances of long-term weight control are enhanced by attending to all aspects of a child's well-being, e.g., physical, emotional and social. Education and role modeling are also important factors in the management of nutrition and promotion of healthier life-styles.

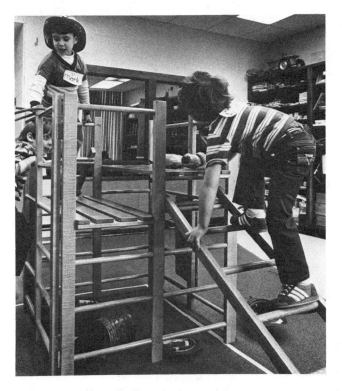

FIGURE 4–8 Increasing children's activity level can help to control their weight.

REFERRALS

The initial step in making successful referrals involves gaining the parent's trust and cooperation. Referrals are of little use unless parents follow through with recommendations. Knowing something about the beliefs, customs, habits, and people of the community can influence the way in which referrals are conducted. For example, mistrust of the medical profession, poverty, job conflicts, religious beliefs, a lack of transportation or education will certainly affect a parent's response.

Meeting with the child's parents or calling them on the telephone are usually the most effective methods for making referrals. If such personal contacts with parents are not possible, a well-written letter is also appropriate. Parents should be given copies of any screening test results or anecdotal notes which they can forward to the specialist who will be further evaluating the child. This gesture will improve the efficiency of the referral process. Also, a teacher who is familiar with local services, such as hospitals, clinics, health departments, medical specialists, private and public service agencies and various sources of funding can be very helpful to parents in obtaining the comprehensive medical care and assistance which the child requires.

Follow-up contacts with parents should be made again in several weeks to determine if further diagnostic testing or treatments have been completed. Any results or recommendations which might affect the child's experiences in school can also be shared at this time. Knowledge of this information enables child care providers to make any necessary adjustments in the instructional program or learning environment. Follow-up contacts can be used to reinforce the positive influences of preventive health care on children's performance and convey to parents a genuine interest in their child's well-being.

SUMMARY

Teachers and care providers play an important role in the health assessment of young children. In addition to their skillful observations, teachers have access to a variety of health information concerning each child. Permanent health records provide a rich source of background and current information which can be useful in identifying potentially handicapping conditions. Results obtained from routine screening procedures, e.g., measures of height and weight, vision, hearing, dental, developmental, can also help to shed light on children's disabilities. Care providers must remember that most routine screening tests have certain limitations and, as a result, a child's performance on such tests must be interpreted carefully.

The process of assessing children's health involves gathering information from a variety of sources. Teachers can initiate the referral process with reasonable assurance when it is based on documented information. Ideally, the reasons for making a referral should be discussed with the child's parents. A follow-up contact is necessary to determine if the recommendations have been carried out.

LEARNING ACTIVITIES

1. List the speech and hearing clinics or facilities in your community. Invite a speaker from one of the programs to talk with the class.

2. Locate and read instructions for administering the Snellen E eye screening test. With another student, practice testing one another.

3. Select one health impairment. Locate all of the resources, services, private and public agencies, clubs and organizations in your community that provide assistance to families for this impairment.

4. Collect samples of child history forms from several centers or day care facilities in your town. Review the types of information that are requested more often. Design your own form.

5. Attend a signing class. Learn to say "hello" and "good-bye" in sign language.

UNIT REVIEW

A. Define the following terms.

   1. audiologist

   2. conductive hearing loss

   3. sensorineural hearing loss

   4. receptive vocabulary

   5. expressive vocabulary

B. Multiple Choice. Select the one best answer.

   1. Amblyopia is the result of
     a. imbalance of the eye muscle
     b. infection
     c. trauma or injury
     d. an unknown cause

   2. Children's health records are useful for
     a. identifying possible problem areas
     b. evaluating the success of treatments
     c. following a child's progress
     d. all of these

   3. A *recognizable* imbalance of the eye muscle is called
     a. hyperopia
     b. myopia
     c. strabismus
     d. none of these

4. Screening procedures most commonly used to evaluate the health of pre-school children include all of the following *except*
   a. vision and hearing
   b. lead poisoning and parasites
   c. height and weight
   d. dental

5. Referrals should be based on
   a. screening test results
   b. teacher observations
   c. parent concerns
   d. all of these

6. Hearing losses are often found in children who
   a. are from poverty families
   b. have allergies and frequent ear infections
   c. are small for their age
   d. live in colder climates

C. Select the screening test that would be recommended for children with the following behaviors, signs, or symptoms. Place the appropriate code letter in each space.
   _H_ Hearing screening
   _V_ Vision screening
   _D_ Developmental screening
   HW Height and weight
   _Dt_ Dental screening
   _S_ Speech
   _N_ Nutrition evaluation

   _____ 1. frequent blinking; often closes one eye to see

   _____ 2. stutters whenever he is tense and in a hurry to speak

   _____ 3. usually listless; appears very small for her chronological age

   _____ 4. stumbles over objects in the classroom; frequently walks into play equipment in the play yard

   _____ 5. very crooked teeth which make his speech difficult to understand

   _____ 6. seems to ignore the teacher's requests; shouts at the other children to get their attention

   _____ 7. awkward; has great difficulty running and climbing; tires easily be-cause of obesity

_____ 8. a five year old who has trouble catching a ball, pedaling a bicycle and cutting with scissors

_____ 9. appears to focus on objects with one eye while the other eye looks off in another direction

_____10. multiple cavities; in recent weeks has not been able to concentrate on any task

_____11. is extremely shy and withdrawn; spends the majority of her time playing alone, imitating the actions of other children

_____12. seems extremely hungry at snack time; always asks for extra servings and takes food left on other children's plates when the teacher isn't looking

_____13. becomes hoarse after shouting and yelling during outdoor time

_____14. arrives at school each morning with potato chips, candy or a cupcake

_____15. a 4½ year old who whines and has tantrums to get his own way

REFERENCES

Allen, K.E.; Rieke, J.; Dmitriev, V.; Hayden, A.H. "Early Warning: Observation as a Tool for Recognizing Potential Handicaps in Young Children." *Educational Horizons* 50(2):43–54, Winter 1972.

Bradley, D. *Language Intervention.* Arlington, VA: ERIC Documents Reproduction Services (ED No. 101–184), 1978.

Brojkovich, H.L. "Snellen's 20/20: The Development and Use of the Eye Chart." *Journal of School Health* 50(8):472–74, August 1980.

Brown, M., and Collar, M. "Research—Effects of Prior Preparation on the Preschooler's Vision and Hearing Screening." *Journal of Maternal/Child Nursing* 7(5):323–28, September/October 1982.

Gray, P.J. "Psst! Can You Hear Me?" *Parents* 59(3):60–68, March 1984.

Haslem, R., and Valletutti, P. *Medical Problems in the Classroom.* Baltimore: University Park Press, 1975.

Haynes, U. *A Developmental Approach to Case-finding.* Washington, DC: U.S. Department of Health, Education and Welfare, Public Health Service, U.S. Government Printing Office (DHEW No. 79-5210).

Lasky, P., and Eichelberger, K. "Implications, Considerations and Nursing Interventions of Obesity in Neonatal and Preschool Patients." *Nursing Clinics of North America* 17(2):199–205, June 1982.

Little, T. "Management of the Obese Child in School." *Journal of School Health* 53(7):440–41, September 1983.

National Health Statistics: NCHS Growth Curves for Children. Series 11, No. 165, U.S. Department of Health, Education and Welfare, Monthly Vital Statistics Report. U.S. Government Printing Office, 1976.

Spodek, B.; Saracho, D.; and Lee, R. *Mainstreaming Young Children.* Belmont, CA: Wadsworth Publishing Co., 1984.

Vision Screening In Schools. New York: National Society for the Prevention of Blindness.

Wilson, P.; Bower, R.; and Eller, B. "Childhood Obesity: Prevention and Treatment." *Young Children* 39(1):21–27, November 1983.

Additional Readings

Adams, J.; Evans, G.; and Roberts, E. "Diagnosing and Treating Otitis Media With Effusion." *Maternal/Child Nursing* 9(1):22–28, January/February 1984.

Johnson, J.; Spellman, C.; Cress, P.; Sizemore, A.; and Shores, R. "The School Nurses' Role in Vision Screening for the Difficult-to-Test Student." *Journal of School Health* 53(6):345–49, August 1983.

Orloske, A., and Luddo, J. "Environmental Effects on Children's Hearing." *Journal of School Health* 51(1):12–14, January 1981.

Unit 5

CONDITIONS AFFECTING CHILDREN'S HEALTH

Terms to Know

alignment	hormone
anemia	dehydration
endocrine	hyperactivity
seizures	syndrome

Objectives

After studying this unit, you will be able to:
- Describe seven chronic conditions that affect children's health.
- List the symptoms of seven chronic health conditions.
- State the factors that make chronic health problems difficult to identify in young children.
- Describe good body mechanics for sitting, standing, and lifting.
- Identify the care provider's role in dealing with chronic health problems.

More important than the occasional illnesses young children experience are the chronic or long-term health problems. Often, chronic conditions go unrecognized because their signs and symptoms are less obvious than those of most acute illnesses. Some chronic health problems such as sickle cell anemia and diabetes may be present from the time of birth. Other chronic conditions such as fatigue and seizures may develop slowly so their appearance is difficult to detect; the child may not even realize that something is wrong. The closeness of parents may also make it more difficult for them to recognize and accept chronic health problems in their child.

Undiagnosed and untreated chronic health conditions can interfere with the development of early learning skills. Teachers and care providers should work with parents to identify children who have existing health problems. These children should then be referred to the appropriate health professionals for comprehensive evaluation and treatment.

FATIGUE

Most children experience periods of fatigue and listlessness from time to time. Growth spurts, late bedtimes, a morning of strenuous outdoor play, or recovery from a recent illness may account for these occasional incidences. However, when a child shows repeated or continuous signs of fatigue, parents and teachers should be concerned.

Typically, preschool children have remarkable vigor, enthusiasm, and interest in daily activities. Chronic fatigue is not a normal condition for children of this age. Possible causes of chronic fatigue include:

- poor nutrition
- chronic infection
- periods of rapid growth
- insufficient hours of rest and sleep
- medications
- *anemia*
- *endocrine* (hormonal) disorders
- allergies
- lead poisoning

Careful evaluation of the child's personal habits and life-style may reveal a reason for chronic fatigue. A complete medical examination can detect any existing health problems. If no definite reasons can be found, there are several steps parents and care providers can take to improve the child's general well-being:

- better dietary habits
- moderate exercise and activity
- increased rest, e.g. naps, earlier bedtimes, brief periods of rest during the day
- alternating periods of activity and rest

Teachers and care providers can also incorporate many of these remedies into daily classroom routines.

POSTURE

Good posture and correct body *alignment* are necessary for many of the physical activities in which children engage, such as walking, jumping, running, skipping, standing, sitting and balancing. Many problems related to poor posture can be avoided by helping young children develop good postural habits from the beginning.

Orthopedic problems (those relating to skeletal and muscular systems) are not common among preschool children. However, there are several conditions which warrant early diagnosis and treatment:

- abnormal or unusual walking patterns, e.g., limping, pigeon-toed
- bowed legs
- knock-knees
- flat feet
- unusual curvature of the spine
- one extremity (arm or leg) shorter than the other

Some irregularities of posture disappear spontaneously as young children mature. For example, it is not uncommon for infants and toddlers to have bowed legs or to later walk slightly pigeon-toed. As they approach three or four years of age, these problems often correct themselves. If these conditions persist beyond the age of four, they should be evaluated by health professionals. Early detection and treatment can prevent many long-term or permanent deformities.

Good posture is an excellent topic for classroom discussions, demonstrations, rhythm and movement activities, games, and art projects, Figure 5–1.

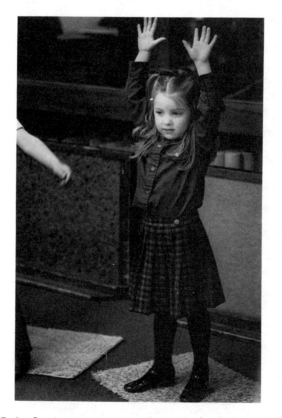

FIGURE 5–1   Good posture is an excellent topic for rhythm and movement activities.

Concepts and techniques that children learn can be shared with parents so they are reinforced at home (Curtis 1982). Parent newsletters can include suggestions for good posture, children can illustrate basic posture concepts in pictures, and parents can be invited to attend a class demonstration of good body alignment.

Although the act of sitting and standing seem quite natural, it is important that children learn the following good body mechanics:

- Sit squarely in a chair with the back against the back of the chair and both feet flat on the floor.
- Sit on the floor with legs crossed in front or with both legs extended out to one side. (Children who repeatedly sit in a "W" position risk the chance of developing serious problems later in life, Figure 5–2. These children need frequent reminders to assume a correct sitting position: "Let's all sit with our legs crossed like this.")
- Stand with the shoulders square, the chin up and the chest out. Distribute body weight evenly over both feet to avoid placing added stress on one or the other hip joints.
- Lift and carry heavy objects using the stronger muscles of the arms and legs rather than the weaker muscles of the back. Get close to the object to be

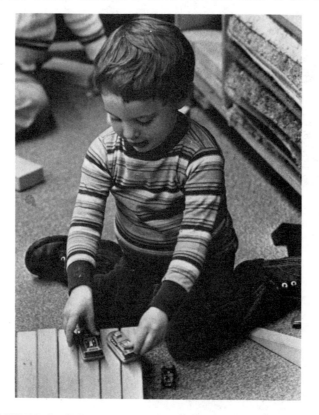

FIGURE 5–2 Children should not sit with legs in a "W" position.

lifted. Stand with the feet slightly apart to give a wider base of support, and stoop down to lift rather than just bend over.

DIABETES

The incidence of diabetes among preschool children is low. However, teachers and care providers should be familiar with the signs, symptoms, and treatment for diabetes. When diabetes occurs in young children, it is more difficult to control. Growth, unpredictable changes in activity levels, poor eating habits, and frequent exposure to respiratory infections challenge the successful management of the juvenile diabetic (Peterson 1975).

Diabetes is a chronic health problem that occurs when the body does not produce enough insulin. Insulin is a *hormone.* Its major function is to aid in the storage of sugars and starches ingested in the diet and later to release this as energy to the body cells. Absence or inadequate amounts of insulin allow sugar to circulate freely in the blood stream rather than be stored and released when needed. A high level of sugar in the blood is called hyperglycemia or diabetic coma. Without medical treatment, this condition gradually worsens and can eventually lead to convulsions and death. Early signs of diabetes include:

- weight loss
- fatigue
- frequent urination
- *dehydration*
- excessive thirst and hunger
- frequent infections
- slow healing
- itching and dry skin

It is important that teachers and care providers be aware of any diabetic children in their classrooms. In addition to the potential dangers of undiagnosed diabetes, there are also complications associated with its treatment. Most diabetic children must take daily injections of insulin. A dose that is too small or too large requires different emergency treatment (see Unit 11).

Valuable information can be gathered by meeting with parents before the diabetic child begins to attend a school or child care center. Parents can alert teachers to changes in their child's behavior and appearance that may signal impending complications. The teacher also needs to be informed of dietary restrictions and management so they can be followed carefully while the child is at school. Telephone numbers and names of contact persons should also be reviewed with parents from time to time.

Equipped with this knowledge, a teacher is in a better position to recognize and cope with emergencies. This can be a source of comfort to the parents of a diabetic child for often they feel uneasy about leaving their child in the care of others. Teachers are also in a unique position to help diabetic children accept their condition and learn to lead well-adjusted lives.

SEIZURES

It is not uncommon to have children who experience *seizures* in a preschool classroom. Unlike many other chronic health problems, mention of terms such as seizures, convulsions, or epilepsy arouse feelings of fear and anxiety in many persons, including teachers. Prior knowledge and planning enable teachers and care providers to react with skill and confidence when working with children who experience these health problems, Table 5–1.

The term seizure describes a cluster of symptoms rather than a particular disease. Seizures are caused by abnormal electrical impulses within the brain. This abnormal activity leads to involuntary or uncontrollable movements of various body parts. Their intensity varies, depending on the type of seizure. Some seizures involve only a momentary lapse of attention or interruption of thought while others may last several minutes and cause vigorous, spasmotic contractions of the entire body. Temporary loss of consciousness, frothing, and loss of bowel and bladder control may also accompany some types of seizures.

The exact cause of a seizure is often difficult to determine. However, several conditions are known to initiate seizure activity in young children:

- fevers that are high or rise rapidly
- brain damage
- infections that affect the central nervous system, such as meningitis or encephalitis

TABLE 5–1   How Teachers Can Help a Child Who Experiences Seizures

1. Be aware of any children with seizure disorders in the classroom. Find out what the child's seizures are like, if medication is taken to control the seizures, and whether the child is limited in any way by the disorder.

2. Know emergency first aid measures. Develop guidelines for staff members to follow whenever a child has a seizure; review the guidelines periodically.

3. Use the presence of an epileptic child in the classroom as a learning experience for other children. Provide simple explanations about what epilepsy is; encourage children to ask questions and express their feelings. Help children learn to accept those who have special problems.

4. Gain a better understanding of epilepsy and seizure disorders. Read books and articles, view films and talk with health professionals and parents.

5. Obtain and read the following books and pamphlets that are written for children. Share them with children in the classroom.
   - *All About Epilepsy*. Epilepsy Foundation of America, 4351 Garden City Drive, Landover, MD 20785.
   - Bookbinder, S. R. *Mainstreaming: What Every Child Needs to Know About Disabilities*. Exceptional Parent Press, 296 Boylston Street, Third Floor, Boston, MA 02116.
   - Silverstein, A. *Epilepsy*. Philadelphia: J. B. Lippincott Co., 1975.
   - Young, M. *What Difference Does It Make, Danny?* London: Andre Deutsch Limited, 1980.

- tumors
- head injuries
- lead, mercury and carbon monoxide poisoning
- hypoglycemia (low blood sugar)
- drug reactions

Heredity has also been suggested as a possible cause. In many cases, the exact cause may never be known.

Seizures are generally classified according to the pattern of symptoms the child presents (Peterson 1975; Chow 1979). The most common types of seizures are:

- petite mal
- grand mal
- jacksonian
- psychomotor

Care providers may be the first to notice the subtle, abnormal behaviors exhibited by children with petite mal seizures. This type of seizure is characterized by momentary losses of attention, including:

- repeated incidences of daydreaming
- staring off into space
- a blank appearance
- brief fluttering of the eyes
- temporary interruption of speech or activity
- twitching or dropping of objects

Petite mal seizures are characterized by a brief ten to thirty seconds loss of consciousness. The child suddenly stops the activity in which it is engaged and resumes it after the seizure subsides. Parents should be informed of the teacher's or care provider's observations and encouraged to contact the child's physician.

In contrast to the mild nature of petite mal seizures, there is seldom any doubt when a child has a grand mal seizure. Convulsive movements usually involve the entire body, often making them frightening to the observer. Most children experience an aura or warning immediately before a seizure begins. This warning may be in the form of a certain sound, smell, taste, sensation or visual cue. Sudden rigidity or stiffness is followed by a loss of consciousness and generalized muscular contractions. When the seizure ends, children usually awaken briefly. They may complain of headache or dizziness before falling asleep for a period of several hours.

The involuntary convulsive movements of a jacksonian seizure begin at the tip of an extremity and travels toward the extremity's connection to the body. The child does not always lose consciousness with this type of seizure. Spontaneous episodes of unusual behavior are a feature of psychomotor seizures. The behavior is considered unusual because it is inappropriate for the circumstances. For example, a child may burst out in sudden hysterical laughter, utter unintelligible sounds, run around in circles or cry out without apparent reason. It is also common to experience an aura before this type of seizure begins. Although there is usually not a total loss of consciousness during the seizure, children may appear drowsy or confused for one to two minutes after the attack and should be encouraged to rest for a short time.

Most seizures can be controlled with medication. It is vital that children take their medications every day, even after seizures are under control. Initially, children may experience some side effects to these drugs such as drowsiness, nausea and dizziness. However, these problems usually disappear after a short time.

Each time a child experiences a seizure, parents should be notified. Also, any time seizures change in character or begin to recur after having once been under control, parents should be informed and encouraged to contact the child's physician. Informing parents enables the parents to keep accurate records of seizure activity and to monitor medical treatment. Teachers and care providers should also complete a brief, written report documenting their observations following each seizure. The report should include a description of:

- events preceding the seizure
- time length of the seizure
- type and location of convulsive movements
- additional observations, e.g., breathing difficulties, loss of bowel or bladder control, skin color
- condition of the child following the seizure, e.g., injuries, length of sleep, complaints of headache

Completed reports should be filed in the child's permanent health folder. This information can be very useful to the child's physician for diagnosing a seizure disorder and evaluating the effectiveness of medications.

Teachers are important figures in helping young children develop positive attitudes toward persons who experience seizures. The teacher's reactions and displays of genuine acceptance can teach respect and understanding for persons with special problems.

ALLERGIES

Allergies are the greatest single cause of chronic health problems among young children. It is believed that allergies affect as many as one in every four children. The severity of allergic conditions range from symptoms that are only mildly annoying to those that are disabling and severely restrict a child's activity.

A substance capable of triggering an allergic reaction in an individual is called an allergen. Most children are not bothered by these substances. However, because the allergic child's immune system is more sensitive, an allergic reaction takes place whenever they come in contact with a particular allergen (Baker 1980).

Allergic reactions are generally classified according to the body site where symptoms most commonly occur:

- ingestants—cause digestive upsets and respiratory problems. Common examples include foods such as milk, citrus fruits, eggs, wheat, chocolate and oral medications.
- inhalants—affect the respiratory system causing a runny nose, cough, wheezing, and watery eyes. Examples include pollens, molds, dust, and animal dander.
- contactants—frequently cause skin eruptions such as rashes, hives and eczema. Common contactants include soaps, cosmetics, dyes, fibers, medications placed directly on the skin, and some plants, e.g., poison ivy and poison oak.
- injectables—result in respiratory, digestive, and skin disturbances. Examples of injectables include insect bites, especially those of bees, wasps and hornets, and medications that are injected directly into the body.

In addition to the acute distress experienced during allergic reactions, these children often do not feel well much of the time (Voignier 1980). To understand how allergies affect them, a simple comparison can be made with the generalized discomfort felt during a cold or case of intestinal flu. Certainly, no child can fully benefit from any learning experience under such conditions. For these reasons, allergies may be an important contributing factor in many behavior and learning problems, including disruptive behaviors, hyperactivity, chronic fatigue, disinterest, irritability and poor concentration.

Care providers can be instrumental in recognizing the early signs of allergic conditions in young children. Daily observations and anecdotal records can help detect patterns of repetitive symptoms that may otherwise be blamed on just the usual childhood illnesses (Marks 1974). Some common signs and symptoms of allergic disorders include:

- frequent colds and ear infections
- chronic congestion, e.g., runny nose, cough or throat clearing
- headaches
- frequent nosebleeds
- unexplained stomachaches
- hives, eczema or other skin rashes
- wheezing or shortness of breath
- intermittent or permanent hearing losses
- reactions to foods or medications
- dark circles beneath the eyes
- mottled tongue
- frequent rubbing, twitching or picking of the nose
- chronic redness of the throat
- swollen eyelids
- irritability

At present, there are no known cures for allergic conditions. Sensitivities are thought to be inherited and are seldom outgrown. However, the types and numbers of substances to which a child is allergic can change periodically. This may give the impression that an allergy has disappeared, only to resurface and become troublesome again at some later time.

Symptoms and complications of allergies are generally less severe and easier to control if they are identified early. Treatment is aimed primarily at limiting a child's exposure to annoying allergens. In some instances, steps can be taken to completely remove these substances from the child's environment. For example, milk and milk products can be totally eliminated from the child's diet, or a dog kept outdoors. In other cases, only the amount of exposure can be controlled, as in allergies to dust or pollens. Smoking should also be discouraged around children with allergies because it can aggravate and intensify their problems. Left untreated, allergies can lead to more serious chronic health problems, including chronic bronchitis, permanent hearing loss, asthma or emphysema.

Antihistamines, decongestants and bronchodilators are commonly used to treat the symptoms of respiratory allergies. However, a major drawback is that medication provides only temporary relief and may make children drowsy. Children taking any of these drugs should be closely supervised, especially during outdoor times and activities that involve risk. Allergy shots (desensitizing therapy) are sometimes used when other forms of treatment have proven unsuccessful.

Most allergic conditions are not life threatening. However, *bee stings, sensitivities to medications, and asthma attacks can lead to death.* In these emergency situations, a child can quickly go into shock and experience extreme difficulty breathing. Prompt medical treatment is necessary to save the child's life.

The emotional effects of allergies on children's lives are often overlooked. Frequently, these children are protected from many everyday experiences in order to avoid the risk of unpleasant reactions. They are continually reminded to be cautious so that exposure to offending allergens is limited. In some cases, severe allergies may actually place limits on a child's level of physical activity. Eventually, such feelings can lead to fear, withdrawn behaviors and maladjustment problems.

It is important that children not be allowed to use their allergies as a means of gaining attention or special privileges. Instead, they must learn to become independent and self-confident in coping with their problems. Teachers can help children make adjustments in their daily life-styles. Also, parenting classes and individual counseling can teach parents the skills they need to help children achieve these goals.

HYPERACTIVITY

The term *hyperactivity* is often used inappropriately to label children who are actually behaving within normal limits (Weiss 1979). Preschool children are, by nature, exceedingly energetic, curious, impatient, and restless, Figure 5–3.

Much confusion surrounds the problems of hyperactivity including its symptoms, causes and treatment. The terms hyperkinesis, hyperactivity, minimal brain dysfunction, and learning disability are often used interchangeably to de-

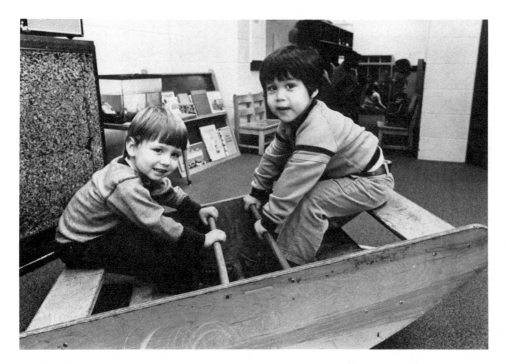

FIGURE 5–3   Preschool children are naturally energetic and curious.

scribe the same condition. Recent attempts to more clearly define hyperactivity refer to it as "a *syndrome* of attention and behavior disturbances that may improve when stimulant-type drugs are administered" (American Psychiatric Association 1981).

Unlike many other health disorders, there are few exact symptoms of hyperactivity. This fact makes it very difficult to establish a clear-cut diagnosis. Some of the behaviors typically used to describe the hyperactive child include:

- explosive
- inattentive
- fidgety
- aggressive

- defiant
- forgetful
- easily frustrated
- clumsy

In many cases the decision that a child is hyperactive is based purely on a combination of personal beliefs and observations. Currently, there are no specific medical tests available for accurately diagnosing the disorder. However, it is known that boys are affected more often than girls.

Recently, the American Psychiatric Association set forth guidelines to aid in the process of identifying hyperactive children. They have suggested that the following behavior patterns be observed and documented for at least one full year before clearly determining that a child is hyperactive:

- excessive levels of motor activity based on the child's age
- limited attention span; easily distracted and forgetful
- repeated incidences of impulsive behavior; aggressive and easily frustrated
- poor motor coordination
- disturbances of sleep

There is no one simple method for treating hyperactivity. Each child requires an individualized approach. Often a combination of methods is used, some of which are considered to be controversial.

One common approach involves prescribing stimulant or antidepressive-type medications for children. Interestingly, in children who are truly hyperactive, these drugs have an effect that is opposite of what might be expected. Rather than increasing their activity level, the drugs often have a calming effect.

The medical profession has been criticized for its over use of medications to treat hyperactive children. Drugs are felt to be an easy way out for parents, doctors and teachers and are often prescribed before other forms of therapy are tried. There are several undesirable side effects associated with these medications, including depression of children's appetite and growth, sleeplessness, listlessness and a stuporlike state. Furthermore, medication seldom cures the child's problem behaviors. The symptoms of hyperactivity will usually return once drug therapy is discontinued. However, medication can be beneficial for some children when it is used over a short period of time and in combination with other forms of therapy.

Success has been achieved with behavior modification techniques and special education to treat hyperactive children. This effectiveness can be attributed to the fact that each method deals directly with the child's problem behaviors. Through carefully planned and controlled experiences, children can learn behaviors that are acceptable and appropriate. Some basic principles include:

- Creating a structured environment. The degree of structure depends on the type and severity of the child's problems. For example, structure for one child may involve restricting the number of furnishings in a classroom to a single table and chair. For another child, structure may be achieved by limiting the number of choices, e.g. choosing between only two toys or activities.
- Establishing a daily routine that is consistent. Hyperactive children function best when things are familiar, including a routine that is the same from day to day.
- Giving directions that are clear and easy for the child to follow. Let the child know exactly what is expected. "Andy, I want you to put the toys in this basket." The use of repetition is also important.
- Offering praise and positive reinforcement. This is an effective means for gaining children's cooperation. It also encourages them to attempt and complete even simple tasks. "Good work, Nel. You have found three of the red beads."
- Providing experiences that are challenging, yet, within the skill and tolerance level of the hyperactive child. Thus, a child can experience frequent success and avoid repeated frustration and failure.

- Providing opportunities for developing new interests, especially physical activities where children can channel excess energy.

Using these techniques with young children may help lessen the development of serious emotional problems that often accompany hyperactivity. Self-confidence improves as children are successful and no longer see themselves as "always bad" or "failures" at whatever they do.

Dietary management has also been suggested as a treatment for hyperactivity (Kolata 1982). The controversial Feingold diet, introduced during the 1970s, linked artificial colors, flavors and foods containing an aspirin-related compound to the uncontrollable behaviors associated with hyperactivity. Feingold reported that when foods with these additives were omitted from the child's diet, behavior improved dramatically.

Many authorities continue to question Feingold's theories and results. However, like many other forms of therapy, what works for one child does not necessarily work for another. If parents recognize this fact beforehand, they are less likely to be frustrated if dietary changes do not produce the results they hoped for. However, there is certainly no harm in feeding children foods that are nutritious and additive free.

SICKLE CELL ANEMIA

Sickle cell anemia is an inherited disorder of the blood that is found primarily in the Black population (Whaley 1979; Richardson 1983). It sometimes occurs in those of Mediterranean, Middle Eastern, Turkish or Puerto Rican descent. Approximately ten percent of Blacks carry the trait for sickle cell anemia but do not necessarily experience symptoms of the disease themselves; these people are called carriers, Figure 5–4. When two adults with the sickle cell trait marry, there is a chance that some of their children will be born with the actual disease, while others will only be carriers.

The abnormal formation of red blood cells in sickle cell anemia causes chronic health problems for the child. Red blood cells form in the shape of a comma or sickle, rather than their normal round shape. As a result, blood flow throughout the body is slowed and occasionally blocked. Symptoms of the disease do not usually appear until sometime after the child's first birthday.

Clumping of deformed blood cells results in periods of acute illness called crises. A crisis can be triggered by infection, injury, strenuous exercise or dehydration. Symptoms of a sickle cell crisis include fever, severe abdominal and leg pain, vomiting, and ulcers (sores) on the arms and legs. Children must usually be hospitalized during a crisis. Between flare-ups, they may be free from any acute symptoms. However, because of chronic infection and anemia, these children are often small for their age and tire easily.

At present there is no known cure for sickle cell anemia. However, genetic counseling offers prospective parents who are carriers the chance to decide whether or not they want to risk having children. Also, screening programs are

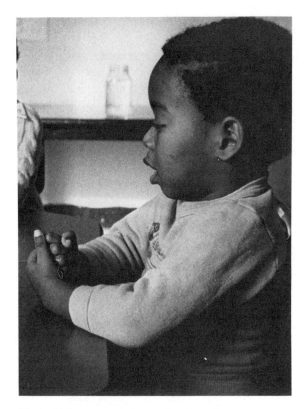

FIGURE 5-4 Many Black children carry the trait of sickle cell anemia but do not have symptoms of the disease themselves.

now available to enable parents to obtain early diagnosis and medical care for infants with sickle cell disease.

LEARNING ACTIVITIES

1. Locate and read at least three children's books written about a chronic health disorder or disease. Prepare a bibliography card for each book and use the cards to begin a file of books for children on related topics.

2. Interview three preschool teachers. Find out what types of allergies they encounter most often and how they manage these problems in the class-room. Develop a simple, five-day snack menu for a child who is allergic to milk and milk products, chocolate, and eggs.

3. Divide into several small groups. Practice good posture techniques for sit-ting, standing, walking, and lifting. Prepare a lesson plan for teaching two of these techniques to a group of preschool and school-aged children.

4. Invite a speaker from the nearest chapter of the Feingold Association. Read at least one of the following articles beforehand and be prepared to ask questions:

Feingold, B.F. "Hyperkinesis and Learning Disabilities Linked to Artificial Food Flavors and Colors." *American Journal of Nursing* 75:797, May 1975.

Herbert, W. "Hyperactivity—Diet Link Questions." *Science News* 121:53, January 23, 1982.

Kolata, G. "Consensus on Diets and Hyperactivity." *Science* 215:958, February 19, 1982.

Meister, K.A. "Do Food Additives Cause Hyperactivity?" *American Baby* 43:10, April 1981.

Oace, S.M. "Diet and Hyperactivity." *Journal of Nutrition Education* 13:5, March 1981.

Robinson, L.A. "Food Allergies, Food Additives and the Feingold Diet." *Pediatric Nurse* 6:38, November/December 1980.

UNIT REVIEW

A. Define the following terms.

1. chronic

2. orthopedic problem

3. allergen

4. insulin

5. hyperglycemia

6. allergic reaction

B. Read the case study and fill in the blanks with a word(s) selected from the following list.

breathing	headache
sleep	anticonvulsants
seizure	affected
informed	consciousness
aura	written report
grand mal	time length
permanent health file	

While climbing up the playhouse ladder, Jamie let out a sudden shriek, released her grip and fell to the ground. Her teacher quickly ran to see what had happened. Jamie lay on the ground unconscious, her arms and legs jerking. The teacher realized that Jamie was having a _____, and that it was probably a _____ type. A warning or _____ usually precedes this kind of seizure.

Jamie's teacher stood back and watched until the muscular contractions ended. In addition to the loss of consciousness, the teacher also carefully noted the exact _____ of the seizure, the parts of the body _____, and whether Jamie had any difficulty _____. Later, this information would be included in a _____ which would be placed in the child's _____.

When Jamie regained _____ she complained of a _____. The teacher encouraged her to _____ for a short while. Meanwhile, Jamie's parents were _____ of her seizure. Her mother explained that the doctor had recently prescribed a new medication and was trying to regulate the dosage. The most common group of medications used to treat seizure disorders are _____.

C. Briefly answer the following questions.

1. List four possible causes for fatigue in young children.

2. Describe the proper way for children to sit on the floor and in a chair.

3. Why has the use of medication to treat hyperactive children stirred so much controversy?

4. List five common symptoms of early diabetes.

5. Distinguish between petite mal and grand mal seizures.

6. Why are many chronic health problems difficult to identify in the young child?

REFERENCES

American Psychiatric Association: Diagnostic Manual for Mental Disorders. Vol. IV. Washington, DC: American Psychiatric Association, 1981.

Baker, B., and Baker, C. "Difficulties Generated by Allergies." Journal of School Health 50(10):583, December 1980.

Chow, M.; Durand, B.; Feldman, M.; and Mills, M. Handbook of Pediatric Primary Care. New York: John Wiley and Sons, 1979.

Curtis, S. The Joy of Movement. New York: Teacher's College Press, 1982.

Kolata, G. "Consensus on Diets and Hyperactivity." Science 215(4535):958–59, February 19, 1982.

Marks, M. "Recognition of the Allergic Child At School: Visual and Auditory Signs." Journal of School Health 44(5):227–85, May 1974.

Richardson, E., and Milne, L. "Sickle-cell Disease and the Childbearing Family: An Update." *Journal of Maternal/Child Nursing* 8:417–22, November/December 1983.

Voignier, R., and Bridgewater, S. "Allergies in Young Children." *Young Children* 35(4):67–70, May 1980.

Weiss, G., and Hechtman, L. "The Hyperactive Child Syndrome." *Science* 205(28):1348–54, September 1979.

Whaley, L., and Wong, D. *Nursing Care of Infants and Children.* St. Louis, MO: C.V. Mosby Co., 1979.

Medical Problems In the Classroom. Edited by Raymond Peterson and J. Cleveland. Springfield, MO: Charles C. Thomas Publishers, 1975.

Additional Reading

Brumer, R.L., and Vorhees, C.V. "Food Colors and Behavior." *Science* 212(4494):578–79, May 1, 1981.

Haslam, Robert, and Valletutti, Peter. *Medical Problems in the Classroom.* Baltimore: University Park Press, 1975.

Kaercher, D. "New Findings About Hyperactive Children." *Better Homes and Gardens,* March 1983.

White, Judy E., and Owsley, Vicki B. "Helping Families Cope With Milk, Wheat and Soy Allergies." *Maternal/Child Nursing* 8:423–28, November/December 1982.

Section

THREE

ENVIRONMENTAL HEALTH AND SAFETY

Unit 6
CREATING A SAFE ENVIRONMENT

Terms to Know

environment	accreditation
compliance	regulation
cognitive	notarized
licensing	

Objectives

After studying this unit, you will be able to:
- *State the relationship between environment and a child's growth and development.*
- *State the purpose of licensing requirements.*
- *List the necessary steps for securing a license to operate a child care program.*
- *Describe ways of making a child's environment safe.*

Children's growth and development are influenced by their *environment*. Growth is enhanced by love, good nutrition, shelter, medical care and protection from harm. New experiences and planned challenges foster intellectual development while social interaction and communication skills promote psychological development.

Preschool teachers and child care providers must continuously be aware of the significant role played by environment. Consequently, they should make every attempt to create physical, *cognitive* and psychological environments that have positive effects on children's growth and development, Figure 6–1.

Licensing standards established by individual states represent an attempt to encourage and ensure child care environments that are safe and healthful for young children (*Young Children* November 1983). Center Accreditation Project (CAP), a new nationwide system of voluntary *accreditation* for early childhood centers and schools is also nearing the final stages of development. The National

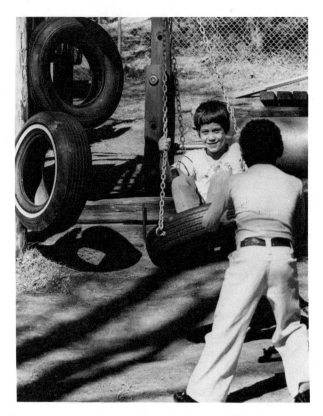

FIGURE 6-1   Environments can have a positive effect on children's growth and development.

Association for the Education of Young Children (NAEYC), the major professional organization for individuals working in the field of early childhood education, supports excellence in child care and has established the National Academy of Early Childhood Programs (the Academy) to administer the CAP program. The accreditation program has as its major goal the identification of outstanding child care centers and the improvement of education for young children. Concerns for children's health and safety are a top priority.

Considerable efforts are currently being directed toward heightening parents' awareness of features that make up good quality child care. Particular attention should be given to:

- physical facilities
- program philosophy, e.g., developmental and educational objectives
- group size
- staff/child ratios
- activities, e.g., planned and unplanned, age appropriate, stimulating
- health related services
- nutritious meals

Various forms of media, including television, radio, newspapers and popular magazines, are helping disseminate this information to the public. Information and referral services already prevalent in many cities assist parents in locating child care services matched to their individualized needs. As an added benefit, the demands of informed parents may eventually force child care programs to improve their standards as competition for quality facilities and programs becomes more intense.

LICENSING

The mothers of nearly one-half of all preschool children in the United States are currently employed outside of the home (*Report on Preschool Programs* May 1984). The number of single parent families has also increased dramatically. As a result, greater demands for child care have brought about a significant increase in the variety and number of preschools and child care programs. However, quality has not always accompanied this rapid expansion.

A system of careful monitoring is necessary to ensure that safe facilities and quality programs are established for young children. State licensing standards provide some assurance that programs have met certain basic requirements. However, these standards are only minimal and vary considerably from one state to another.

Licensing requirements serve a twofold purpose. First, they protect children's psychological well-being by regulating the quality of child care environments and educational programs. Second, licensing *regulations* offer a measure of protection to child care personnel and established programs. Centers are often less vulnerable to charges of negligence if they adhere to basic licensing standards.

Early attempts to regulate child care facilities dealt primarily with the sanitary and safety conditions of large institutions. However, current licensing regulations go beyond strict concern only for the safety of physical settings. Today, the qualifications of care providers and the quality of educational programs planned for young children are also recognized as important. Programs are expected to meet certain predetermined standards.

At present, all states have established some method for licensing child care programs. One agency in each state is invested with the legal authority to conduct inspections and issue licenses to child care and preschool programs. This agency is also responsible for developing licensing standards and methods for enforcing *compliance*. As a result, many differences in licensing standards and degree of enforcement are apparent from state to state. Also lacking in this plan is any method for making certain that individual states are indeed carrying out their responsibilities.

In addition to meeting state licensing regulations, child care programs receiving federal funds must also conform to special supplemental guidelines (U.S. Department HEW 1981). Governmental requirements adapted in the spring of

1981 apply to all child care centers funded through Title XX of the Social Security Act. Separate regulations also exist for all Head Start programs.

Licensing requirements only define minimal standards that must be met by programs in order to care for young children. These guidelines serve a twofold purpose. First, they protect children's physical and psychological well-being by regulating the quality of child care environments and, in some cases, educational programs, Figure 6–2. Second, licensing regulations offer a measure of protection to child care personnel and established programs. Centers are less vulnerable to charges of negligence if they adhere to basic licensing standards.

Determining licensing requirements that will adequately protect young children's health and safety, yet are realistic enough for individuals and centers to achieve, is a challenging task. Some people believe that too much control or standards that are set too high will reduce the number of available child care facilities. The licensing process is also costly for state agencies to administer and often difficult to enforce. Lowering standards may be a tempting option. On the other hand, many parents and professional child care providers favor stricter regulations to ensure high-quality child care facilities and services.

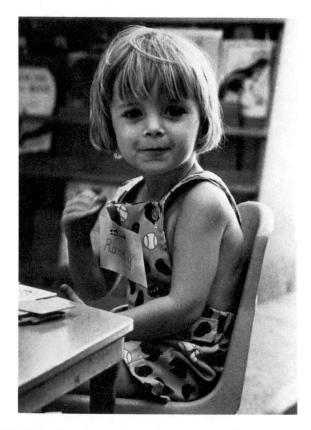

FIGURE 6–2   Licensing regulations help to protect children's well-being.

Despite the controversy, licensing of child care programs is necessary. Ideally, licensing standards should adequately safeguard children but not be so overly restrictive that qualified individuals and centers who are interested in providing a much needed service are eliminated. The development of separate licensing requirements for home child care services and center-based programs may be one logical solution to this dilemma (Adams 1984).

Obtaining a License

Becoming licensed permits an individual to conduct a child care program on a regular basis. As mentioned earlier, the process for obtaining a license differs from one state to another. However, the steps described here are representative of the procedure that is generally involved. In some cases, the process may require considerable time and effort, especially if major renovations need to be made in the proposed facility.

Persons interested in operating a child care program should first contact their state or local agency responsible for issuing such licenses. Questions can also be answered at this time regarding the applicant's eligibility and specific requirements that must be met.

In addition to complying with state licensing regulations, child care facilities must also be in accordance with local laws and ordinances. Zoning codes must be checked carefully to determine whether or not the location of a child care center is permissible in a particular neighborhood. Often this requires meeting with local planning authorities and reviewing proposed floor plans.

Buildings that house child care programs must also pass a variety of inspections to be sure they meet fire, safety and sanitation codes. These inspections are usually conducted by personnel from the local fire and public health departments. From these inspections, it is possible to determine what, if any, renovations are necessary in order to comply with licensing regulations. In most cases, these are relatively simple; in other cases, it may not be feasible or economical to complete all of the required changes.

After these steps have been completed, the licensing office should again be contacted. Formal application can be made at this time for a permanent license. Copies of the program's plans and policies are then submitted to the licensing authorities for review. Final approval includes an on-site inspection of the facilities to see that all requirements and recommendations have been satisfied.

ENVIRONMENTAL STANDARDS

Each child care program is unique. This uniqueness is both important and desirable as it fulfills many different types of needs for parents and young children. Licensing regulations attempt to assure children's health and safety in such a diverse range of settings.

Building Facilities

In a time of increasing demand for child care and shrinking budgets, the selection of a building appropriate for preschool and child care programs often requires a creative approach. It would be ideal to plan and design a facility specifically for this purpose. However, few programs have sufficient funds to accomplish such a project. Instead, it is frequently necessary to locate preschool and day-care services in existing buildings. Unused classrooms in public schools, older houses, unoccupied stores, church basements, or places of business such as factories or hospitals can usually be modified or remodeled to make them suitable for infant and child care. This type of work can be expensive and may actually be impractical in certain instances. However, it is sometimes possible to use the talents of willing parents to help complete at least a small portion of the work.

How much space a school or center needs depends to some extent on the type of child care program and services that will be offered. Thirty-five square feet of usable floor space per child is considered an absolute minimum for adequate child care (*Young Children* May 1983). Teachers and care providers often find even this amount of space crowded and difficult to work in. Additional space may be needed to accommodate large indoor play structures or special equipment for children with physical handicaps. Ground floor levels are always preferable for infants and preschool-aged children, although basement areas can be used for several hours at a time provided there are at least two exits.

The arrangement of space, or basic floor plan, should be examined carefully to determine the ease of conducting specific activities (Thomson 1983). For example, the traffic flow should allow ample room for children to arrive and depart without disturbing others who are playing. Small rooms that lack storage space, good lighting, accessible bathrooms or adequate outdoor play areas are inconvenient and frustrating for both the staff and children.

Location is also an important factor to consider when selecting a site. Buildings chosen for child care programs must first meet local zoning requirements. These ordinances often make it difficult to locate preschools and child care centers in residential neighborhoods where often they are most needed. Child care facilities should preferably be located away from sources of excessive noise, heavy traffic and other safety hazards, such as railroad tracks, airports and busy streets.

One of the most important licensing requirements that must be met pertains to fire safety codes. Although these codes may take extra effort to satisfy, they are critical in terms of children's safety. Older buildings and those not originally designed for infants and young children may require extensive changes before they pass inspection. Rooms that children occupy must have a minimum of two exits, one of which leads directly outdoors. All doors leading out of a classroom should be hinged so they swing out of the room, Figure 6–3. Programs located above ground level should also have an enclosed stairwell.

Smoke detectors are invaluable in any child care setting, but are especially important where infants and young children will be sleeping. Additional fire safety

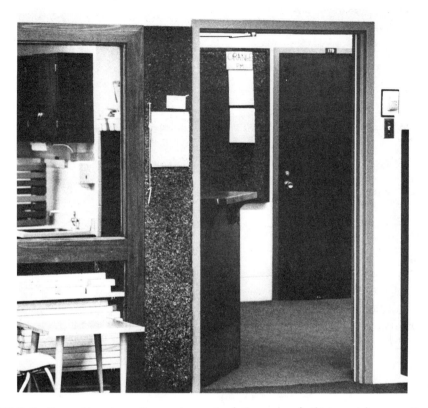

FIGURE 6-3 Doors hinged so they swing out of the room facilitate quick evacuation in emergencies.

precautions include flame-retardant floor coverings and draperies, and having at least one multipurpose fire extinguisher available. The staff should be trained to plan and conduct fire drills, Table 6-1.

Heating and cooling systems should be in good operating condition and able to maintain room temperatures between 68°F and 85°F year round. Rooms occupied by young children should not have hot radiators, pipes, furnaces or fireplaces exposed where children can come in contact with them.

Adequate bathroom facilities are also necessary. They should be accessible to both indoor and outdoor play areas. Installation of child-sized fixtures, including sinks, toilets and towel racks, allow children to take care of their own needs, Figure 6-4. If only adult-sized fixtures are available, foot stools, large wooden blocks or platforms make it easier for children to independently use the fixtures. However, these aids must be carefully anchored to the floor to prevent children from slipping or falling. One toilet and sink should be available for every 10 to 12 children. In centers that serve children with physical handicaps, bathrooms and equipment should be designed to accommodate their special needs. A separate bathroom area should be available for adults and staff members.

TABLE 6–1 How to Conduct a Fire Drill

Develop an evacuation plan
- Plan at least one alternate escape route from every room.
- Post a written copy of the plan by the door of each room.
- Inform new personnel.

Assign specific responsibilities
- Designate someone to call the fire department. Be sure to give the fire department complete information: name, address, approximate location of the fire inside the building, whether or not anyone is inside.
- Designate several adults to assemble children and lead them out of the building.
- Designate one adult to take a flashlight and the notarized emergency cards or class list.
- Designate someone to turn off the lights and close the doors to the rooms.

Establish a meeting place
- Once outside, meet at a designated location so that everyone can be accounted for.
- DO NOT GO BACK INTO THE BUILDING!

Practice fire evacuation drills
- Conduct drills at least once a month; have some of these be unannounced.
- Practice alternate routes of escape.
- Practice fire evacuation safety, e.g., feel closed doors before opening them, select an alternate route if hallway or stairwells are filled with smoke, stay close to the floor (crawl) to avoid heat and poisonous gases, learn the stop-drop-roll technique.
- Use a stopwatch to time each drill and record the results; work for improvement.

Handwashing facilities located near toilets and sleeping areas encourage good handwashing habits. Hot water temperatures should be maintained between 105°F and 120°F to prevent children from being accidentally burned. The use of individual paper towels and cups improves sanitation and limits the spread of communicable illness among young children. Smooth surfaces on walls and floors facilitate cleaning. Fixtures such as mirrors, light switches and towel dispensers placed within children's reach, and good lighting and bright paint create a functional and pleasant atmosphere in which young children can learn to help care for themselves.

Low windows and glass doors should be constructed of safety glass or plastic to prevent serious injuries if they are broken. Colorful pictures or decals placed at children's eye level also help to discourage children from accidently walking into the glass.

Good lighting is essential in classrooms and hallways. Rooms that are sunny and bright are inviting and attractive to both teachers and young children. Natural light from windows and glass doors is one of the most desirable ways to supply rooms with light. Sunlight costs nothing to use and has a positive psychological effect.

Proper arrangement of artificial lighting is equally as important as the amount of brightness it produces. Areas of a room that are used for close activi-

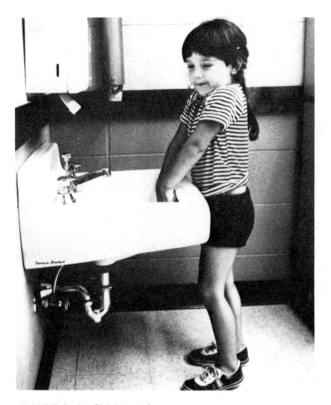

FIGURE 6-4 Child-sized fixtures encourage independence.

ties, such as reading centers or art tables, require more lighting. Fluorescent lights are ideal for this purpose because they give off greater amounts of soft light than incandescent bulbs. Although fluorescent lighting is more costly to install, it uses less electricity to operate.

Furniture and equipment should be selected carefully. Children are likely to receive fewer injuries if chairs and tables are appropriately proportioned. Quality is also an important feature to consider. Furniture should be sturdy so that it can withstand hard use by groups of children. Items with sharp corners or edges should be avoided. Bookcases, lockers, pianos and other heavy objects should be anchored securely to the wall or floor to prevent children from pulling them over. Tall bookshelves should be replaced or cut in half to make them more child size.

Materials used for wall and floor coverings should be easy to clean. Vinyl floor coverings are popular choices for use in child care centers for this reason. However, they do become very slippery when wet. Care must be taken to wipe up spills immediately or to place rugs or newspapers in areas where floors are likely to get wet. Often a combination of carpeted and tiled areas is most satisfactory because it provides soft, warm surfaces where children can sit as well as surfaces that can easily be cleaned.

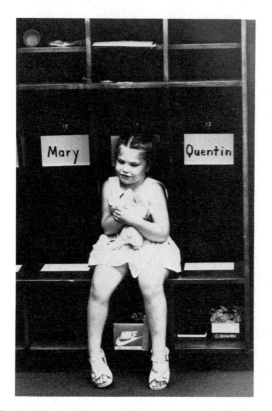

FIGURE 6-5   Each child should have a personal space or cubby to store belongings.

Each child should have an individual storage space, cubby or locker where personal belongings and outdoor clothing can be stored, Figure 6-5. A child's private space is particularly important in group settings. It has the psychological benefit of being something that belongs to only that child, whereas most other objects in the classroom are expected to be shared. Individual lockers help minimize the loss of prized possessions; they also help to control the spread of some communicable illnesses.

Other licensing requirements aimed at improving the safety of a child care facility include having locked cabinets available for storing medicines and other potentially poisonous substances, e.g., cleaning products, paints, gasoline, Figure 6-6. A safety checklist is shown in Table 6-2. All electrical outlets should be covered with safety caps, which can be purchased in most grocery or hardware stores. However, caps are only a temporary solution because they are frequently removed and lost. Conventional outlets can be replaced by an electrician with specially designed safety receptacles to make them safe permanently.

For emergency use, a telephone should be located conveniently in the building. A list of emergency phone numbers, including the fire department, police, ambulance and poison control center should be placed nearby.

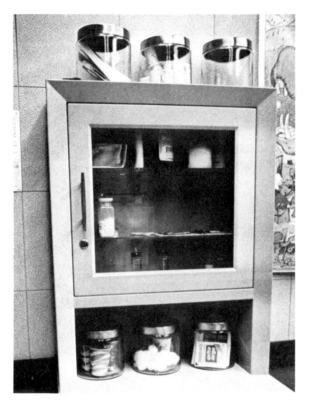

FIGURE 6-6   Locked cabinets should be used to store medicines and poisonous substances.

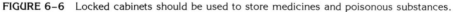

Outdoor Play Areas

The outdoors presents an exciting environment for an endless array of imagi-native activities and opportunities (Stone 1970). For maximum use, play areas should include a variety of surfaces. Large, open areas encourage active play such as running or tossing balls, while protected, hard surfaces allow children to ride bikes and play outside despite inclement weather. Trees add a natural touch and provide shade from hot summer sun.

Safety is a primary goal of licensing regulations that pertain to outdoor play areas. Minimum space requirements for outdoor play yards range from 75–100 square feet per child. Ideally, play areas should be located adjacent to the child care facility or within a very short walking distance. Traveling even short dis-tances to play grounds with young children requires considerable time and effort and often discourages spontaneous outdoor play.

A fence, at least four feet high with a latched gate, should surround the play yard to prevent children from wandering away. Periods of outdoor play are also less stressful for teachers and staff if the entire area is enclosed.

TABLE 6–2   Safety Checklist

	DATE CHECKED	PASS/ FAIL	COMMENTS
Indoor Areas			
1. A minimum of 35 square feet of *usable* space is available per child			
2. Room temperature is between 68–85°F			
3. Rooms have good ventilation			
a. windows and doors have screens			
b. mechanical ventilation systems in working order			
4. There are two exits in all rooms occupied by children			
5. Carpets and draperies are fire-retardant			
6. Rooms are well lighted			
7. Glass doors and low windows are constructed of safety glass			
8. Walls and floors of classrooms, bathrooms, and kitchen appear clean; floors are swept daily, bathroom fixtures are scrubbed at least every other day			
9. Tables and chairs are child size			
10. Electrical outlets are covered with safety caps			
11. Extension cords are in good repair			
12. Smoke detectors are located in appropriate places and in working order			
13. Furniture, activities and equipment are set up so that doorways and pathways are kept clear			
14. Play equipment and materials are stored in designated areas; they are inspected frequently and are safe for children's use			
15. Large pieces of equipment, e.g., lockers, piano, bookshelves, are firmly anchored to the floor or wall			
16. Cleaners, chemicals and other poisonous substances are locked up			
17. If stairways are used:			
a. a handrail is placed at children's height			
b. stairs are free of toys and clutter			
c. stairs are well lighted			
d. stairs are covered with a nonslip surface			
18. Bathroom areas:			
a. toilets and washbasins are in working order			
b. one toilet and washbasin available for every 10–12 children; potty chairs provided for children in toilet training			
c. water temperature is no higher than 120°F			
d. powdered or liquid soap is used for handwashing			
e. individual or paper towels are used for each child			
f. diapering tables or mats are cleaned after each use			
19. At least one fire extinguisher is available and located in a convenient place; extinguisher is checked annually by fire-testing specialists			
20. Premises are free from rodents and/or undesirable insects			

	DATE CHECKED	PASS/ FAIL	COMMENTS
21. Food preparation areas are maintained according to strict sanitary standards			
22. At least one individual on the premises is trained in emergency first aid; first aid supplies are readily available			
23. All medications are stored in a locked cabinet or box			
24. Fire and storm/disaster drills are conducted on a monthly basis			
Outdoor Areas			
1. Play areas are located away from heavy traffic, loud noises and sources of chemical contamination			
2. Play areas are located adjacent to premises or within safe walking distance			
3. Play areas are well drained			
4. Bathroom facilities and drinking fountain easily accessible			
5. A variety of play surfaces, e.g., grass, concrete, sand are available; there is a balance of sunny areas and shady areas			
6. Play equipment is in good condition, e.g., no broken or rusty parts, missing pieces, splinters, sharp edges, frayed rope			
7. Selection of play equipment is appropriate for children's ages			
8. Soft ground covers present in sufficient amounts under large, climbing equipment; area is free of sharp debris			
9. Large pieces of equipment are stable and anchored in the ground			
10. Equipment is placed sufficiently far apart to allow a smooth flow of traffic and adequate supervision			
11. Play areas are enclosed with a fence at least four feet high, with a gate and a workable lock			
12. There are no poisonous plants, shrubs, or trees in the area			
13. Chemicals, insecticides, paints and gasoline products are stored in a locked cabinet			
14. Grounds are maintained on a regular basis and are free of debris; grass is mowed; broken equipment is removed			
15. Wading or swimming pools are always supervised; water is drained when not in use			

Safety must be a major consideration when outdoor equipment is selected and placed in play yards. Choices should be based on:

- amount of available play area
- ages and developmental levels of children
- variety of learning experiences provided
- quality and safety of construction

Large pieces of equipment and portable climbing structures should be firmly anchored in the ground with metal pins or cement. Play equipment should be arranged carefully so that all pieces can be seen and easily supervised. Swings and climbing structures should be located away from hard surfaces such as asphalt and concrete to prevent children from being seriously injured if they should fall, Figure 6–7. Surface materials placed under play equipment should be relatively soft and resilient. Bark chips, finely chopped rubber, sand, grass, or mats are good choices.

Some of the safest and most inviting pieces of outdoor play equipment are not necessarily the modern, highly technical structures designed by manufacturers. Few structures are more attractive and safe for young children than a simple sandbox, bucket of water, collection of old boxes, crates, tires or boards, a tent fashioned from an old sheet, a wagon, or a set of large wooden building blocks that can tease their imagination for hours. The play yard itself provides endless opportunities for a wide variety of activities, including a small garden, a marching band, "camping trips," leaves for art projects or just watching the clouds change shape. These alternatives are especially valuable if resources and storage space are limited.

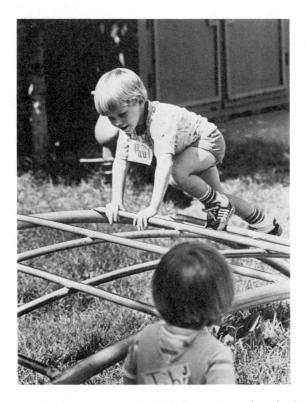

FIGURE 6–7 Climbing structures should be located away from hard surfaces.

Wading or swimming pools can also be an interesting addition to outdoor play yards. However, they do require extra supervision and safety precautions. Whenever children are in the water, there should be extra adults in attendance; at least one adult should have a good knowledge of water safety procedures and lifesaving techniques. Children's swimming activities are safer and easier to monitor if the numbers of children are also limited. Safety rules should be carefully explained to the children and strictly enforced. Pool water should be disinfected prior to each use. Inexpensive water-quality test kits are available from stores where pool supplies are sold. Permanent pools or natural bodies of water should be fenced in or drained to prevent accidental drownings.

Inspecting outdoor play areas on a daily basis helps to identify hazardous conditions before a child is hurt. Equipment with broken parts, jagged or sharp edges, loose screws or bolts, or missing pieces should be removed. Surface materials under equipment should be checked periodically to be sure that amounts are adequate. Sharp sticks, broken glass or other debris that might harm young children should be removed. Great care should also be exercised to identify and eliminate poisonous vegetation, including shrubs, trees and flowers, Table 6–3.

Staff Qualifications

Perhaps one of the weakest areas in many state licensing regulations pertains to staff qualifications (*Young Children* July 1983). Emphasis is usually placed on the safety of physical settings, while staff requirements such as years of experience, educational preparation and personal qualities are often lacking or poorly defined. Where requirements for child care providers and teachers exist, they tend to differ a great deal from state to state. Often the nature of the child care program itself determines the qualifications of the teaching staff.

Staff qualifications are critical to quality preschools and child care. Unfortunately, an individual 18 years of age or older with a high school diploma satisfies the educational requirement in some states. However, the range of training and educational options in the area of early childhood education is diverse, and includes:

- personal experiences (child rearing)
- on-the-job training
- CDA (Child Development Associates credential)
- one-year vocational training
- two-year associate degree
- four-year bachelor degree
- advanced graduate training (M.A. and Ph.D.)

Ideally, all directors and head teachers should have a CDA (Child Development Associate) credential or a two-year associate arts degree with specialized training in early childhood. However, in many areas of the country, teachers and child care providers with such preparation are in short supply.

TABLE 6-3   Common Poisonous Vegetation

VEGETATION	POISONOUS PART	COMPLICATIONS
Bittersweet	Berries	Causes a burning sensation in the mouth. Nausea, vomiting, dizziness and convulsions.
Buttercup	All parts	Irritating to the digestive tract. Causes nausea and vomiting.
Castor Bean	Beanlike pods	Extremely toxic. May be fatal to both children and adults.
Daffodil, hyacinth, narcissus, jonquil	Bulbs	Nausea, vomiting and diarrhea. Can be fatal.
Iris	Underground roots	Digestive upset causing nausea, vomiting and diarrhea.
Lily-of-the-Valley	Leaves and flowers	Nausea, vomiting, dizziness and mental confusion.
Mistletoe	Berries	Extremely toxic. Diarrhea and irregular pulse.
Poinsettia	Leaves	Very irritating to throat, mouth and stomach. Can be fatal.
Rhubarb	Raw leaves	Can cause convulsions, coma and rapid death.
Sweet Pea	All parts, especially the seeds	Shallow respirations, possible convulsions, paralysis and slow pulse.
Black Locust Tree	Bark, leaves, pods and seeds	Causes nausea and weakness, especially in children.
Cherry Tree	Leaves and twigs	Can be fatal. Causes shortness of breath, general weakness and restlessness.
Golden Chain Tree	Beanlike seed pods	Can cause convulsions and coma.
Oak Tree	Acorns and leaves	Eating large quantities may cause poisoning. Gradually causes kidney failure.
Rhododendron	All parts	Causes vomiting, convulsions and paralysis.
Wisteria	Seed pods	Causes severe diarrhea and collapse.
Yews	Berries and foliage	Foliage is very poisonous and can be fatal. Causes nausea, diarrhea, and difficult breathing.

Paraprofessionals can be a valuable source of additional staff to help relieve shortages of child care personnel. They may be aides who work for wages or unpaid volunteers. Paraprofessionals should receive a brief, but intensive, orientation and training period before they begin to work in the classroom. Preparing staff members in this manner enables them to be more productive and successful when they start working with children.

Staff/child ratios are determined by individual states and only reflect the minimal number of adults considered necessary to protect children's well-being

(Collins 1983). However, quality learning experiences, personalized child care and conditions that favor children's health and safety require more adult care providers than is usually recommended. Programs based on these objectives often will have lower staff/child ratios.

Ideally, staff ratios for high-quality child care should include one full-time adult care provider for every 9–10 children who range in age from three to six years. Programs serving children with disabilities should have one teacher or adult care provider for every 4–7 children, depending on the age group and severity of children's handicaps. If children younger than two and one-half years are included in a preschool or child care program, the staff/child ratio should be lowered to one full-time staff member per 3–5 children. In the event of illness or sudden resignations, centers can avoid being caught short of staff by maintaining a list of substitute care providers.

Recent research data suggests that small group size and low staff/child ratios improve the quality of child care programs. However, low ratios do not always guarantee that children will be safer (Ruopp 1978; Hildebrand 1984). Much depends on the supervisory skills of individual care providers.

Licensing standards in many areas require teachers and adult care providers to attend a variety of professional meetings, training sessions, and workshops throughout the year. Exposure to new concepts, ideas and approaches promotes continued professional growth and competence. Contact with other members of the profession also provides teachers and child care providers with opportunities for discussing common problems and sharing ideas and unique solutions.

The ability to relate well to children as well as other adults, such as parents, staff members, and professional personnel, is important for teachers and adult care providers. Warmth, patience, sensitivity to children's needs and respect for individual differences are also desirable qualities all child care providers should possess. The ability to plan, organize and make decisions is also essential for success. Teachers and care providers who enjoy good health are better able to cope with the physical and emotional demands of long, action-packed days. These qualities are important not only because they make a teacher a better teacher or care provider but also because they can have a positive effect on children's growth and development.

Group Size and Composition

When a license is issued to a child care center, family day-care home, or preschool, it defines specific conditions or limits under which the program is allowed to operate. These conditions usually identify the:

- ages of children that can be enrolled
- total group size
- maximum enrollment limits
- special populations of children to be served, e.g., physically handicapped, nonhandicapped, children with behavior problems, mentally retarded

For example, a preschool program may be licensed to provide two half-day sessions for children 3–5 years of age, with a maximum enrollment of 18 children per session. A home day-care program might be licensed to accept only six children, ages birth to two years.

Group size is recognized as an important factor in providing quality child care (*Young Children* May 1983). Therefore, restrictions are often placed on group size. This figure is determined by the amount of available space, ages, and special populations of children being served and the number of available adult care providers.

A description of group composition as defined by the licensing agency should be included in a center's admission policies. The ages, special populations, and total numbers of children that a program will accept must be clearly stated to avoid future misunderstandings.

Program Content

The value of early stimulation and learning experiences is well documented. Because many children spend the majority of their waking hours in various child care arrangements, it is important that opportunities for learning be included.

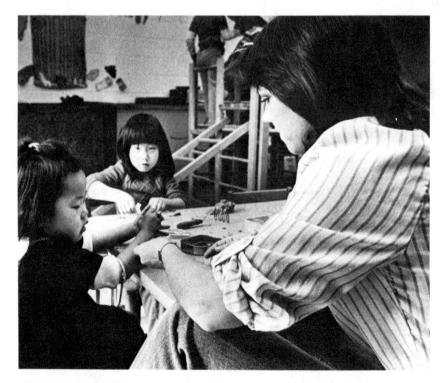

FIGURE 6–8 Children's fine and gross motor skills are developed through carefully planned activities.

Educational and recreational activities should be planned to meet children's developmental needs in the areas of:

- fine and gross motor skills, Figure 6–8
- language acquisition
- social skills
- problem-solving
- self-care skills
- emotional development

In addition to providing developmentally appropriate learning experiences for young children, the arrangement of their daily schedules and routines is also important to plan carefully. The organization of various activities can affect children's physical stamina as well as their attitudes. Fatigue and lack of interest can often be avoided by planning activities that provide alternating periods of rest and activity. For example, a long walk outdoors might be followed by a teacher-produced flannel board story or puppet show. A copy of daily schedules should be posted where they can easily be read by parents.

Health Services

Concern for children's health and well-being is a fundamental part of any child care program (Weiser 1982). Only when children are healthy can they fully benefit from learning experiences and opportunities. Therefore, basic health services offered by child care programs should reflect their commitment to the philosophy of preventative health care for young children. Licensing regulations related to health services are primarily concerned with:

- written policies
- children's medical records
- provisions for first aid and emergency care
- preparations for emergencies and disasters
- plans for health and safety education

Again, there are many differences in the types of policies and records that each state requires. However, there are certain basic policies related to children's health that every preschool and child care program should develop and maintain. (These policies were identified and described in an earlier unit.)

Licensing authorities carefully review all health and safety records for completeness. The most essential health and safety records that every center should keep on file include:

- children's health assessments
- attendance
- emergency contact information
- developmental profiles
- adult health assessments
- fire and storm drills

- accident and injuries
- health observations

Licensing personnel are also interested in how schools and child care programs are meeting their responsibilities to provide first aid and emergency care services. Every center should have at least one staff member who is trained in first aid techniques. This person should be responsible for administering any necessary medical treatment. However, it is preferable for all staff members to have completed such training so they can respond immediately to any emergency.

EMERGENCY CONTACT INFORMATION

Child's Name_____   Date of Birth_____

Address_____   Home Phone_____

Mother's Name_____   Business Phone_____

Father's Name_____   Business Phone_____

Name of other person to be contacted in case of an emergency:

1._____ Address_____

   Relationship (sitter, relative, friend, etc.)_____ Phone_____

2._____ Address_____

   Relationship (sitter, relative, friend, etc.)_____ Phone_____

Authorization is hereby given for the Child Development Center Staff to release the above named child to the following persons, provided proper identification is first established (list *all* names of authorized persons, including immediate family):

1._____ Relation:_____

2._____ Relation:_____

3._____ Relation:_____

Physician to be called in an emergency:

1._____ Phone_____ or_____

2._____ Phone_____ or_____

I, the undersigned, authorize the staff of the Child Development Center to take what emergency medical measures are deemed necessary for the care and protection of my child enrolled in the Child Development Center program.

_____   _____
(Signature of Parent or Guardian)   Signature witnessed by:
                                             (Notary)

_____   _____
(Signature of Parent or Guardian)   The above statement sworn
                                             before me on:

                                             _____

                                             _____

FIGURE 6-9   An emergency contact information form.

Notarized permission forms, similar to the one shown in Figure 6–9, listing the name, address, and telephone number of the child's physician should be completed by parents when the child is first enrolled. This measure grants child care providers the authority to administer or secure emergency medical treatment. A list of emergency telephone numbers, e.g., ambulance, fire department, police, should also be placed in a convenient location for quick reference. Advanced arrangements should be made so that a vehicle is always available for transportation in the event of a medical emergency.

A special room or quiet area in an existing room should be available for times when children become ill. An area separate from the other children is necessary both to provide privacy for a child who is sick or injured, and to protect other children from illnesses that could be contagious. Medical supplies and equipment can be stored in or near this area so they are readily available.

Child care programs are also expected to develop a set of plans and guidelines for emergency preparedness, Table 6–4. These plans should describe the actions that will be taken to protect children's safety in the event of fire, severe storms or major disasters. Persons from local fire and police departments, Red Cross, and Civil Defense are usually quite willing to assist with this planning. Parents should be encouraged to read through these guidelines so they will feel more reassured and also, hopefully, use the information to develop similar plans in their own homes.

Transportation

Some child care centers and preschools provide transportation for children to and from their homes, or occasionally for field trips. Whenever motor vehicles are used to transport young children, special safety precautions are necessary.

First, the driver of any vehicle must be a responsible individual and possess a current license appropriate for the number of passengers that will be transported. Parents whose children will ride on a regular basis should become familiar with the driver so they feel more confident. Written permission should be obtained from each parent before allowing children to be transported.

Second, vehicles should be equipped with restraints that are appropriate for the age of each child:

- an infant bed or carrier for infants up to nine months of age
- a child-sized car seat or harness for children nine months to two years

TABLE 6–4 Principles of Emergency Preparedness

1. Don't panic—stay calm!
2. Be informed. Tune in a local station on your battery-powered radio
3. Get to a safe place. Develop and practice an appropriate disaster plan.
4. Keep a first aid kit and flashlight handy.
5. Learn basic emergency first aid.

- a vehicle seat belt for children two to five years of age
- a vehicle seat belt and shoulder harness for children who are at least 55–58 inches in height

Children must be buckled in for every trip even though it may be a time-consuming process.

Motor vehicles used to transport children must be in good repair. Periodic inspections of all safety and mechanical features ensure the vehicle's safe performance. An ABC-type fire extinguisher should be fastened in the front of the vehicle where it is readily available for emergencies. Liability insurance should be purchased to cover the vehicle, driver, and maximum number of passengers it will be carrying.

Whether parents or child care programs are responsible for transporting children, additional precautions can be taken to improve children's safety. Special off-street areas can be designated for the purpose of loading and unloading young children. If conditions do not allow schools to make this safety measure available, more emphasis must be placed on safety education. Parents should be reminded from time to time to have children get into and out of the car door closest to the curb rather than directly out into the street. Also, having an adequate number of parking spaces available helps to reduce traffic hazards around school areas.

It is not an uncommon practice for child care programs to occasionally ask parents to provide transportation for off-site field trips. However, this practice is quite risky and has the potential for creating many serious problems in the event of an accident. Centers have no guarantee that privately-owned vehicles or individual drivers meet the standards and qualifications previously discussed. As a result, centers are vulnerable to unnecessary lawsuits and charges of negligence. Instead, various forms of public transportation can be safely substituted. These systems have taken the necessary precautions to ensure passengers' safety.

SUMMARY

The quality of children's environments can influence their physical growth as well as their intellectual and psychological development. Consequently, care must be given to planning and providing settings that are both enriching and safe for young children.

Careful regulation of child care facilities and programs is necessary. Individual states are responsible for developing specific licensing standards and methods for enforcing these standards. Unfortunately, the standards are only minimal requirements and seldom support optimal conditions. Licensing standards and procedures for obtaining a license vary from state to state. Programs receiving federal funds must meet additional standards over and above those set by state licensing agencies.

Licensing regulations help to ensure safe facilities and learning programs that are planned for young children. They also extend protection to parents, young children and child care providers who adhere to them. Controversy continues over how much control is necessary.

Although procedures for securing a license differ in each state, many of the basic steps are similar. Generally, there are requirements regarding an applicant's age and educational preparation. Buildings selected for child care programs must meet local zoning regulations in addition to fire, safety and sanitation codes. A review of staff qualifications, program content and policies is also conducted before final approval is granted. Additional areas of concern in the licensing process include a center's provisions for health services, transportation guidelines and sanitary food service.

LEARNING ACTIVITIES

1. Develop a safety checklist that can be used by child care providers or parents to inspect outdoor play areas for hazardous conditions. Using your list, conduct an inspection of two different play yards, or the same play area on two separate occasions.

2. Contact the local licensing agency for your area. Make arrangements to accompany licensing personnel on an on-site visit of a child care facility. Be sure to review licensing regulations beforehand. Observe to see how a licensing inspection is conducted. In several short paragraphs, describe your reactions to this experience.

3. Often licensing personnel are viewed as unfriendly or threatening authority figures. However, their major role is to offer guidance and help teachers and child care providers create safe environments for children. Role play how the following situations might be handled during a licensing visit. Keep in mind the positive role of licensing personnel, e.g., offering explanations, providing suggestions, planning acceptable solutions and alternatives.

   • electrical outlets not covered

   • all children's toothbrushes found stored together in a large plastic bin

   • open boxes of dry cereals and crackers in kitchen cabinets

   • an adult-sized toilet and wash basin in the bathroom

   • a swing set located next to a cement patio

   • incomplete information on children's immunization records

   • a care provider who prepares snacks without first washing his or her hands

4. Organize a class debate on the topic of minimal vs. quality standards for child care facilities.

5. Send for information about the Child Development Associate program (available from the Child Development Consortium, 1341 G. Street, NW, Suite 802, Washington, DC 20005). After reading the materials, write a brief summary describing the program.

6. Contact the U.S. Consumer Product Safety Commission (Washington, DC 20207) and check the product safety of at least eight playground items.

UNIT REVIEW

A. Multiple Choice. Select the best answer.

1. The minimum educational requirement for preschool teachers is
   a. special training in early childhood education
   b. a high school diploma
   c. graduate work in child development
   d. accreditation from CDA

2. Bathroom facilities for preschool children should have
   a. one toilet and one wash basin for every five to seven children
   b. child-sized fixtures
   c. carpeted floors
   d. hot water temperatures no higher than 135°F

3. Potentially poisonous substances should be
   a. labeled "Poison"
   b. stored in locked cabinets
   c. stored on a high shelf out of children's reach
   d. none of the above

4. Minimum space requirements per preschool-aged child for an outdoor play area is
   a. 35 square feet
   b. 50 square feet
   c. 75–100 square feet
   d. over 100 square feet

5. Health services are an essential part of any early childhood program because they
   a. protect and promote children's health
   b. provide for emergency and first aid care
   c. include health and safety education as part of the preventive health care approach
   d. all of the above

6. Schools can help to reduce traffic accidents by
   a. having parents transport the children
   b. eliminating field trips
   c. prohibiting parking in front of the building
   d. including traffic safety education for children

7. To be suitable for preschool or child care programs, buildings should
   a. have a cooling system
   b. be located away from excessive noise and traffic
   c. have a minimum of 50 square feet of space per child
   d. have safety glass in all windows

8. Staff ratio for high-quality child care for children ages 3 to 6 is one full-time adult care provider for every
   a. 3 to 5 children
   b. 4 to 7 children
   c. 9 to 10 children
   d. 12 children

B. Briefly answer the following questions.

1. How does environment affect a child's growth and development?

2. What steps are generally involved in obtaining a license to operate a child care program?

3. Why is it important for each child to have a personal locker or cubby?

4. Name three features that help to make an outdoor play yard safe for young children?

5. List four conditions that identify group composition?

6. What two purposes do licensing requirements serve?

C. Match the definition in column I with the term in column II.

Column I	Column II
1. local ordinance that indicates what type of facility shall be in an area	a. regulation
2. rule dealing with procedures	b. minimal standards
3. method of action that determines present and future decisions	c. staff qualification
4. witnessed form that indicates the signature that appears on the form is really that of the person signing the form	d. notarized permissions
5. skills possessed by the people responsible for the operation of a business	e. policy
6. meeting the least possible requirements	f. zoning code

REFERENCES

Adams, Diane, and Mann, Judy. "Family Day Care Registration: Is It Deregulation or More Feasible State Public Policy?" *Young Children* 39(4):74–77, May 1984.

Collins, Raymond C. "Child Care and the States: The Comparative Licensing Study." *Young Children* 38(5):3–11, July 1983.

"Dramatic Changes in Families Make Child Care Necessary." *Report on Preschool Programs,* May 1, 1984.

Hildebrand, Verna. *Management of Child Care Centers.* New York: Macmillan Publishing Co., 1984.

"Progress Report on the Center Accreditation Project." *Young Children* 39(1), November 1983.

Ruopp, Richard R., et al. *Children at the Center, Final Report of the National Day Care Study,* Vol. 1. Washington, DC: Department of Health, Education and Welfare, 1978.

Stone, Jeanette. *Play and Playgrounds.* Washington, DC: National Association for Education of Young Children, 1970.

Thomson, Carolyn L., and Ashton-Lilo, Jennifer. "A Developmental Environment for Child Care Programs." In *Early Childhood Education: Special Environmental, Policy and Legal Considerations.* Rockville, MD: Aspen Publications, 1983.

"Three Components of High-Quality Early Childhood Programs: Administration, Staff Qualifications and Development, and Staff-Parent Interaction." *Young Children* 38(5):53–58, July 1983.

"Three Components of High-Quality Early Childhood Programs: Physical Environment, Health and Safety, and Nutrition." *Young Children* 38(4):51–56, May 1983.

U.S. Department of Health, Education and Welfare. *Summary Report of the Assessment of Current State Practices in Title XX Funded Day Care Programs: Report to Congress.* Washington, DC: Day Care Division Administration for Children, Youth and Families, Office of Human Development Services, 1981.

Weiser, M.G. *Group and Education of Infants and Toddlers.* St. Louis, MO: C.V. Mosby Co., 1982.

Additional Reading

Caldwell, Bettye. "NAEYC Adopts Child Care Licensing Position." *Young Children* 39(2):49–51, January 1984.

Class, Norris, and Orton, Richard. "Day Care Regulation." *Young Children* 35(6):12–17, September 1980.

Conger, F., et al. *Child Care Aide Skills.* New York: McGraw-Hill Book Co., 1979.

Day Care: Serving Preschool Children. DHEW #74–1057. Washington, DC: U.S. Department of Health, Education and Welfare.

Harms, Thelma, and Clifford, Richard. *Early Childhood Environmental Rating Scale.* New York: Teachers College Press, 1980.

Pamphlets

Home/Environmental Safety

Home Safe: A Child's Eye View, P.O. Box 1114, Carrollton, TX 75006.

Home Safety, Kinder Gard Corporation, Dallas, TX 75234.

Open The Door To Safety, National Safety Council, 444 North Michigan Ave., Chicago, IL 60611.

Poison Perils In the Home, National Safety Council, 444 North Michigan Ave., Chicago, IL 60611.

Safety Education Data Sheets, National Safety Council, 444 North Michigan Ave., Chicago, IL 60611.

Disaster Preparedness

Coping with Children's Reaction to Earthquakes and Other Disasters, Family Earthquake Drills, Earthquake Safety Checklist, Federal Emergency Management Agency, Washington, DC 20472

Get Out Fast, National Fire Safety Council, Jackson, MI.

Learn Not To Burn Curriculum, National Fire Protection Association, 470 Atlantic Avenue, Boston, MA 02210.

Teaching Poison Prevention in Kindergarten and Primary Grades, Public Health Services, U.S. Department of Health and Human Services, Division of Accident Prevention, Washington, DC 20201.

Tornado, Superintendent of Documents, U.S. Government Printing Office, Washington, DC 20402

Unit 7

SAFETY MANAGEMENT

Terms to Know

accident   prevention
liability   supervision
negligence   incidental learning

Objectives

After studying this unit, you will be able to:
- List the most frequent causes of accidental death among preschool children.
- Describe several reasons why preschool children are more likely victims of accidents.
- Describe the four basic principles of accident prevention.
- State two types of negligence.

Accidents are the leading cause of death and permanent disabilities among preschool children. Accidents are also responsible for many nonfatal injuries that are costly in terms of time, energy and medical costs. Curiosity and impulsive behaviors often lead young children into new and unexpected dangers. At the same time, children are not always able to anticipate the possible consequences of their actions because they lack an adult's maturity, experience and intellectual sophistication. Parents, teachers and child care providers must, therefore, take extra precautionary measures to provide environments and activities that are safe for preschool children, Figure 7–1.

Providing for the protection and safety of children placed in their care is a primary concern that administrators, child care providers and teachers in the field of early childhood education face. This task is especially challenging and demanding because of the ages of children involved. Their normal developmental characteristics and limited past experiences make it necessary for adults to establish and practice high standards of safety.

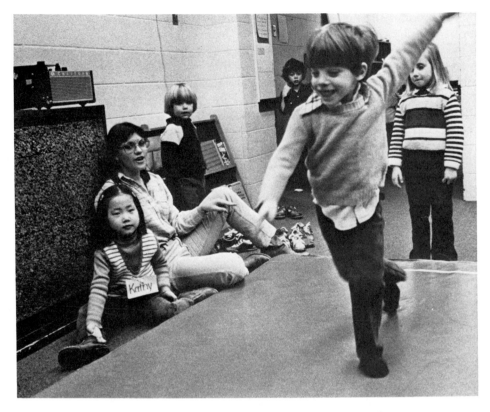

FIGURE 7–1   Parents expect child care facilities to be safe.

WHAT IS AN ACCIDENT?

The term *accident* refers to an unplanned or unexpected event. For example, children seldom plan on getting a finger pinched when they close a door or being hit by a car when they dash out into a street. In terms of safety, the word accident frequently implies or suggests that some form of injury or harm has also resulted.

Young children are involved in many different kinds of accidents. The most common causes of death, in order of rank from most to least common, are:

- motor vehicles—as pedestrians and passengers
- burns—from fireplaces, appliances, stoves, chemicals, electrical outlets
- drownings—in swimming pools, bathtubs, sinks, ponds
- falls—from stairs, play equipment, furniture, windows
- poisoning—from aspirin and other medicines, cleaning products, insecticides, and cosmetics

In addition to the common causes of accidents, there are a number of interesting facts that can be useful in planning for children's safety. Boys are more likely to be involved in accidents than girls (Solomons 1982). This may be due in part to their more active and aggressive behavior. Also, their play frequently involves more physical contact and roughhousing (Matheny 1980). Fatigue also seems to be an important contributing factor. Accidents are more likely to occur toward the end of the day when children and care providers are tired.

In group child care settings, more children are injured during outdoor activities, Table 7–1. At home, the majority of accidents take place indoors, Table 7–2.

TABLE 7–1 Percent of Children's Injuries by Type of Equipment

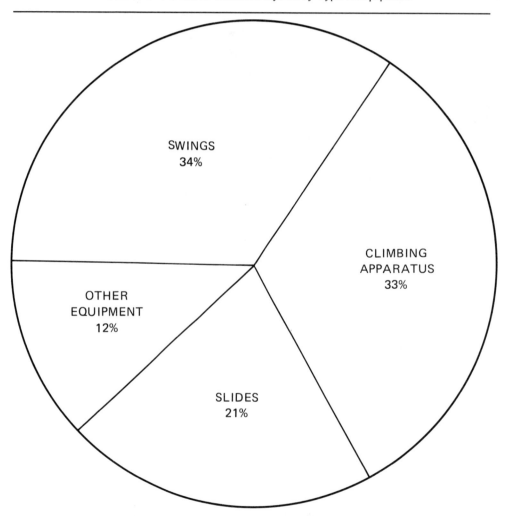

Source: Adapted from National Recreation and Park Association Study, 1978.

TABLE 7-2   How Children Died in Home Accidents

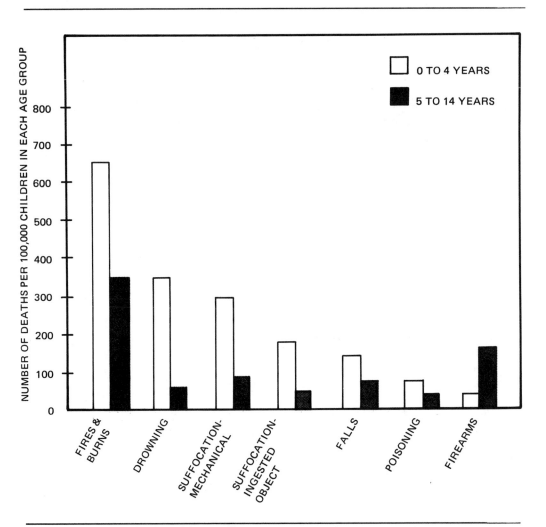

Source: 1983 National Safety Council Accident Facts.

ACCIDENT PREVENTION

Accident *prevention* is based on the ability of parents and teachers to accurately assess children's developmental skills and to be able to anticipate their actions. This information can be used for planning and organizing children's environments and activities, selecting appropriate play equipment, establishing rules, supervising their work and play, and developing safety education programs.

Accident prevention requires continuous awareness and implementation of safe practices. Teachers, child care providers, and parents must always consider the element of safety in everything they do with young children. This includes the environments they create, the selection of equipment, and individual activities (Aronson 1983). To new or busy teachers or parents this may seem overly time-consuming and unnecessary. However, if the teacher or parent is new or busy, it is even more important to focus attention on children's safety. Any amount of effort is worthwhile even if it spares only one child from injury!

In many communities, local building codes and licensing regulations provide standards that influence the quality and safety of child care centers and homes. In addition to these requirements, the following four basic safety principles can be used by teachers, care providers and parents as guidelines for setting up environments that are safe for young children:

- advanced planning
- establishing rules
- careful supervision
- safety education

It is not possible to prevent all accidents. Regardless of how much care is exercised, there will always be some circumstances that are beyond a teacher's or care provider's control. No amount of planning can prevent a child from suddenly releasing a grip on climbing equipment or a foot from slipping on dry pavement. However, a teacher who conscientiously implements safety principles can significantly reduce the number and seriousness of school-related accidents.

Advanced Planning

Considerable thought and careful planning should go into the selection of equipment and activities that are appropriate for preschool children (Herbert-Jackson 1978; Machado 1984). Choices must take into account the children's skill levels and developmental abilities. Teachers should plan activities and select play equipment that encourages curiosity, exploration and a sense of independence without endangering children's safety (Frost 1982). Advanced planning allows teachers to help children expand their current level of skills and safely acquire new skills.

Planning for children's safety requires that teachers and care providers recognize the risks or hazards that are involved in each activity and setting. Many problems can be avoided quite simply if teachers take the time to examine the materials, methods and equipment they present to children. This process includes thinking through each step of an activity before allowing children to begin. Advanced planning means being prepared for the unexpected and developing specific safety rules for each activity. It is important that teachers and care providers develop the unique skill of anticipating children's often unpredictable behaviors, Figure 7–2.

Organization is a basic ingredient of advanced planning. Teachers must know what they are doing before they begin a project with young children. They must be familiar with each step that is involved and have all the necessary materials gathered and ready for use before starting. Anytime a teacher forgets supplies or is unsure of how to proceed, the chances of an accident occurring greatly increase. Foresight also enables teachers to substitute safe alternatives for those of questionable risk.

Examination of accident records can be very useful during the planning stage (Kinne 1982). For example, if teachers begin to recognize a pattern in the type of injuries children receive, steps can be taken to alter the way an activity is conducted. If children are repeatedly injured on a particular piece of outdoor play equipment, a cause should immediately be sought. Plans should be made to modify either the rules, amount of supervision, or the equipment itself so that it will be safe for children to use.

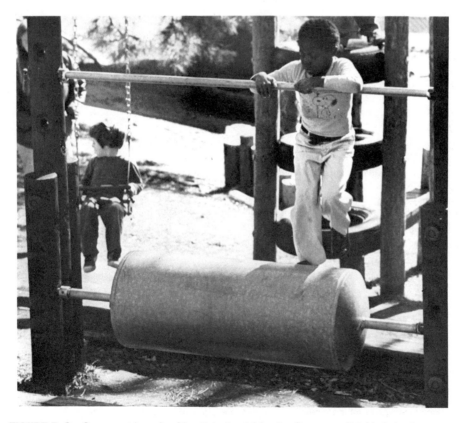

FIGURE 7–2   Care providers should anticipate children's often unpredictable behaviors.

Establishing Rules

Rules are statements of what is considered to be acceptable behavior as it relates to the welfare of an individual child, concern for group safety, and respect for shared property, Table 7–3. Rules can help children learn appropriate ways to use play equipment and interact with each other by defining the limits of safe behavior.

Teachers and care providers can use rules to encourage children's appropriate behavior by stating them in positive terms, e.g., "Slide down the slide on your bottom, feet first, so you can see where you are going." To be most effective, rules should be stated clearly and in terms that are simple enough for even very young children to understand. Children are generally more willing to accept rules if they are given a clear explanation of the reasons why such rules are necessary.

TABLE 7–3   Rules for Safe Use of Play Equipment

CLIMBING APPARATUS

Rules for children
- Always hold on with both hands.
- No pushing or shoving.
- Look carefully before jumping off equipment; be sure the area below is clear of objects and other children.
- Be extra careful if equipment or shoes are wet from snow or rain.

Rules for care provider
- Inspect equipment before children begin to play on it. Check for broken or worn parts and sharp edges; be sure the equipment is firmly anchored in the ground.
- Be sure surface material under equipment is adequate and free of sharp stones, sticks and toys.
- Limit the number of children on climber at any one time.
- Always have an adult in direct attendance when children are on the equipment.
- Supervise children carefully if they are wearing slippery-soled shoes, sandals, long dresses or skirts, mittens, bulky coats or long scarves.

SLIDES

Rules for children
- Always use the ladder or stairs to climb up; do not crawl back up the slide.
- Slide down in a sitting position, feet first.
- Hold on to the sides with both hands.
- Make sure the area at the bottom of the slide is clear of other children and toys before sliding down.

Rules for care provider
- Inspect slide carefully before children play on it. Check for stability and for loose or sharp parts; be sure there is sufficient surface material at the bottom of the slide.
- Check metal slides for excessive heat or cold.
- An adult should always be in direct attendance when children are using the slide.

There are no universal safety rules that teachers and care providers can adopt. Each classroom or child care program must develop their own safety guidelines and rules based on the:

- population of children being served
- individual facilities and equipment (indoor and outdoor)
- number of adults available for supervision
- type of activity involved

It is often necessary to establish more precise rules and limits with young or difficult to manage children. Different pieces of equipment and whether they are being used in classroom or home settings also affect the types of rules that are essential for safety.

When parents or teachers establish rules, they must also be sure that they are enforced. Unless children are consistently expected to obey rules, they quickly learn that rules have no meaning. However, a teacher must never threaten children or make them afraid in order to get them to comply. Rather, children should be praised whenever they demonstrate appropriate safety behaviors. For example, a teacher might recognize a child's efforts by saying, "Carlos, I liked the way you rode your bike carefully around the other children who were playing," or "Tricia, you remembered to lay your scissors on the table before getting up to leave." Through repeated positive verbal encouragement, children soon learn that these behaviors are both acceptable and desirable.

Occasionally, a child will misuse play equipment or not follow directions. A gentle reminder concerning rules is usually sufficient. If this approach fails and the child continues to behave inappropriately, then the teacher or care provider must remove the child from the activity or area. A simple statement such as, "I cannot allow you to hit the other children," lets the child know that this is not acceptable behavior. Permitting the child to return later to the same activity conveys confidence in the child's ability to learn the proper way.

Rules never replace the need for careful adult *supervision,* Figure 7–3. Preschool children have a tendency to forget rules very quickly, especially when they are busy playing or are very excited about what they are doing. Rules should allow enough freedom so that children can work and play, yet remain within the boundaries of safety.

Rules should be realistic for preschool-aged children. They should not be so overly restrictive that children are discouraged or afraid to explore and experiment with their environment. Gradually, as children learn to recognize danger and establish their own standards for protecting themselves, the need for extensive rules is lessened.

Careful Supervision

Parents and teachers of young children are faced with many responsibilities. Their supervisory role is, perhaps, one of the most important of these duties. Children depend on the guidance of responsible adults to help them learn appropriate safety behaviors. The younger the children, the more protective this super-

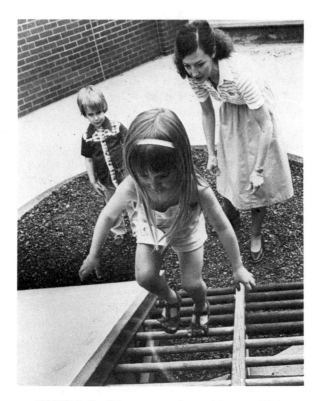

FIGURE 7–3   Rules never replace adult supervision.

vision must be. As children gain additional coordination, skill, and experience in handling potentially dangerous situations, adult supervision can become less restrictive.

The amount of adult supervision that is necessary is also directly related to the type of activity, Figure 7–4. For example, a cooking project that requires the use of a hot appliance must be more carefully supervised than a "dress-up" center containing play clothes. In outdoor play areas, some pieces of play equipment may be more hazardous than others. Teachers should station themselves near these structures so they can watch children more closely.

The number of children a teacher can safely manage is also affected by the nature of the activity. One adult can oversee a game of Farmer-in-the-Dell, while a field trip to the fire station requires several adults. **Caution:** Never leave children unattended for any length of time. If a teacher must leave an area, it should be supervised by another adult or the activity stopped until the teacher returns.

Occasionally, there are children in a classroom or child care group who are physically aggressive or who engage in behaviors that could possibly bring harm to themselves or other children. A teacher can be held liable by the courts if an accident or injury is caused by the actions of a child known to have such a reputation. Teachers are expected to supervise such children more closely. Their

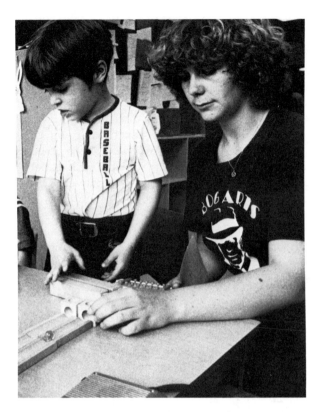

FIGURE 7-4 The amount of teacher supervision necessary is directly related to the type of activity.

responsibility goes beyond merely issuing a warning to the child to stop—they must intervene and actually stop the child from continuing the dangerous activity even if it means physically removing the child from the area.

For safety purposes, the adult/child ratio for both indoor and outdoor settings is generally defined by state regulations. However, there are considerable differences in abilities to supervise and manage children's activities and behaviors. Some teachers are less effective at controlling unruly or disruptive children. In these situations, it may be necessary to have more than the required number of adults available to monitor children's play.

Safety Education

One of the prime methods for avoiding accidents and injuries is through safety education. It is most desirable to begin informal safety training with children as soon as they understand the meanings of words. The earlier children learn about safety, the more naturally they will develop the attitudes and respect that lead to lifelong patterns of safe behavior.

Much safety education takes place through *incidental learning* experiences. Preschool children who already show many safe attitudes and practices can be valuable role models for the other children. Their comments and actions can have a strong influence on other children's behaviors. For example, several children may be jumping from the top of a platform rather than climbing down the ladder. Suddenly, one child yells, "You shouldn't be doing that. You could get hurt!" As a result, the children stop and begin to use the ladder instead. Examples of improper behavior can also be used effectively for teaching young children about safety. When children stand up on a swing or run with sharp objects in their hand, teachers can use these opportunities to explain why such actions are not appropriate. Suggestions can also be made for safer alternatives. Often learning of this type is more meaningful to the young child.

Teachers and child care providers should not overlook their own safety in their concern for children. It is easy for adults to be careless when they are under stress or have worked long, hard hours. Sometimes, in their zealous attempts to help children, teachers take extraordinary risks; it is at such times that even greater caution must be exercised.

IMPLEMENTING SAFETY PRACTICES

Much of the responsibility for maintaining a safe environment belongs to teachers and child care providers. Their daily, intimate contact with children gives them an advantageous position for identifying many problem areas. However, safety must be a concern of all school personnel, including support staff such as aides, cooks, janitors, secretaries and bus drivers. One person may spot a safety hazard that had previously gone unnoticed by others.

Safety must be a continual concern. Each time teachers arrange a classroom, add new play equipment, plan an activity, or take children on a field trip or walk they must first stop to assess whether or not there is any risk involved for the children. Even differences in groups of children can affect the types of safety problems that occur and the kinds of rules that are necessary. For example, extra precautions may be needed when children with handicaps, chronic health problems, or behavior problems are present.

Toys and Equipment

Many injuries can be prevented by carefully selecting toys and equipment that are appropriate for young children (Community Playthings 1981). The ages, interests, behavioral characteristics, and level of motor skills of the children serve as useful guidelines when choosing toys and equipment, Table 7–4 and 7–5. Accidents are more likely to occur when children try to use educational materials and play equipment that are intended for older children. Rings that are too large for small hands to grip, steps on ladders that are spaced too far apart for young children to climb, or climbing equipment that is too tall are examples of unsafe play equipment.

TABLE 7-4 Guidelines for Selecting Toys and Play Equipment

1. Carefully consider children's ages, interests and developmental abilities; check manufacturer's label for recommendations.
2. Choose fabric items that are washable and labeled flame-retardant or nonflammable.
3. Look for quality construction; check durability, good design, stability, absence of sharp corners or wires.
4. Select toys that are made from nontoxic materials.
5. Avoid toys and play materials with small pieces that a child could accidentally choke on.
6. Select toys and equipment that are appropriate for the amount of available play and storage space.
7. Avoid toys with electrical parts.
8. Choose play materials that children can use with minimal adult supervision.

The amount of available classroom or play yard space will also influence choices. Large pieces of equipment or toys that require spacious room for their use will be a constant source of accidents if they are set up in areas that are too small.

Quality is also very important to consider. The construction of toys or equipment should be examined carefully and not purchased if they have:

- sharp wires or edges
- small pieces that might come loose, e.g., buttons, "eyes", screws
- moving parts that can pinch fingers
- inappropriate size
- unstable bases or frames
- toxic paints and materials

TABLE 7-5 Appropriate Toy Choices for Infants and Toddlers

INFANTS	TODDLERS
nonbreakable mirrors	peg bench
cloth books	balls
wooden cars	records
rattles	simple puzzles
mobiles	large building blocks
music boxes	wooden cars and trucks
plastic telephone	dress-up clothes
balls	bristle blocks
toys that squeak	large wooden beads to string
blocks	picture books
nesting toys	nesting cups
teething ring	pull toys
washable, stuffed animals	plastic dishes, pots and pans
	riding toys
	simple musical instruments, such as drums, bells, triangle, tambourine

- defective parts
- inability to hold up under hard use
- possibility of causing electrical shock

The construction and finish on equipment that is to remain outdoors should be checked to be sure it can withstand unfavorable weather conditions. Whenever secondhand equipment is purchased, extreme care should be taken to look it over very thoroughly.

Toys and play equipment should be inspected on a daily basis. They should be in good repair and free of splinters, rough edges and broken or missing parts. Ropes on swings or ladders should be checked routinely and replaced if they begin to fray. Large equipment should be checked frequently to be sure that it remains firmly anchored in the ground.

Regularly scheduled maintenance of toys and play equipment ensures their safety and helps them to last longer. Play equipment that is defective or otherwise unsafe for children to use should be removed promptly until it can be repaired. Items that cannot be repaired should be discarded.

Special precautions are necessary whenever large equipment or climbing structures are set up indoors. This type of equipment should be placed in an open area away from furniture or objects that could injure the children. Mats, foam pads, or large cushions placed around and under structures that are any distance above the floor will protect children from getting hurt if they accidently fall. Rules for the safe use of such equipment should be clearly explained to the children before they use it. At least one adult should be in a position of direct attendance when children are using this equipment, Figure 7–5.

Safety is a prime concern whenever new equipment, toys or educational materials are introduced into a classroom or outdoor setting. Initially, rules are developed and should be limited to those that protect children's well-being. Too many rules may dampen children's enthusiasm for using new equipment and restrict their inventiveness. Also, if more than one new item is to be introduced, it is best to do this over a period of time so that children are not overwhelmed by multiple sets of rules.

Classroom Activities

Safety must also be a major concern when teachers select and plan activities for young children. Many teachers and child care providers are sensitive to the need for safety awareness in outdoor settings. However, there is often a more relaxed attitude and effort where indoor activities are concerned. This false sense of security may result from the belief that fewer accidents take place while children are indoors. Although this is true in group child care settings, it is no excuse for overlooking strict safety precautions. The potential for accidental injury is present in most classroom activities. Even wooden building blocks can be dangerous if children use them incorrectly.

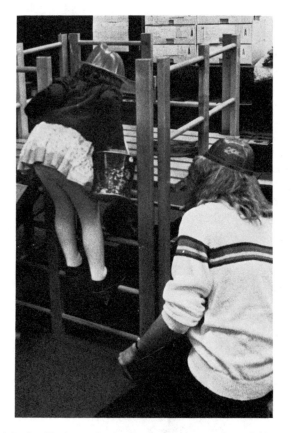

FIGURE 7-5 An adult should always be in direct attendance when children are using climbing structures.

It is more difficult to provide a concise checklist for evaluating the safety of classroom activities. However, there are several guidelines that teachers and child care providers can follow when they select and conduct learning activities. Teachers should ask themselves the following questions.

- Is the activity appropriate for preschool children?
- What are the possible risks involved?
- What special precautions are needed to make an activity safe?

After these questions have been answered, the next step involves applying the basic principles of safety, e.g., advanced planning, formulating rules, deciding on the type of supervision that is necessary, and instituting an educational program.

Extra safety precautions and more precise planning are necessary for some types of activities. This is especially true for activities that involve:

- pointed or sharp objects such as scissors, knives, and woodworking tools, e.g., hammers, nails, saws

- pipes, boards, blocks or objects made of glass
- electrical appliances, e.g., hot plates, radio, mixers
- hot liquids, e.g., wax, syrup, oil, water
- cosmetics or cleaning supplies

For added safety, a separate area can be set aside for any activity that involves dangerous materials. Boundaries can be established with portable room dividers or a row of chairs.

The number of children participating in an activity at any one time can also be restricted. Some activities may need to be limited to as few as one child. Limiting the number of children improves a teacher's ability to effectively supervise a given space. Color-coded necklaces can be used to control the number of children in an area at any one time. This system also makes it easy for children to determine if there is space available for them.

The condition of all electrical appliances should be checked very carefully before they are used. Be sure that the plugs are intact and cords are not frayed.

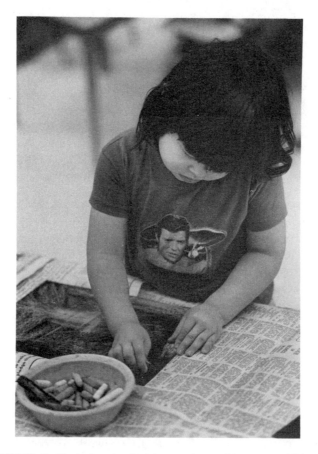

FIGURE 7-6 Nontoxic art materials must be used by young children.

Appliances must never be used near a source of water, including sinks, wet floors or large pans of water.

When children will actually be operating an electrical appliance, it should be set on a low table or the floor so that it is easy for them to reach. Equipment that is placed any higher than children's waist level is dangerous. Teachers should continuously remind children to stand back away from machinery with moving parts to prevent their hair, fingers or clothing from getting caught or burned. Special precautions such as turning the handles of pots and pans toward the back of the stove or hot plate should be taken whenever hot liquids or foods are involved. Always detach cords from the electrical outlet, never the appliance. Safety caps should be promptly replaced in all electrical outlets when the project is completed.

Safety must also be a concern in the selection of art media and activities. Art materials, such as paints, glue, crayons and clay must always be nontoxic when they are used by young children, Figure 7–6. It is also preferable to avoid using dried beans, peas, toothpicks, berries or beads that are very small in size in art activities. Children often stuff these small objects into their ears or nose or swallow them in an instant. It is better to use fabric pieces, dried leaves or grasses, styrofoam, packing materials, yarn, or ribbon for children's art creations. Some safe substitutions for hazardous art materials are provided in Table 7–6. Proper storage of liquid paints and glue is also an important consideration. Plastic containers should always be used in place of glass bottles, jars, or dishes that could break.

Special precautions should be taken in classrooms with hard-surfaced or highly-polished floors. Spilled water, paint, or other liquids and dry materials such as beans, rice, sawdust, flour or cornmeal cause these floors to be very slippery. Spills should be cleaned up promptly. Newspapers or rugs spread out on the floor help prevent children from slipping and falling.

Environments and activities that are safe for young children are also less stressful for the adults who work in these situations. When classrooms or care facilities and play yards are free of potential hazards, teachers and care providers can concentrate on selecting safe activities and providing quality supervision.

LEGAL IMPLICATIONS

Safety generates more concern than any other aspect of early childhood education. Recent lawsuits, legal decisions, and increased public awareness have added to a feeling of uneasiness. As demand for child care services continue to grow, interest in regulating programs and facilities has also increased. Parents want, and have a right, to be assured that facilities are safe. Parents expect schools and child care centers to be responsible for the safety of their children.

Persons who teach and care for young children should be aware of the legal

TABLE 7–6   Safe Substitutes for Hazardous Art Materials

UNSAFE SUBSTANCES	SUBSTITUTES
Clay in dry form. Dry powder contains silica which is easily inhaled and may damage the lungs.	Clay in wet form only. Wet clay cannot be inhaled.
Glazes that contain lead.	Poster paints or water-based paints.
Solvents such as turpentine, benzene, toluene, rubber cement and its thinner.	Use water-based paints and glues.
Cold water or commercial fabric dyes.	Food coloring or natural vegatable dyes made from onion skins, parsley, nuts, cranberries, etc.
Permanent markers which may contain toluene or other toxic solvents.	Water-based markers.
Instant papier machés that may contain asbestos fibers or lead pigments.	Use black and white newspaper and white paste or flour and water.
Aerosol sprays such as paints and lacquers.	Water-based paints and brushes for splatter techniques.
Powdered tempera paints. Their dusts may contain toxic pigments.	Use only nontoxic paints. Purchase liquid paint or mix powders in a well-ventilated area, preferably wearing a dust mask.
Pastels or chalk that create dust.	Crayons or oil-based cra-pas.
All photographic chemicals.	Use blueprint paper and sun to make prints.
Epoxy or other solvent-based glues.	Water-based white glue or library paste.
Solvent-based silk screen and other printing inks.	Paper stencils and water-based inks.

Adapted with permission from the Art Hazards Information Center, 5 Beckman Street, New York, NY 10038.

issues and responsibilities that affect their positions. There are several reasons why this is essential. First, children of preschool age are considered too young to be capable of protecting themselves from potential harm. As a result, adults are expected, by law, to provide for their safety. Second, the incidence of injury and accident is known to be high among preschool children. Third, it helps teachers, administrators and child care providers to protect themselves against possible legal action. The combination of immaturity and the unpredictable behavior of young children necessitates careful safety management.

The most important legal concerns for teachers and care providers center around the issue of liability (Scott 1983; Treadwell 1980). The term *liability* refers to the legal obligations and responsibilities, especially those related to safety, that are accepted by administrators, teachers and child care providers when they agree to care for children. Failure to carry out these duties in an acceptable manner is considered *negligence.*

Negligence often results from questionable safety practices and management. For legal purposes, negligent acts are generally divided into two categories according to the circumstances and the resulting damages or injuries. The first category includes situations in which a teacher or care provider fails to take precautionary measures necessary to protect children from danger. Standards for determining what is necessary are based on what precautionary measures most people with comparable training would take in a similar situation. A person who does not take the proper precautions could be considered negligent. A lack of adequate supervision, play equipment that is defective or in need of repair, and allowing children to engage in harmful activities such as throwing rocks or standing on swings are some examples of this form of negligence.

The second category of negligent acts includes situations in which the actions or decisions of a teacher or child care provider involve a risk to the children. An example of this type of negligence might be a teacher making arrangements to have children transported in private vehicles that are not insured, or planning classroom activities that allow children to use poisonous chemicals or sophisticated electrical equipment without careful supervision.

Prevention is the best method for ensuring the safety of young children and avoiding difficult legal problems and lawsuits. However, there are several measures that provide additional protection to child care programs and their staff.

Teachers and child care providers are legally responsible for their actions. Despite careful attempts at providing safe conditions for children, staff members may be accused of negligence. For this reason, it is wise for every administrator, teacher, and child care provider to obtain personal liability insurance. Such policies can be purchased from most private insurance companies and through the National Association for the Education of Young Children (NAEYC). Accident insurance, purchased on individual children who are enrolled, also affords preschool and child care programs extra protection.

Administrators and staff should not hesitate to seek legal assistance on issues related to child care and education. Legal advice can be a valuable source of protection. Preschool and day-care programs might want to consider selecting a member of the legal profession to fill a position on their board of directors or advisory council.

Careful examination of job descriptions before accepting employment offers teachers and child care providers an additional measure of protection against future legal problems. Potential employees should be sure they have the appropriate training and skills to perform required duties. For example, if teachers are expected to administer first aid to injured children, then they should complete a first aid course before they begin to work.

Accurately maintained records, particularly accident reports, are also an added source of legal protection, Figure 7-7.

ACCIDENT REPORT FORM

Child's name_____   Date of accident_____
Parent_____   Time_____AM_____PM
Address_____   Parent notified_____AM___PM

Description of injuries_____
_____

Action taken at home or center (first aid)_____
_____

Doctor consulted_____   Address_____
Doctor's diagnosis_____
_____

Number of days missed from the child care facility as a result of the accident_____

Adult in charge when accident occurred_____
Description of activity, location in facility and circumstances, immediately before and at the
time of the accident.

_____
_____
_____
_____
_____
_____

What corrective measures could be taken to eliminate such accidents in the future?

_____
_____

Report prepared by_____   Date_____

FIGURE 7-7 Accident form for recording serious injuries (Courtesy of the Kansas Department of Health and Environment, Bureau of Adult and Child Care Facilities).

Information contained in these reports can be used in court as evidence to prove a teacher's or school's innocence against charges of negligence. A thorough report should be completed for each accident that occurs, regardless of how minor or unimportant it may seem to be at the time. This is very important because the results of some injuries are not always immediately apparent. There is also the possibility that complications may develop at a later date. A special form such as the one shown in Figure 7–8 can be used for this purpose. These forms should be filled out by the person who saw the accident and administered first aid treatment. Accident records are considered legal documents and should be kept on file at the child care center for a period of at least five years.

SUNNY DAYS CHILD CARE CENTER
Record of Children's Accidents

Date and Time	Child's Name	Nature of Child's Injuries	How the Accident Occurred	Observed By	Type of First Aid Treatment Administered	By Whom

FIGURE 7-8   A sample accident record form.

SUMMARY

The normal characteristics and nature of young children demand that safety be a major concern of all teachers, child care providers and parents. Because accidents are the leading cause of death for young children, every effort must be taken to prevent accidents. This obligation requires much time, deliberate effort, and careful planning.

Aside from the moral obligations teachers have to protect children's safety, parents also expect this type of treatment from professional child care personnel. Liability is the term used to describe the legal aspect of this responsibility. Two types of negligence may be proven by the courts: failure to take adequate precautionary safety measures, and intentional acts or decisions that involve elements of risk.

In addition to practicing principles of safety, child care personnel can provide some protection for themselves by purchasing personal liability insurance, reading job descriptions carefully before accepting a new job, filling out accident reports when children are injured, and seeking professional legal assistance when necessary. Prevention is always the preferred method for ensuring the safety of young children.

Accident prevention is based on four basic principles: advanced planning, establishing rules, careful supervision, safety education. One of the teacher's and care provider's most important functions is implementing these principles in classrooms and outdoor play areas. Specific guidelines should be followed carefully for the selection and presentation of toys, equipment and various activities.

LEARNING ACTIVITIES

1. Visit a preschool play yard or public playground. Select one piece of play equipment and observe children playing on or with it for at least 15 minutes. Make a list of actual or potential dangers that could result from improper use. Develop a set of workable safety rules for children to follow.

2. Role play how a teacher might handle a child who is not riding a tricycle in a safe manner.

3. Imagine that you have been asked to purchase outdoor play equipment for a new child development center. Make a list of safety features you would look for when you make your selections. Write to several companies for equipment catalogues. Using the catalogues, select basic outdoor equipment to furnish the play yard of a small child care center that has two classes of 15 children each and a budget of $1000.

4. Develop a fire evacuation plan for a child care facility with which you are familiar. If this is not feasible, develop an evacuation plan for your present classroom and building, the dormitory where you live or your own home.

UNIT REVIEW

A. Complete the following crossword puzzle.

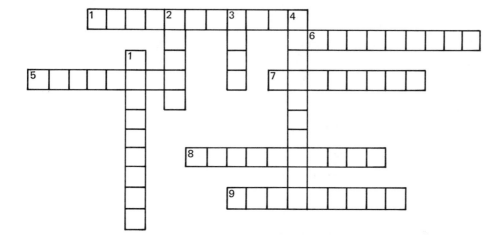

Across

1. Watching over children's safety.
5. A basic ingredient of advanced planning involves the ability to _____.
6. The process of learning safe behaviors.
7. Accident prevention involves advanced _____.
8. The best method for ensuring children's safety is _____.
9. The ability to anticipate children's actions.

Down

1. Legal responsibility for children's safety.
2. Limits which define safe behavior.
3. Environments that are free of potential hazards are _____.
4. Failure to safeguard children's safety.

B. Fill in the blanks with one of the words listed below.

removed	accidents	anticipate
legal	responsible	safety principles
supervision	safety education	safety
inspected		

1. Broken play equipment must be _____ immediately from a classroom or play yard.

2. The leading cause of death for preschool children is _____.

3. Adults must be able to _____ children's actions as part of advanced planning.

4. Parents expect teachers and child care providers to be _____ for their child's safety.

5. Basic _____ _____ include advanced planning, establishing rules, careful supervision and safety education.

6. Accident records are _____ records.

7. A continuous concern of teachers and child care providers is _____.

8. Rules never replace the need for adult _____.

9. Toys and play equipment should be _____ daily.

10. A prime method for avoiding accidents is through _____ _____.

REFERENCES

Aronson, S. "Injuries In Child Care." *Young Children* 38(6):19–20, September 1983.

Criteria for Selecting Play Equipment. Rifton, NY: Community Playthings, 1981.

Frost, J. L., and Henninger, Michael L. "Making Playgrounds Safe for Children and Children Safe for Playgrounds." In *Curriculum Planning for Young Children.* Edited by Janet Brown. Washington, DC: National Association for Education of Young Children, 1982.

Herbert-Jackson, Emily; O'Brien, Marion; Porterfield, Jan; and Risley, Todd. *The Infant Center.* Baltimore, MD: University Park Press, 1978.

Kinne, Marilyn. "Accidents." *Journal of School Health* 52(9):564–65, November 1982.

Machado, Jeanne. *Early Childhood Practicum Guide.* Albany, NY: Delmar Publishers Inc., 1984.

Matheny, A.P. "Visual-Perceptual Exploration and Accident Liability in Children." *Journal of Pediatric Psychology* 5:343–51, 1980.

Scott, Carol L. "Injury In the Classroom: Are Teachers Liable?" *Young Children* 38(6):10–18, September 1983.

Solomons, H.; Larkin, J.; Snider, B.; and Paredes-Rojas, R. "Is Day Care Safe for Children?" *Children's Health Care* 10(3):90, Winter 1982.

Treadwell, L.W. *The Family Day Care Provider's Legal Handbook.* Oakland, CA: Bananas, 1980.

Additional Reading

Adams, P.K., and Taylor, M.K. "Liability: How Much Do You Really Know?" *Day Care and Early Education,* Spring 1980.

Aikman, W.F. *Day Care Legal Handbook: Legal Aspects of Organizing and Operating Day Care Programs.* Urbana, IL: ERIC Clearinghouse on Early Childhood Education, 1977.

Anker, D.; Foster, J.; McLane, J.; Sobel, J.; and Weissbound, B. "Teaching Young Children As They Play." *Young Children* 9(5), March 1974.

Frost, J., and Klein, B. *Children's Play and Playgrounds.* Boston, MA: Allyn and Bacon, Inc., 1979.

Kramer, Anne, and Parks, Ruth. *The Buyer's Guide to Children's Toys and Games.* Babylon, NY: Pilot Industries, 1983.

McKenzie, J.F., and Williams, I.C. "Are Your Students Learning In A Safe Environment?" *Journal of School Health* 52(5):284–85, May 1982.

The Care and Safety of Young Children. New York: Council on Family Health.

Pamphlets

Equipment Safety

A Parent's Safety Guide to Kid Stuff, National Safety Council, 444 North Michigan Ave., Chicago, IL 60611.

Backyard Play Equipment Accidents, National Safety Council, 444 North Michigan Ave., Chicago, IL 60611.

Care and Safety of Young Children, Council on Family Health, Department F., 633 Third Ave., New York, NY 10017.

Let's Learn About Safety, Public Relations Services Department, Eli Lily and Company, 307 East McCarty St., Indianapolis, IN 46206.

Choosing Toys For Children, Toy Manufacturers of America, Inc., 200 Fifth Avenue, New York, NY 10010.

Safety Sampler—Hazards of Children's Products, U.S. Consumer Products Safety Commission, Washington, DC 20207.

The Swing That Swung Back, U.S. Consumer Products Safety Commission, Washington, DC 20207.

Think Play Safety, U.S. Consumer Product Safety Commission, Washington, DC 20207.

Toys and Playground Equipment, National Safety Council, 444 North Michigan Ave., Chicago, IL 60611.

Your Child's Safety, Metropolitan Life Insurance Company, 1 Madison Avenue, New York, NY 10010.

Section

FOUR

HEALTH AND SAFETY EDUCATION

EDUCATIONAL EXPERIENCES FOR YOUNG CHILDREN

Terms to Know

attitudes	retention
values	evaluation
criteria	inservice
objective	spina bifida
concept	giardiasis

Objectives

After studying this unit, you will be able to:
- Explain the four principles of instruction.
- Develop a lesson plan for teaching health and safety concepts.
- Explain the importance of including parents in children's learning experiences.
- List five health/safety topics that are appropriate for toddlers, and five that are appropriate for preschool-aged children.

Many of today's health problems are self-imposed. Communicable illnesses no longer threaten lives as they once did. Instead, poor eating habits, lack of exercise, failure to follow safety practices, increased stress, and substance abuse (alcohol, drugs and tobacco) are lessening the quality of children's health (U.S. Department of Health, Education and Welfare 1979).

The early years are formative years. Children spend much of their time gathering information and imitating the practices of others. It is also a time when children are more receptive to new ideas, changes and suggestions. Many health/safety attitudes and habits established during this period will be carried over into adulthood. Consequently, early childhood is an ideal time to help children acquire the basic health/safety information, skills, and attitudes necessary both now and in future years. The key to improvement lies with education (Kolbe 1982). Education involves a sharing of information, ideas, *attitudes, values* and skills. The desired outcomes of this learning process are positive changes in behavior.

One of the major goals of health/safety education is to encourage the use of newly acquired knowledge and skills in daily living situations. For children, this means helping them to assume greater responsibility for making decisions related to health and safety, and becoming more involved in their own health care.

THE ROLE OF PARENTS IN HEALTH AND SAFETY EDUCATION

Seldom is anyone more influential than a child's family (Reiber 1983). Many of children's health/safety habits and beliefs are acquired from their parents. The number of hours children spend in their home environments during the first few years of life often encourages health/safety behaviors patterned after those of family members.

Preschool teachers and child care providers can significantly enrich the health/safety knowledge, values and practices of young children. Much of what children learn at home takes place through incidental learning. That is, teaching is usually spontaneous and occurs in conjunction with daily routines and activities. Understanding the rationale for desired behaviors is not always a prime consideration.

In contrast, teachers know that it is important for children to understand the principles behind their actions. Instruction and learning experiences are, therefore, planned to provide young children with a component of understanding. It is also important to work together with parents and encourage them to include explanations when teaching new skills or reinforcing values and habits. For children to attain the ultimate goal of health/safety education programs, that is, to make choices and decisions that will maintain or improve the quality of their lives, they must understand the reasons and purposes for their behavior.

One way to increase understanding is to include parents in children's educational programs. Information about the health/safety concepts children receive in school can be shared with parents and actually enhance what the child learns at home. Most parents welcome additional information and ideas for expanding children's knowledge and learning experiences.

Successful parent education is built on involvement, Figure 8-1. There are many resourceful ways teachers can involve parents in children's health/safety instructional programs, including:

- newsletters
- parent meetings
- observations
- participation in class projects, demonstrations, films, lectures

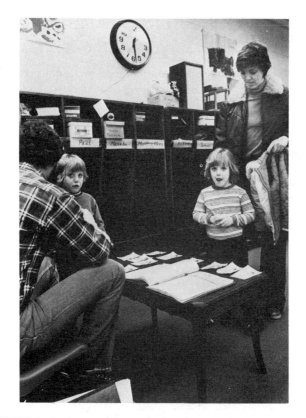

FIGURE 8-1   Successful parent education is built on involvement.

- assisting with field trips, health assessments, or making special arrangements
- preparing and presenting short programs on special topics

Parent involvement and cooperation encourage greater uniformity of health/ safety information and practices between the child's home and school. Frustration that often stems from a child being told to do things differently at school and home can be minimized. Other advantages of sharing health/safety instruction with parents include:

- better understanding of children's needs and development
- improved parental esteem
- expanded parental knowledge and outlook
- reinforcement of children's learning
- strengthening good parenting skills
- improved communication between home and school

The resources and efforts of parents, children and teachers can be united to bring about long-term improvements in health and safety for everyone.

THE ROLE OF TEACHER INSERVICE PROGRAMS IN HEALTH AND SAFETY EDUCATION

Teachers and child care providers are expected to conduct educational programs in health and safety as part of children's early learning experiences. Yet, few teachers are prepared to take on such responsibilities. Most teachers have only limited formal training in health and safety instruction. Consequently, *inservice* education for early childhood educators can improve their teaching skills, especially as they relate to matters of health and safety.

Inservice education should be an ongoing process of expanding and updating teachers' information and skills. Many excellent topics can be presented, including:

- teachers and the law
- emergency preparedness
- identifying child abuse
- advances in health screening
- review of sanitary procedures
- relaxation techniques
- parent education
- disease updates
- information on specific health problems, e.g., epilepsy, *spina bifida, giardiasis*
- review of first aid techniques

It is important that all levels of personnel, aides, volunteers, support staff, teachers and care providers, among others, be included in these educational opportunities. However, the different roles and educational backgrounds of these people requires that information and materials be presented in a manner that is meaningful to everyone involved.

PRINCIPLES OF INSTRUCTION

Opportunities to help children develop health awareness and bring about desired changes in their behavior present exciting challenges for preschool teachers and child care providers. Carefully planned educational experiences prepare children to be responsible, healthy adults. The challenge becomes one of developing long-range goals and plans that will systematically teach children basic health concepts and skills.

Topic Selection

Long-range planning is essential in any educational program, including health/safety education. However, too often health/safety instruction is approached in a haphazard fashion. Topic selection is left to individual teachers rather than according to any organized plan.

There are several *criteria* teachers and child care providers can use to aid in the selection of appropriate health/safety topics for young children. Once such a list is compiled, long-range instructional programs can then be developed. *Concepts* that have been left out can easily be identified and included in a revised plan. This process ensures that children will receive instruction in all essential areas.

Most importantly, topics should be selected to meet children's immediate needs and interests (Davis 1983). The types of health and safety problems vary with children's ages as well as with any special needs, e.g., physical impairments, learning disabilities, different cultural backgrounds and language, giftedness. Ideally, potential problems should be dealt with before they arise. Isolated facts and concepts are meaningless to young children as well as quickly forgotten. Children must see the relevance and usefulness of information to be motivated to action.

The age-group of children also requires special consideration when topics are being selected. Practices and concepts should be matched not only to children's ages, but also to their particular stage of development, Figure 8-2. The principle

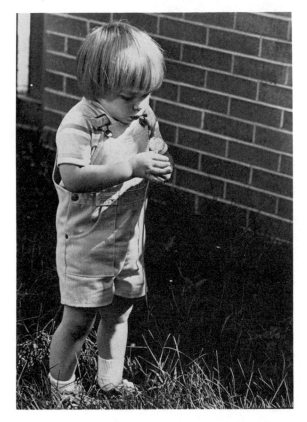

FIGURE 8-2   Blowing away a dandelion that has gone to seed can demonstrate how germs travel through the air in a manner meaningful to a toddler.

that children learn when they are ready certainly is critical to the success of health/safety education. For example, teaching three and four year olds how to brush teeth and wash hands correctly can contribute to their sense of independence. However, health issues such as drug and alcohol abuse do not meet any of a young child's immediate needs.

Learning experiences should also be selected for their ability to improve the quality of children's lives. Children need to understand the value of making healthful decisions and following good health and safety practices. They must be able to see the ultimate rewards or benefits for behaving in a safe and healthy manner. A simple explanation is needed, e.g., "Washing your hands gets rid of germs that can make you sick. When you aren't sick, you can come to school and be part of the fun things we do."

There are many appropriate health/safety concepts that can be introduced into the early childhood curriculum. Toddlers enjoy learning about:

- body parts
- growth and development
- nutritious food
- social skills/positive interaction, e.g., getting along with others
- the five senses
- personal care skills, e.g., brushing teeth, handwashing, bathing, toilet routines, dressing
- friendship
- developing self-esteem and positive self-concepts
- cooperation
- exercise/movement routines
- safe behaviors

Topics of interest to preschool children include:

- growth and development
- dental health
- safety and accident prevention, e.g., home, playground, traffic, poison, fire
- community helpers
- poison prevention
- mental health, e.g., fostering positive self-image, feelings, responsibility, respecting authority, dealing with stress
- cleanliness and good grooming
- good posture
- food and good nutrition
- the values of rest and relaxation techniques
- families
- exercise/movement activities
- control and prevention of illness
- manners
- environmental health and safety

School-age children are eager to explore topics in greater detail, including:

- personal appearance
- dental health
- food and nutrition
- consumer health, e.g., taking medicines, understanding advertisements, labels, quackery
- factors affecting growth
- mental health, e.g., personal feelings, making friends, family interactions, getting along with others
- roles of health professionals
- communicable illnesses
- safety and accident prevention, e.g., bicycle, pedestrian, playground and home safety, first aid techniques
- coping with stress
- avoiding strangers/protection against sexual abuse
- physical fitness.

Objectives

The ultimate goal of health and safety education is the development of positive knowledge, behavior and attitudes. Learning is demonstrated by children's ability to make good decisions and carry out health and safety practices that maintain or improve their present state of health. *Objectives* describe the exact quality of change in knowledge, behavior, attitude or value that can be expected from the learner upon completion of the learning experiences (Oberteuffer 1972).

Objectives serve several purposes:

- as a guide in the selection of content material
- to identify desirable changes in the learner
- as an aid in the selection of appropriate learning experiences
- as an evaluation or measurement tool

To be useful, objectives must be written in clear and meaningful terms; for example, "The child will be able to identify appropriate clothing to wear for three different types of weather conditions." The key word in this objective is "identify." It is a specific behavioral change that can be evaluated and measured. In contrast, the statement, "The child will know how to dress for the weather," is too vague and difficult to accurately measure. Additional examples of precise and measurable terms include:

- draw
- list
- discuss
- explain
- select
- write
- recognize

- describe
- identify
- answer
- demonstrate
- match
- compare

Specific and measurable objectives are a bit more difficult to develop for learning experiences that involve values, feelings and/or attitudes. Results may not be immediately apparent. Instead, it must be assumed that children's actions and behavior will at some point reflect what they have actually learned.

Classroom Instruction

How a teacher or health care provider conveys health and safety information, skills and values to children depends on the instructional method that is selected. This component is one of the most challenging and creative in the educational process (Read 1980). When deciding on a method, teachers should consider:

- presenting only a few, simple concepts or ideas during each session
- limiting presentations to a maximum of 15 minutes per session for preschool children; longer sessions are appropriate for older children
- class size, age group, type of materials being presented and available resources
- emphasizing the positive aspects of concepts; avoid confusing combinations of do's and don'ts, good and bad
- ways to involve children as participants
- opportunities for repetition (to improve learning)
- ways to use encouragement and positive reinforcement to acknowledge children's accomplishments

There are a variety of methods that can be used to present health/safety instruction, including:

- adult-directed vs. group discussions
- audiovisuals, e.g., films, records, models, specimens, cassettes
- demonstrations and experiments
- teacher-made displays, e.g., posters, bulletin boards, booklets
- printed resource material, e.g., pamphlets, posters, charts (See Table 8–1 for ways to evaluate printed resource material.)
- guest speakers
- personal example

Methods that actively involve young children in learning experiences are the most desirable, Figure 8–3. It is easier to attract and hold the attention of the children if they participate in an activity. Such methods are also more appealing to young children and increase learning and *retention* of ideas. Examples of some methods that actively involve children in learning include:

- dramatic play, e.g., dressing up, hospital, dentist office, restaurant, traffic safety, supermarket
- field trips, e.g., visits to a hospital, dental office, exercise class, supermarket, farm
- art activities, including posters, bulletin boards, displays, pictures or flannel boards created by children

TABLE 8–1 How To Evaluate Printed Resource Material

Look for materials that:
- are prepared by authorities or a reliable source
- contain unbiased information; avoid promotion or advertisement of products
- present accurate, up-to-date facts and information
- involve the learner, e.g., suggested projects, additional reading
- are thought provoking, or raise questions and answers
- are attractive
- add to the quality of the learning experience
- are worth the costs involved

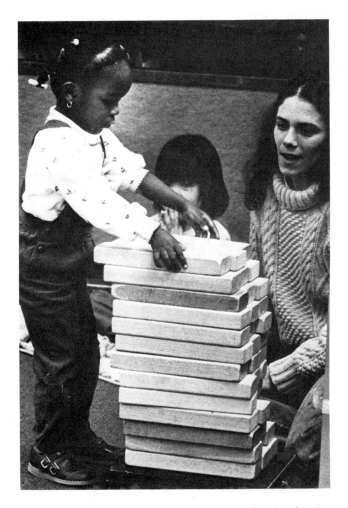

FIGURE 8–3 This care provider is involving her young student in a learning activity.

- actual experiences, e.g., handwashing, brushing teeth, grocery shopping, cooking projects, growing seeds, animal care
- puppet shows, e.g., care when you are sick, protection from strangers, health checkups, good grooming practices
- games and songs
- guest speakers, e.g., firefighters, dental hygienists, nurses, aerobics or dance instructor, nutritionist, poison control staff, mental health professionals.

Combinations of these approaches may also be very useful for maintaining interest among children, especially when several sessions will be presented on a similar topic or theme.

Evaluation

Ongoing *evaluation* is an integral part of the educational process. It is also an important step during all stages of health/safety instruction. Evaluation provides feedback concerning the effectiveness of instruction. It reveals whether or not students have learned what a teacher set out to teach. Evaluation procedures also help teachers and care providers determine the strengths, weaknesses and areas of instruction that need improvement (Oberteuffer 1972).

Evaluation is accomplished by measuring positive changes in children's behavior. The goals and objectives established at the onset of curriculum development are used to determine whether or not the desired behavior changes have been achieved. Do children remember to wash their hands after using the bathroom without having to be reminded? Do children check for traffic before dashing out into the street after a runaway ball? Do children brush their teeth at least once daily? Are established rules followed by children when they are alone on the playground? In other words, evaluation is based on demonstrations of change in children's behaviors. Many of these changes can simply be observed. However, written tests may also be an appropriate method for evaluating learning in older children.

Evaluation must not be looked upon as a final step. Rather, it should add a dimension of quality throughout the entire instructional program. The following criteria may be used for the evaluation process:

- Do the objectives identify areas where learning should take place?
- Are the objectives clearly stated and realistic?
- Were children able to achieve the objectives?
- Was the instructional method effective? Were children involved in learning experiences?
- What suggestions for improvement could be made the next time the lesson is presented?

Evaluation should be a nonthreatening process. Results of an evaluation can be used to make significant improvements in the way future health/safety programs are presented to children. It then becomes a tool that teachers, care providers and other professionals can use to improve communication of health/safety knowledge and skills to young children.

LESSON PLANS

A teacher's day can be filled with many unexpected events. Lesson plans encourage advanced planning and organization. They can also improve the efficiency of classroom experiences because teachers and care providers are better prepared and more likely to have instructional materials ready.

A written format for lesson plans is often as individualized as are teachers. However, basic features that lesson plans for health/safety instruction should contain include:

- subject title or concept to be presented
- specific objectives
- materials list
- step-by-step learning activities
- evaluation and suggestions for improvement

Lesson plans should contain enough information so they can be used by another person, such as a substitute teacher, classroom aide or volunteer. The objectives should clearly indicate what children are expected to learn. A description of materials, how they are to be used, and safety precautions required for an activity are also necessary information to include. Following are several examples of lesson plans.

Lesson Plan #1

TITLE: Germs and Prevention of Illness
CONCEPT: Sneezing and coughing release germs that can cause illness.
OBJECTIVES:
- Children will be able to identify the mouth and nose as major sources of germs.
- Children will cover their coughs and sneezes without being reminded.
- Children will be able to discuss why it is important to cover coughs and sneezes.

MATERIALS LIST: Two balloons and a small amount of confetti.
LEARNING ACTIVITIES:
- Fill both balloons with a small amount of confetti. When the activity is ready to be presented to children, carefully inflate one of the balloons by only blowing into the balloon. **Caution:** Remove your mouth from the balloon each time before inhaling. When it is inflated, quickly release pressure on the neck of the balloon, but do not let go of the balloon itself. Confetti will escape as air leaves the balloon, imitating

germs as they leave the nose and mouth during coughs and sneezes. Repeat the procedure. This time, place your hand over the mouth of the balloon as the air escapes (as if to cover a cough or sneeze). Your hand will prevent most of the confetti from escaping into the air.

- Discuss the differences in the two demonstrations with the children:
  "What happens when someone doesn't cover their mouth when they cough?"
  "How does covering your mouth help when you cough or sneeze?"
- Include a discussion of why it is important to stay home when you are sick or have a cold.
- Have several books available for children to look at and discuss:
  Clean Enough by Kevin Henkes. New York: Greenwillow Books, 1982.
  Germs Make Me Sick by Parnell Donahue. New York: Knopf, 1975.
  Phoebe Dexter Has Harriet Peterson's Sniffles by Laura J. Numeroff. New York: Greenwillow Books, 1977.
  Morris Has A Cold by Bernard Wiseman. New York: Dodd, Mead & Co., 1978.

EVALUATION:
- Children can describe the relationship between germs and illness.
- Children can identify coughs and sneezes as a major source of germs.
- Children voluntarily cover their own coughs and sneezes, Figure 8–4.

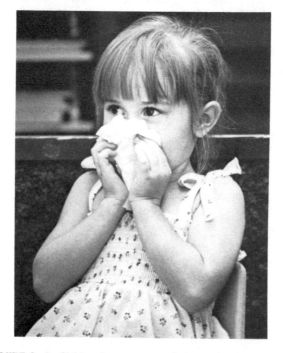

FIGURE 8–4 Children learn to cover their coughs and sneezes.

Lesson Plan #2

TITLE: Handwashing

CONCEPT: Germs on our hands can make us sick and/or spread illness to others.

OBJECTIVES:

- Children can describe when it is important to wash their hands.
- Children can demonstrate the handwashing procedure without assistance, Figure 8–5.
- Children will value the concept of cleanliness as demonstrated by voluntarily washing their hands at appropriate times.

MATERIALS LIST: Liquid or bar soap, paper towel, sink with running water.

LEARNING ACTIVITIES:

- Present the fingerplay, "Bobby Bear and Leo Lion." Have children gather around a sink to observe the handwashing procedure as it is demonstrated.

    "One bright, sunny morning, Bobby Bear and Leo Lion (make a fist with each hand, thumbs up straight), who were very good friends,

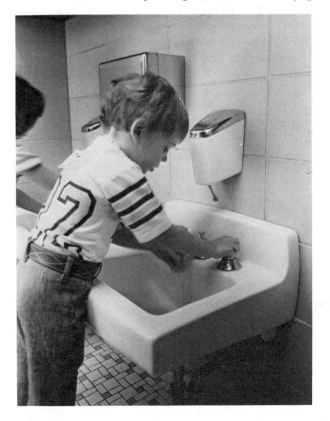

FIGURE 8–5 Good handwashing technique is important for children to learn.

decided to go for a long walk in the woods (move fists in walking motion). They walked and walked, over hills (imitate walking motion raising fists) and under trees (imitate walking motion lowering fists) until they came to a stream where they decided to cool off.

Bobby Bear sat down on a log (press palm of hand on faucet with adequate pressure to release water) and poured water on Leo Lion and Leo Lion danced and danced under the water (move hand and fingers all around underneath the water) until he was all wet. Then it was Bobby Bear's turn to get wet, so Leo Lion (hold up other fist with thumb up) sat down on a log (press palm of hand on faucet with adequate pressure to release water) and Bobby Bear danced and danced under the water until he was all wet (move other hand under water).

This was so much fun that they decided to take a bath together. They found some soap, picked it up (pick up bar of soap), put a little on their hands (rub a little soap on hands), then laid it back down on the bank (place soap in dish on side of sink). Then they rubbed the soap on their fronts and backs (rub hands together four or more times) until they were all soapy.

After that, Bobby Bear jumped back on his log (press faucet) and poured water on Leo Lion until all his soap was gone (move hand under water). Then Leo Lion jumped back on his log (press other faucet) and poured water on Bobby Bear and rinsed him until all his soap was gone (move other hand under water).

Soon the wind began to blow and Bobby Bear and Leo Lion were getting very cold. They reached up and picked a leaf from the tree above (reach up and take a paper towel from the dispenser) and used it to dry themselves off (use paper towel to dry both hands). When they were all dry, Bobby Bear and Leo Lion carefully dropped their leaves into the trash can (drop paper towel into wastebasket). They joined hands (use fists, thumbs up and joined; walking motion, rapidly) and ran merrily back through the woods."[1]

- Review the handwashing procedure with small groups of children at a time. Ask simple questions and encourage all children to contribute to the discussion.

  "When is it important to wash our hands?"

  "What do we do first? Let's list the steps together."

  "Why do we use soap?"

  "Why is it important to dry our hands carefully after washing them?"

- Help children understand why it is important to wash their hands, especially after blowing their noses, playing outdoors, using the bathroom, and before eating. (Teachers and care providers must set a good example by *always* remembering to wash their hands before handling food.)

[1]The authors would like to acknowledge Rhonda McMullen, a former student and graduate of the Early Childhood Program, University of Kansas, for sharing her delightful story and creative ways with young children.

Set up a messy art activity, e.g., fingerpaint, clay, glue. Have children look at their hands before and after washing them. Point out the value of washing hands carefully.

- Read and discuss with the children several of the following books:

  Clean As a Whistle by Aileen Fisher. New York: Cromwell, 1969.

  Dirty Feet by Steven Kroll. New York: Parents' Magazine Press, 1980.

  Harry The Dirty Dog by Gene Zion. New York: Harper and Row, 1956.

  I Hate To Take A Bath by Judith Barrett. New York: Four Winds Press, 1975.

  Messy by Barbara Bottner. New York: Delacorte Press, 1979.

  No More Baths by Brock Cole. New York: Doubleday, 1980.

  Swampy Alligator by Jack Gantos. New York: Windmill/Wanderer Books, 1980.

  The Messy Rabbit by Ruth Nivola. New York: Panetheon Books, 1978.

  The Sticky Child by Malcolm Bird. New York: Harcourt Brace Jovanovich, 1981.

- Observe children washing their hands from time to time to make sure they continue to follow good procedures.

EVALUATION:

- Was the fingerplay effective for demonstrating the handwashing technique?
- Can children wash their hands correctly and alone?
- Do children wash their hands at the appropriate times, without being prompted?

Lesson Plan #3

TITLE: Dressing Appropriately for the Weather

CONCEPT: Clothing helps to protect our bodies

OBJECTIVES:

- When given a choice, children will be able to match appropriate items of clothing with different kinds of weather, e.g., rainy, sunny, snowy, hot, cold.
- Children will be able to perform two of the following dressing skills: button a button, snap a snap, or zip up a zipper.
- Children will demonstrate proper care and storage of clothing by hanging up their coats, sweaters, hats, etc., at least two out of three days.

MATERIALS LIST: Items for a clothing store, such as clothing, cash register, play money, mirror; old magazines and catalogues containing pictures of children's clothing, paste and paper or newspaper; buttons, snaps and zippers sewn on pieces of cloth; dolls and doll clothes; books and pictures.

LEARNING ACTIVITIES:
- Read and discuss with the children several of the following books:

  The Cat's Pajamas by Ida Chittum. New York: Parent's Magazine Press, 1980.

  What Will I Wear? by Helen Olds. New York: Knopf, 1961.

  What Should I Wear? by Pamela Rowland. Chicago: Children's Press, 1975.

  The Emperor's New Clothes by Hans Christian Andersen. New York: Four Winds Press, 1977.

  How Do I Put It On? by Shigeo Watanabe. New York: Collins, 1979.

- Help children set up a clothing store. Provide clothing for both boys and girls. Include items that could be worn for different types of weather conditions. Talk about the purpose of clothing and how it helps to protect our bodies. Help children identify qualities in clothing that differ with weather conditions, e.g., short sleeves vs. long sleeves, light colors vs. dark colors, lightweight fabrics vs. heavyweight fabrics, etc.

- Have children select two different seasons or weather conditions. Give children old magazines or catalogues from which they can choose pictures of appropriate clothing. Display completed pictures where parents can see them.

- Provide children with pieces of cloth on which a button, zipper and snap have been sewn. Working with a few children at a time, help each child master working these items. Have several items of real clothing available for children to practice putting on and taking off.

EVALUATION:
- Children can select at least two appropriate items of clothing for three different types of weather.
- Children can complete two of the following skills—buttoning a button, snapping a snap, zipping a zipper.
- Children hang up their personal clothing, e.g., hats, coats, sweaters, raincoats, at least three out of four days.

Lesson Plan #4

TITLE: Dental Health
CONCEPT: Good dental care helps to keep teeth healthy.
OBJECTIVES:
- Children will be able to identify at least two functions that teeth serve.
- Children can name at least three foods that are good for healthy teeth.
- Children can describe three ways to promote good dental health.

MATERIALS LIST: Order pamphlets on dental health and proper dental care from:

American Dental Association
Bureau of Dental Health, Education and Audio-Visual Services
211 Chicago Avenue
Chicago, IL 60611 (Preschool to sixth grade)

Colgate-Palmolive Company
300 Park Avenue
New York, NY 10010

Lever Brothers Company
390 Park Avenue
New York, NY 10022 (Kindergarten to sixth grade)

Public Health Service
Washington, DC 20201
(Order PHS Publication #1483, "Research Explores Dental Decay")
Old magazines, paper, glue, and string; selected snack food items.

LEARNING ACTIVITIES:
- Distribute pamphlets. Discuss the information with children. Talk about the purposes teeth serve, e.g., chewing, formation of word sounds, spacing for new teeth, shaping of the jaw and face, a pretty smile.
- Discuss ways children can help to keep their teeth healthy, e.g., daily brushing with a fluoride toothpaste; regular dental checkups; eating nutritious foods and snacks (especially raw fruits and vegetables); avoiding chewing on nonfood items, e.g., pencils, spoons, keys; limiting sweets.
- Help children construct "good food" mobiles. Use old magazines to cut out pictures of foods that are good for healthy teeth. Paste pictures on paper, attach with string or yarn and tie to a piece of cardboard cut in the shape of a smile.
- Have children help plan snacks for several days; include foods that are both nutritious and good for the teeth.

EVALUATION
- Children can identify at least two functions that teeth serve.
- Children can name at least three foods that are good for healthy teeth.
- Children can describe three good dental health practices that help to keep teeth healthy.

Lesson Plan #5

TITLE: Toothbrushing
CONCEPT: Teeth should be brushed every day to stay white and healthy.
OBJECTIVES:
- Children can state appropriate times when teeth should be brushed.
- Children can demonstrate good toothbrushing technique.
- Children can describe one alternate method for cleaning teeth after eating.

MATERIALS LIST: 1 white egg carton per child, cardboard, pink construction paper; several old toothbrushes, cloth, and grease pencil.

LEARNING ACTIVITIES:
- Invite a dentist or dental hygienist to demonstrate toothbrushing to the children. Ask the speaker to talk about how often to brush, when to brush, how to brush, alternate ways of cleaning teeth after eating, what type of toothpaste to use, and care of toothbrushes. This may also be a good opportunity to invite parents to visit so they can reinforce toothbrushing skills at home.
- Help children construct a set of model teeth from egg cartons, Figure 8-6. Cut an oval approximately 14 inches in length from lightweight cardboard; crease oval gently along the center. Cut the bottom portion of an egg carton lengthwise into two strips. Staple egg-carton "teeth" along the small ends of the oval. Glue pink construction paper along the edges where "teeth" are fastened to form "gums." Also cover the backside of the oval with pink construction paper. Use a grease pencil to mark areas of plaque on the teeth. Cover the head of an old toothbrush with cloth and fasten. With the toothbrush, have children demonstrate correct toothbrushing technique to remove areas of plaque (grease pencil markings).
- Send a note home to parents and request that children bring a clean toothbrush to school. Practice toothbrushing, step-by-step with small groups of children.
- Older children will enjoy designing posters or bulletin board displays that reinforce good dental hygiene.

EVALUATION:
- Children can identify times when teeth should be brushed.
- Children can demonstrate good toothbrushing technique.
- Children can correctly identify at least one alternate method for cleaning their teeth after eating.

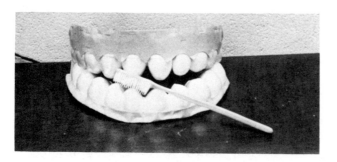

FIGURE 8-6 A set of "egg-carton" teeth.

Lesson Plan #6

TITLE: Understanding Feelings (Mental Health)
CONCEPT: Feelings affect the state of one's mental as well as physical well-being.
OBJECTIVES:
- Children will be able to name at least four feelings or emotions.
- Children can express their feelings in words.

MATERIALS LIST: Old magazines, glue, paper; large, unbreakable mirror; shoe boxes.
LEARNING ACTIVITIES:
- Read and discuss with the children several of the following books:
  Feelings by Richard Allington and Kathleen Cowles. Milwaukee: Raintree Children's Books, 1980.
  How I Feel by June Behrens. Chicago: Children's Press, 1973.
  Robbers, Bones and Mean Dogs by Barry and Velma Berkey. Reading, MA: Addison-Wesley Publishers, 1978.
  The Me I See by Barbara Hazen. Abingdon: Nashville, 1978.
  I Hate It by Miriam Schlein. Chicago: Albert Whitman and Co., 1978.
  Why Am I Different? by Norma Simon. Chicago: Albert Whitman and Co., 1976.
  Sometimes I Like to Cry by Elizabeth Stanton. Chicago: Albert Whitman and Co., 1978.
  Feeling Angry by Sylvia Root Teater. Elgin, IL: Children's World, 1976.
  Sometimes I Hate School by Carol Barkin and Elizabeth James. Milwaukee: Raintree Publishing, Ltd., 1975.
- Have children sit in a circle on the floor. Discuss the fact that children and adults have many different kinds of feelings. Stress that many of these feelings are normal and that it is important to learn acceptable and healthy ways of expressing them. Ask children, one at a time, to name a feeling, e.g., happy, sad, tired, bored, special, excitement, surprise, fear, lonely, embarrassed, proud, angry. Have children act out the feeling. Encourage children to observe the expressions of one another. Help children learn to recognize these feelings. "Have you ever seen someone look like this?" "Have you ever felt like this?" "What made you feel like this?" Talk about healthy and acceptable ways of coping with these feelings.
- Place an unbreakable mirror where children can see themselves. Encourage them to imitate some of the feelings they have identified and observe their own facial expressions.
- Make a collage of feelings using pictures of people from old magazines. Help children identify the feelings portrayed in each picture.
- Construct "I Am Special" boxes. Have children decorate old shoe boxes with pictures of things that reflect their individuality, such as

favorite foods, activities, toys, etc. Have children fill their boxes with items that tell something special about themselves; for example, a hobby, favorite toy, photograph, souvenirs from a trip, pet, picture of their family. Children can share their boxes and tell something special about themselves during "Show and Tell" or large group time.

- Older children can be involved in role play. Write out problem situations on small cards; for example, "you and another child want the same toy," "someone knocks down the block structure you just built," "another child pushes you," "a friend says they don't like you anymore." Have pairs of children select a card and act out acceptable ways of handling their feelings in each situation. Discuss their solutions.

EVALUATION:
- Children can name at least four different feelings or emotions.
- Children begin using words rather than physical aggression to handle difficult or emotional situations.

Lesson Plan #7

TITLE: Safety in Cars
CONCEPT: Good safety rules are important to follow in and around vehicles.
OBJECTIVES:
- Children will wear an appropriate seat belt restraint (seat belt for children over three years of age, safety car seat for children under three years of age), Figure 8–7 and 8–8.
- Children can name at least one important safety rule to follow in and around cars.
MATERIALS LIST: Order pamphlets about seat belt restraints and car safety from:

      American Automobile Association
      8111 Gatehouse Road
      Falls Church, VA 22042
              OR
      All State Insurance Company, F–3
      Northbrook, IL 60062

- Prepare photographs of children demonstrating the following safety rules:
  a. Always hold an adult's hand when going to and from the car; never dash ahead.
  b. Always get in and out of a car on the curbside.
  c. Open and close car doors properly. Place both hands on the door handle to reduce the possibility of getting fingers caught in the door.
  d. Sit in the car seat; never ride standing.

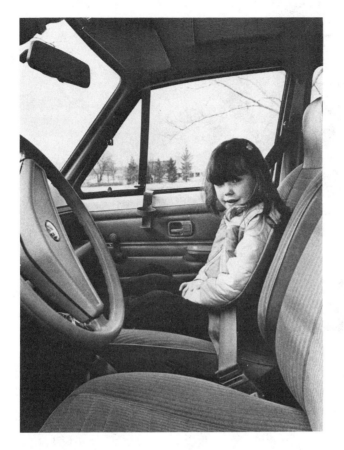

FIGURE 8–7 Seat belts should be worn by children over three years of age.

    e. Put on seat belt or use safety car seat.

    f. Lock all car doors before starting out.

    g. Ride with arms, legs, head and other body parts inside the car.

    h. Don't play with controls inside of the car.

    i. Ride quietly so as not to disturb the driver.

LEARNING ACTIVITIES:

- Discuss with the children information found in the pamphlets. Stress the importance of wearing seat belts or riding in an appropriate car seat restraint. Later, have children take the pamphlets home to share with parents.

- Mount photographs of safety rules on posterboard or display on a table. Encourage children to identify the safe behavior demonstrated in each picture.

- Use large group time to discuss with the children the importance of each safety rule pictured in the photographs.

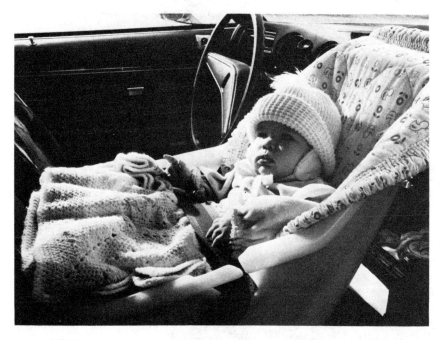

FIGURE 8-8   Safety car seats provide protection for infants and toddlers.

- For dramatic play, use large wooden blocks, cardboard boxes or chairs and a "steering wheel" to build a pretend car. Have children demonstrate the car safety rules as they play.
- Prepare a chart with all of the children's names. Each day, have children place a checkmark next to their name if they wore their seat belt on the way to school.
- Establish a parent committee to plan a "Safe Riding" campaign. On randomly-selected days, observe parents and children as they arrive and depart from the center; record whether or not they were wearing seat belt restraints. Enlist children's artistic abilities to design and make awards to be given to families who ride safely. Repeat the campaign again in several months.

EVALUATION:
- Children can be observed wearing seat belts or sitting in a proper safety car seat.
- Children can name one safety rule to observe when riding in a car.

TEACHER RESOURCES:

"Seat Belts Activity Book" (Teacher's Guide), U.S. Department of Transportation, National Highway Traffic Safety Administration, Washington, DC 20590.

"Don't Risk Your Child's Life!" Physicians for Automotive Safety, 50 Union Avenue, Irvington, NJ 07111 (Enclose a self-addressed, stamped envelope and $.25 for each copy).

Lesson Plan #8

TITLE: Pedestrian Safety

CONCEPT: Young children can begin to learn safe behaviors in and around traffic and a respect for moving vehicles.

OBJECTIVES:
- Children will be able to identify the stop, go, and walk signals.
- Children can describe two rules for safely crossing streets.
- Children will begin to develop respect for moving vehicles.

MATERIALS LIST: Flannel board and characters; cardboard pieces, poster paint, wooden stakes; masking tape, yarn or string; 6-inch paper plates; red, green and yellow poster paint; black marker.

LEARNING ACTIVITIES:
- Discuss rules for safe crossing of streets:
  a. always have an adult cross streets with you (this is a must for pre-school children)
  b. only cross streets at intersections
  c. always look both ways before stepping out into the street
  d. use your ears to listen for oncoming cars
  e. don't walk out into the street from between parked cars or in the middle of a block
  f. ask an adult to retrieve balls and toys from streets
  g. always obey traffic signs
- Introduce basic traffic signs (only those that have meaning to young pedestrians), e.g., stop, go, walk, pedestrian crossing, one-way traffic, bike path, railroad crossing. Help children learn to recognize each sign by identifying certain features, such as color, shape, location.
- Help children to construct the basic traffic signs using cardboard and poster paint. Attach signs to wooden stakes. Set up a series of "streets" in the outdoor play yard using string, yarn or pieces of cardboard to mark paths; place traffic signs in appropriate places. Select children to ride tricycles along designated "streets" while other children practice pedestrian safety.
- Prepare a flannel board story and characters to help children visualize pedestrian safety rules.
- Help children construct a set of stop-go-walk signs. Have each child paint three paper plates—one red, one green, one yellow. On a plain white plate write the word WALK. Fasten all four plates together with tape or glue to form a traffic signal.

EVALUATION:
- Children respond correctly to the signals stop, go, walk.
- Children can state two rules for safely crossing streets. (Puppets can be used to ask children questions).
- Children demonstrate increased caution in the play yard while riding tricycles and other wheeled toys and also as pedestrians.

Lesson Plan #9

TITLE: Poisonous Substances and Prevention of Poisoning

CONCEPT: Identification and avoidance of known and potentially poisonous substances.

OBJECTIVES:
- Children will be able to name at least three poisonous substances.
- Children will be able to describe what the "Mr. Yuk" symbol represents.
- Children can identify at least one safety rule that can help prevent accidental poisoning.

MATERIALS LIST: Old magazines, large sheet of paper, glue; small squares of paper or self-adhesive labels, marking pens.

LEARNING ACTIVITIES:
- Invite someone from the hospital emergency room or Public Health Department to talk with the children about poison prevention.
- Show children pictures of poisonous substances. Include samples of cleaning items, grooming supplies, medicines, perfumes, plants and berries. Show the children a "Mr. Yuk" symbol. Emphasize that children should stay away from any product displaying this label. ("Mr. Yuk" labels can be obtained for $1.00 from the National Poison Center Network, 125 DeSoto Street, Pittsburgh, PA 15213.) Also caution children that not all poisonous substances are identified in this manner.
- Discuss rules for poison prevention:
  a. Only food should be put into the mouth, Figure 8–9.
  b. Medicine is not candy and should only be given by an adult.
  c. An adult should always inform a child that they are taking medicine, not candy.
  d. Never eat berries, flowers, leaves or mushrooms before checking with an adult.
- Have children make their own "Mr. Yuk" labels by drawing a sad face on small pieces of paper or self-adhesive labels. Encourage parents to place the labels on products that are poisonous.
- Make a wall mural for the classroom displaying pictures of poisonous substances. Be sure to include a sampling of cleaning products, personal grooming supplies, medicines, plants, products commonly found in garages, such as insecticides, fertilizers, gasoline, and automotive fluids. Glue pictures of these products on a large sheet of paper. Display the mural where parents and children can look at it.

EVALUATION:
- Children can identify the "Mr. Yuk" label as a symbol of poisonous substances.
- Children can name at least three poisonous substances.
- Children can name at least one safety rule that can help prevent accidental poisoning.

TEACHER RESOURCES:

A Guide to Teaching Poison Prevention in Kindergarten and Primary Grades. Public Health Service, U.S. Department of Health Education and Welfare, Division of Accident Prevention, Washington, DC.

Common Poisonous and Injurious Plants by Kenneth F. Lampe, U.S. Government Printing Office, Washington, DC [HHS Publication No. (FDA)81–7006, $2.75].

Poisonous Plants by Laurence Gadd. New York: Macmillan Publishing Co., 1980.

Your Child and Household Safety. American Academy of Pediatrics, 1801 Hinman Avenue, Evanston, IL 60201.

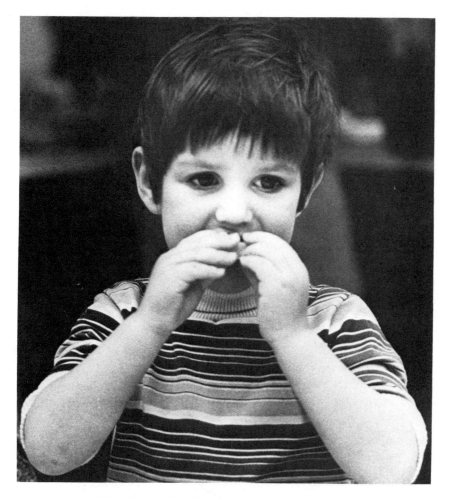

FIGURE 8–9 Only food belongs in children's mouths.

SUMMARY

Poor health practices and habits are responsible for many of today's health problems. However, education can significantly improve the overall quality of children's health. Education creates an awareness of health and provides the necessary information to make wise decisions. Health and safety education encourages individuals to assume responsibility for, and become actively involved in, their own health care. Education promotes good health/safety behaviors that can improve the quality of one's life.

The development of long-range plans for health and safety educational programs ensures that young children will receive comprehensive instruction. Topic selection should be based on children's immediate health needs and interests, age, and the ability to improve the quality of their lives. Objectives identify the changes in children's behavior that can be expected following instruction. They can also be useful for selecting content material, learning experiences, and as an evaluation tool. Instructional methods should include opportunities for children to participate in learning activities. Involvement increases what young children learn and remember. Evaluation determines whether or not desired behavior changes have been achieved.

Including parents in children's education programs encourages consistency between school and home. Parents can reinforce information, skills and values when they are aware of what children have learned. Continuous inservice education also helps teachers and care providers expand and update their information and skills.

LEARNING ACTIVITIES

1. Interview a teacher of toddler or preschool children and a first or second grade teacher. Ask them to describe the kinds of health and safety concepts that are stressed at each group level. Arrange to observe one of the teachers or care providers conducting a health/safety session with children. What were the teacher's objectives? Was the instructional method effective? Did the teacher involve children in learning activities? Were the children attentive? Were the objectives met?

2. Write to several organizations for materials on seat belt restraints and car safety seats. Read and compare the information. Do all statements agree? Do the statements disagree? For whom is the material written, e.g., parents, children, professionals?

3. Develop a lesson plan for a unit to be taught on "What Makes Us Grow?" Include objectives, time length, materials, learning activities, measures for evaluation and any teacher resource information. Exchange lesson plans with another student; critique each other's lesson plan for clarity of ideas, thoroughness and creativity.

4. Select, read and evaluate three children's books from the reference lists provided in this unit.

UNIT REVIEW

A. Select the best answer in each of the following statements.

1. Objectives
   a. measure a teacher's expertise
   b. define instructional methods
   c. describe an open-minded attitude
   d. identify desired behavior changes

2. The early years of a child's life are
   a. unimportant
   b. unproductive
   c. formative
   d. incidental

3. Health and safety learning experiences should
   a. involve children
   b. encourage children to be passive
   c. be spontaneous
   d. be difficult so as to challenge children

4. Evaluation
   a. measures positive changes in behavior
   b. should be a final step in the teaching process
   c. is generally a threatening experience
   d. only determines the quality of instructional methods

5. Inservice educational programs should
   a. be conducted three to four times each year
   b. be developed specifically for classroom teachers
   c. include parents
   d. expand and update information and skills

6. Involving parents in children's health/safety education programs
   a. is frustrating to parents
   b. encourages consistency of information and practices
   c. disrupts teacher/child relationships
   d. all of these

7. Long-range planning for health/safety education
   a. is very difficult
   b. should only take advantage of spontaneous learning opportunities
   c. ensures systematic teaching of basic concepts
   d. not essential

8. Many of today's health problems are
   a. not preventable
   b. the result of poor habits and practices
   c. caused by life-threatening communicable illnesses
   d. unpredictable

B. Matching. Match the definition in column I with the correct term in column II.

Column I	Column II
1. to assess the effectiveness of instruction	a. education
2. favorable changes in attitudes, knowledge and/or practices	b. outcome
	c. positive behavior changes
3. a sharing of knowledge or skills	d. attitude
4. ideas and values meaningful to a child	e. relevance
5. subject or theme	f. topic
6. feeling or strong belief	g. incidental learning
7. occurs in conjunction with daily activities and routines	h. evaluation
8. the end product of learning	

C. Following is a list of suggested health/safety topics. Place an *A* (appropriate) or *NA* (not appropriate) next to each of the statements. Base your decision on whether or not the topic is suitable for preschool-aged children.
_____ dental health
_____ feelings and how to get along with others
_____ primary causes of suicide
_____ consumer health, e.g., understanding advertisements, choosing a doctor, medical quackery
_____ eye safety
_____ the hazards of smoking
_____ how to safely light matches
_____ physical fitness for health
_____ cardiopulmonary resuscitation
_____ the values of rest and sleep
_____ safety at home
_____ animal families

REFERENCES

Davis, Anita P. "Project HITE (Health Individualization and Teacher Education): A Health Curriculum for 3-, 4- and 5-year olds." *Journal of School Health* 53(7):433–34, September 1983.

Kolbe, Lloyd J. "What Can We Expect From School Health Education?" *Journal of School Health* 52(3):145–50, March 1982.

Oberteuffer, Delbert; Harrelson, Orvis A.; and Pollock, Marion B. *School Health*

Education. New York: Harper and Row, 1972.

Read, D., and Greene, W. *Creative Teaching in Health.* New York: Macmillan Publishing Company, 1980.

Reiber, Joan L., and Embry, Lynne H. "Working and Communicating With Parents." In *Early Childhood Education: Special Environmental, Policy, and Legal Considerations* by Elizabeth M. Goetz and K. Eileen Allen. Rockville, MD: Aspen Publications, 1983.

U.S. Department of Health, Education and Welfare. *Healthy People: The Surgeon General's Report on Health Promotion and Disease Prevention.* Washington, DC: Government Printing Office, 1979.

Additional Reading

Adams, L., and Garlick, B., eds. *Ideas That Work with Children.* Vol. II. Washington, DC: National Association for the Education of Young Children, 1979.

Berger, Eugenia H. *Parents As Partners in Education.* St. Louis: C.V. Mosby Co., 1981.

Duryea, Elias J. "Decision Making and Health Education." *Journal of School Health* 53(1):29–32, January 1983.

Elison, Claudia F., and Jenkins, Loa T. *A Practical Guide to Early Childhood Curriculum.* 2d ed. St. Louis: C.V. Mosby Co., 1981.

Fetter, M. "Nonverbal Teaching Behavior and the Health Educator." *Journal of School Health* 53(7):431–32, September 1983.

Machado, Jeanne M., and Meyer, Helen C. *Early Childhood Practicum Guide.* Albany, NY: Delmar Publishers Inc., 1984.

Seefeldt, C. *Curriculum For Preschool Children.* Columbus, OH: Charles E. Merrill Co., 1980.

Weiser, M. *Group Care and Education of Infants and Toddlers.* St. Louis, MO: C.V. Mosby Co., 1982.

FIVE

THE ROLE OF THE CARE PROVIDER IN ILLNESS AND EMERGENCY CARE

COMMUNICABLE
ILLNESS

Terms to Know

acute	digestive tract
communicable	incubation
antibodies	prodromal
immunized	direct contact
contagious	indirect contact
respiratory tract	lymph glands
pathogen	convalescent
susceptible host	

Objectives

After studying this unit, you will be able to:
- Define communicable illness.
- List the three factors which are essential for an infection to be communicable.
- Name four control measures that child care facilities can use to reduce communicable illnesses.
- Identify signs and symptoms of common communicable diseases.

Communicable illnesses are a common health problem preschool teachers and child care providers frequently encounter in their work with children. Some of the contagious diseases typically experienced by infants, toddlers and preschool-aged children include chickenpox, strep throat, head lice, tonsillitis, colds and influenza. Many preventable but often deadly diseases such as smallpox, whooping cough and polio are observed less frequently today. However, their control depends on comprehensive and continuous programs of education, immunization and sanitation (Highberger 1983).

Repeated incidences of illness are common for infants, toddlers and preschool children during their first experiences in group settings. This occurs because young children have not had an opportunity to build up *antibodies* against many of the common communicable illnesses and, therefore, their resistance is often lower. Children with chronic illnesses or handicapping conditions are usually more susceptible to infectious illnesses.

The immature development of the young child's body structures is another contributing factor to the high rate of illness. Since the majority of communicable illnesses involve the *respiratory tract,* it is easy to understand how short distances between a young child's ears, nose and throat are more favorable to infection. Young children's habit of sucking on fingers and putting toys and other objects into their mouths also encourages the rapid spread of illness, Figure 9–1.

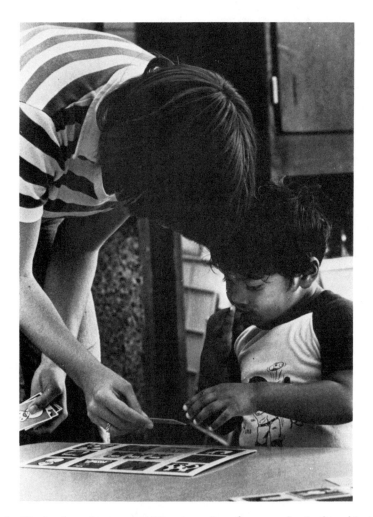

FIGURE 9–1   The tendency for young children to suck on fingers and put other objects into their mouths encourages the spread of illness among this age group.

COMMUNICABLE ILLNESS

A communicable illness is an illness that can be transmitted or spread from one person or animal to another. Three factors are necessary for this process to occur:

- a pathogen
- a susceptible host
- a method for transmission

First, a living *pathogen* or infectious agent, usually a bacteria or virus, must be present and available for transmission. These invisible organisms are specific for each illness and are most commonly located in discharges from the respiratory (nose, throat, lungs) and intestinal tracts of infected persons. Most pathogens require a living host for their survival. One exception, however, is the organism that causes tetanus; it can survive in soil and dust for several years.

Second, there must be a *susceptible host* or person who can be infected with the pathogen. The types of communicable illnesses experienced most often by young children generally enter their new host through either the skin, respiratory tract or *digestive tract*. The route of entry depends on the specific disease involved.

Not every child who is exposed to a particular virus or bacteria will become infected by it. Conditions must be favorable to allow an infectious organism to successfully avoid the body's defense systems, multiply, and establish itself. Children who are well rested, adequately nourished, *immunized* and in a good state of health are generally less susceptible to communicable illnesses. Also, in many instances, a previous case of the same illness affords protection against repeated infections. However, the length of this protection varies with the illness and may range from several days to a lifetime. Children who experience a very mild or subclinical case of an illness or who are carriers of an infection are often resistant to the illness without realizing that they have experienced it.

Third, a method for transmitting the infectious agent from the original source to the new host is necessary to make the communicable process complete. This passage commonly takes place through *direct contact* with another infected person. Whenever an infected child or adult coughs, sneezes or talks, tiny droplets of moisture containing pathogens are expelled through the air, Figure 9–2. Anyone inhaling these airborne droplets will be exposed directly to the infectious organisms. Influenza, colds, meningitis, tuberculosis, and chickenpox are examples of infectious illnesses spread in this manner.

Another form of direct contact involves touching infected areas on another individual, especially with communicable skin conditions such as ringworm, athlete's foot and impetigo. The infectious organisms are transferred directly from an infected host to a new host. In cases of pinworms and hepatitis, the infectious pathogen leaves the human body in blood and feces. These infections are spread directly from one person to another when careful handwashing is not practiced after using the bathroom.

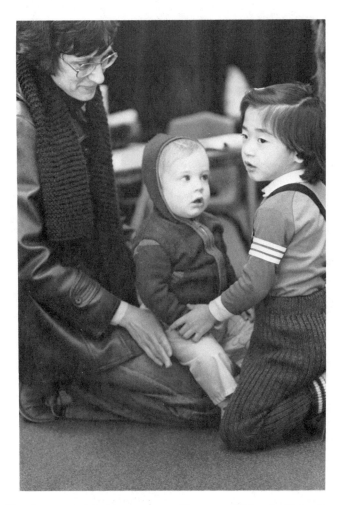

FIGURE 9–2   The close contact that is necessary with young children facilitates the spread of communicable illnesses.

Communicable illnesses can also be transmitted through *indirect contact*. This method involves the transfer of infectious organisms from an infected host to an intermediate object, such as water, milk, dust, food, toys, towels, eating utensils, animals or insects, and finally to the new susceptible host. Recent studies suggest that it may be possible to infect oneself with certain viruses, such as those causing colds and influenza, by touching the moist linings of the eyes and nose with hands contaminated with the infectious agent.

The absence of any one of these factors (pathogen, host, or method of transmission) will prevent the spread of communicable illness. This is an important factor for teachers and care providers to remember in their attempts to control outbreaks of communicable illness in group settings.

STAGES OF ILLNESS

Communicable illnesses follow a fairly predictable progression of stages: incubation, prodromal, acute, convalescence. Since many of these stages overlap, it is often difficult to identify when each one begins and ends.

The *incubation* stage includes the time between exposure to a pathogen and the appearance of the first signs or symptoms of illness. During this period, the infectious organisms enter the body and multiply rapidly in an attempt to overpower the body's defense systems and establish themselves. The length of the incubation stage is described in terms of hours or days and varies for each communicable disease. For example, the incubation period for chickenpox ranges from two to three weeks following exposure, while for the common cold it is thought to be only 12 to 72 hours. Many infectious illnesses are already communicable near the end of this stage. The fact that children are often *contagious* before any symptoms are apparent makes the control of infectious illness in the classroom more difficult, despite teachers' careful observations.

The *prodromal* stage begins when an infant or young child experiences the first nonspecific signs of infection and ends with the appearance of symptoms characteristic of a particular communicable illness. This stage may last from several hours to several days. However, not all communicable diseases have a prodromal stage. Early symptoms commonly associated with the prodromal stage may include headache, low-grade fever, a slight sore throat, a general feeling of restlessness or irritability. Many of these complaints are so vague that they often go unnoticed. However, because children are highly contagious during this stage, care providers and parents must learn to recognize that these subtle changes may signal impending illness.

During the *acute* stage an infant or child is definitely sick. This stage is marked by the onset of symptoms that are typical of the specific communicable illness. Some of these symptoms such as fever, sore throat, cough, runny nose, rashes, enlarged lymph glands are common to many infectious diseases. However, there are usually characteristic combinations and variations of these symptoms which can be used to identify a particular communicable illness. An infant or child continues to be highly contagious throughout this stage.

The *convalescent* or recovery stage follows automatically unless complications develop or the child dies. During this stage, symptoms gradually disappear, the child begins to feel better and usually is no longer contagious.

CONTROL MEASURES

Teachers and child care providers have an obligation and responsibility to help protect young children from communicable illnesses. Preschool classrooms and child care centers are ideal settings for the rapid spread of many infectious conditions. However, a variety of practical control measures are available that teachers and child care providers can implement in their settings to reduce the incidence of communicable illness.

Observations

Perhaps one of the most successful and effective control measures available to preschool teachers and child care providers is that of identifying and removing sick children from the classroom or group environment. This action eliminates the immediate source of infection which is an essential factor in the communicable process. Without a potential supply of infectious pathogens, illness cannot continue to spread unless new cases develop. Early recognition of sick children requires that adults develop a sensitivity to changes in children's normal appearance and behavior patterns. A preschool teacher, who knows that Tony's allergies often cause a red throat and cough in the fall or that Shadra's recent irritability is probably related to her mother's hospitalization would not be alarmed by these observations. However, the same signs and symptoms in other children might warrant concern. From these observations, teachers and child care providers can begin to distinguish between children with potentially infectious illnesses and those whose health problems are explainable and not contagious. It is also important that teachers and care providers be more alert to signs of illness during certain seasons of the year when some diseases are more prevalent.

The process of early identification is simplified by the fact that young children usually look and behave differently when they are not feeling well. Changes in their actions, facial expressions, skin color, sleep habits, appetite, and comments often present valuable warnings of impending illness (Pringle 1982). Children who show any of the following signs of communicable illness, the cause of which is not readily apparent, should be excluded from classroom or group settings:

- unusually pale or flushed skin
- red or sore throat
- enlarged *lymph glands*
- nausea, vomiting or diarrhea
- rash, spots or open lesions
- watery or red eyes
- headache or dizziness
- chills or fever
- achiness
- unusual tiredness

Occasionally, circumstances make it difficult to reach a child's parents or for them to come and take a child home immediately. For these reasons, it is ideal to have a separate room where sick children can be taken to wait and rest. Even a small office can be equipped and used as a temporary sick room. However, someone must be available at all times to stay with the child or at least be able to observe the child from nearby. Infants, toddlers and preschool children must never be left unattended.

In buildings where a separate room is not available for this purpose, sick children can be isolated from the rest of the group by moving them to a corner of the room. Dividers placed around the child will provide privacy as well as minimize distractions and contact with other children.

Policies

Policies offer another distinct method for the control of communicable illnesses. Child development centers and child care facilities should establish specific policies and guidelines. They should clearly define when children should be excluded from the facilities when they are ill, and the length of time they must remain away before being readmitted. Standards should also be set for acceptable immunization levels of entering children, and for actions dealing with those who do not comply. Written policies explaining procedures that will be followed by the child care center when children in attendance become ill should be available to parents. It is also important to adopt a policy regarding the notification of parents whenever children are exposed to communicable illnesses so they can help to observe their child for symptoms, Figure 9–3. Local public health authorities can offer much useful information and assistance to centers and child care providers when they are planning and formulating new policies or are confronted with a communicable health problem.

Successful control of infectious illness in preschool or child care programs depends on carefully preparing and enforcing policies and guidelines concerning communicable illness. Parents who are well informed are much more likely to cooperate with a center's control program. It is also important that every teacher

---

Date_____

Dear Parent:

There is a possibility that your child has been exposed to chickenpox. If your child has not had chickenpox, observe carefully from _____ to _____ (more likely
                                                                        date   date
the first part of this period), for signs of a slight cold, runny nose, loss of appetite, fever, listlessness, and/or irritability. Within a day or two, watch for a spot (or spots) resembling mosquito bites on which a small blister soon forms. Chickenpox is contagious 24–48 hours *before* the rash appears.

If you have any questions, please call the Center before bringing your child. We appreciate your cooperation in helping us keep incidences of illness to a minimum.

FIGURE 9–3 Sample letter to parents indicating their child has possibly been exposed to a communicable disease.

and staff member be familiar with these policies so that enforcement is consistent.

Immunization

Immunization offers permanent protection against many of the preventable
childhood communicable diseases, including diphtheria, tetanus, whooping
cough, polio, measles, mumps, and rubella. However, during the late 1970s,
immunization levels of children under 15 years of age dropped to an all-time low.
In response to this serious decline, massive public education programs, passage
of stricter school immunization requirements and the concerted efforts of federal,
state and local health authorities successfully turned this trend around. Current
figures estimate that 90 percent of school-aged children are immunized against
all preventable childhood diseases (Paskert 1983). However, this rate may not be
as high for infants and preschool children.

Why are some parents so seemingly unconcerned about obtaining immunizations for their children? Perhaps they do not realize how life threatening some
communicable illnesses really are. Others may believe these diseases have been
totally eliminated and are no longer something to worry about. Also, the conve-
nience of modern medicines and techniques has led to a more relaxed attitude
toward serious infections and diseases in general.

Immunization against all preventable childhood diseases is currently required
for school entry in all 50 states and the District of Columbia (Center for Disease
Control 1980). In states where no preschool immunization laws exist, individual
teachers and child care providers can encourage full immunization of every child
according to the recommended standards by establishing strict requirements for
children entering their programs. At the same time, they should continue as a
group to support legislation establishing requirements at the state level.

Vaccines cause children to become immune (no longer susceptible) to invasion by a specific infectious organism. Protective substances called antibodies
are formed by the body in response to the introduction of a specific infectious
organism either in a vaccine or during an episode of the actual illness.

Most babies are born with some immunity, transferred to them from their
mothers, to many communicable diseases. However, the temporary nature of this
immunity makes it very important to begin the immunization process early in a
baby's life. The following immunization schedule is generally recommended by
the American Academy of Pediatrics:

Child's Age	Immunization
2 months	Diphtheria, pertussis, tetanus (DPT) and trivalent oral polio vaccine (TOPV)
4 months	DPT and TOPV
6 months	DPT and TOPV* (*optional dose)
15 months	Measles, mumps, and rubella (MMR)
18 months	DPT and TOPV

4–6 years	DPT and TOPV
12–14 years	DT (diphtheria and tetanus)
Every 8–10 years thereafter	DT

Immunization can be obtained from the child's own physician, the neighborhood immunization clinic, or the local health department. Often there is no charge for immunization at the local health department.

Environmental Control

Modifications made in preschool classrooms or child care environments can have a positive influence on the control of communicable illnesses. Room temperatures, for example, can be adjusted to 68°–72°F. This range of temperatures is less favorable for the spread of contagious illnesses and is also more comfortable for young children. Children's smaller body surfaces make them less sensitive than adults to cooler temperatures.

Rooms occupied by infants and young children should also be well ventilated. Circulating fresh air helps to reduce the concentration of infectious organisms within a given area. Large child care facilities should be equipped with a mechanical ventilating system that is in good operating condition. Fresh air can also be introduced through open doors and windows whenever possible. Screens should cover any open doors or windows to prevent disease-carrying flies and mosquitoes from entering.

The humidity level in rooms should also be checked periodically. This practice is especially important in the winter when rooms must be heated and there are fewer opportunities to let in fresh air. Extremely warm, dry air increases the chances of respiratory infection. Moisture can be added to the air by means of a humidifier built into the central heating system. An alternative method is to run a warm- or cool-mist vaporizer in individual rooms. The cool-mist unit is preferable for use in areas where there are young children because it eliminates the possibility of burns. These units should be emptied, washed out with soap and water and refilled with fresh water each week. Plants or small dishes of water placed around a room will also provide increased humidity.

The physical arrangement of a classroom and grouping of children within it are also effective methods for controlling communicable illness, Figure 9–4. The main objective of these measures is to limit the amount of close contact among children and adults. It is unrealistic and undesirable to try and eliminate all physical contact between children and adults. However, there are some steps that can be taken without destroying this important form of communication for young children.

Crowding at tables or in play areas can be avoided by dividing older children into smaller groups. The use of round tables is preferable because it allows for greater distances between children than do square or rectangular tables. During naptimes, children's rugs or cots can be arranged in alternating directions, head to foot, to prevent them from talking, coughing and breathing in each other's

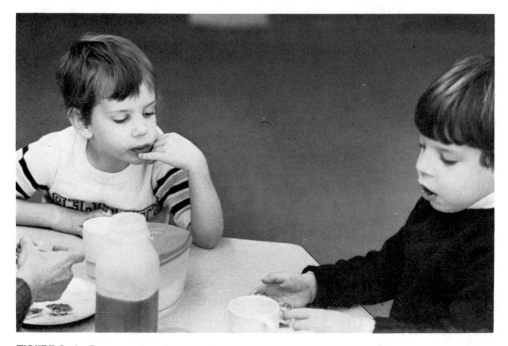

FIGURE 9–4   Room arrangement and grouping of children in order to limit close contact helps to control the spread of communicable illnesses.

faces. Provisions should also be made for children to have individual lockers or cubbys for storage of personal items, such as blankets, coats, hats, toys, toothbrushes and combs.

Precautions for controlling communicable illness are especially important to observe when infants and toddlers are being cared for. Strict sanitary procedures must be followed by all personnel. Play equipment, cribs, mats, and strollers should be wiped off at least twice weekly with a solution of one-fourth cup of chlorine bleach mixed with one gallon of water. Changing tables, toys that infants put in their mouths and eating surfaces should be washed daily.

Careful handwashing is also a special concern with infants and toddlers who are crawling and eating with their hands. Washcloths moistened with soap and water or washing children's hands under running water are the methods of choice. Teachers and care providers must also practice good handwashing technique, Table 9–1. This is especially important before feeding children and after diaper changing.

Education

Preschool teachers and child care providers make a valuable contribution to the control of communicable illness through education. Continuous instruction on subjects such as personal health habits, exercise, and nutrition can be a key

TABLE 9-1 Handwashing Technique

Correct handwashing procedures require only a very short time to be carried out by staff and children.
- Rinse hands under warm, running water.
- Lather hands with soap to loosen and suspend dirt and bacteria.
- Rub hands together vigorously. Friction helps to remove microorganisms and dirt (young children may need help with this step).
- Pay special attention to rubbing soap and water between the fingers and around the nails.
- Rinse off all dirt and soap under running water. Keep hands lower than the elbows to prevent dirty water from running up the arms.
- Dry well with paper towel. Dispose of the paper towel properly after using.
- Keep fingernails short and clean.

factor in improving children's resistance to infectious organisms and shortening the length of convalescence. Topics of special value for young children include:

- appropriate technique and times for handwashing
- proper way for covering coughs and blowing noses
- sanitary use of drinking fountains
- not sharing personal items, e.g., drinking cups, toothbrushes, shoes, hats, towels, eating utensils
- dressing appropriately for the weather
- good nutrition
- the need for rest and exercise

Periodic outbreaks of contagious illness in a group setting provide excellent opportunities for preschool teachers and care providers to review preventive health concepts and practices with children. Learning is more meaningful for young children when a friend or classmate has chickenpox or pink eye. Teachers can also reinforce learning by demonstrating good health practices themselves; children will often imitate teachers' behaviors.

Parents must be included in any educational program that hopes to reduce the incidence of communicable illness. Families should be kept informed of special health practices and problems that are being taught to the children. Preschool teachers and care providers can reinforce the importance of (1) serving nutritious meals and snacks, (2) making sure that children get sufficient rest and exercise, (3) obtaining immunizations for infants and young children, and (4) routine medical and dental supervision. Teachers and parents must work together to control the spread of communicable illness and promote children's health.

COMMON COMMUNICABLE ILLNESSES

Effective control and protection of other children in the classroom requires that preschool teachers and child care providers have a general knowledge and understanding of communicable illnesses. Table 9-2 presents brief descriptions of some of the communicable illnesses common among young children.

TABLE 9-2 Common Communicable Illnesses

COMMUNICABLE ILLNESS	SIGNS AND SYMPTOMS	INFECTIOUS AGENT	METHODS OF SPREAD	INCUBATION PERIOD	LENGTH OF COMMUNICABILITY	CONTROL MEASURES
Chickenpox	Slight fever, irritability, coldlike symptoms. Red rash with blisterlike head, scabs later. Most abundant on covered parts of body, e.g., chest, back, neck, forearm.	Virus	Person to person; through direct contact with secretions from the respiratory tract. Transmission from contact with blisters less common.	2–3 weeks after exposure.	2–3 days prior to the onset of symptoms until 5–6 days after first eruptions. Scabs are not contagious.	Specific control measures: (1) Exclusion of sick children (2) Practice good personal hygiene, especially careful handwashing. Children can return to group care in approximately one week following the onset of last eruptions or when all blisters have formed a dry scab.
Cold Sores (Fever blisters)	Clear blisters usually on face and lips which crust and heal within a few days.	Virus	Direct contact with saliva of infected persons	Up to 2 weeks	Virus remains in saliva for as long as 7 weeks following recovery.	No specific control. Good personal hygiene. Child does not have to be excluded from school.
Conjunctivitis (Pinkeye)	Swelling and redness of the white portion (conjunctiva) of the eye, swelling of the lids, and a yellow discharge from eyes.	Bacteria	Contact with discharge from eyes or upper respiratory tract of an infected person; through contaminated fingers.	1–3 days	Throughout active infection; several days up to 2–3 weeks.	Antibiotic treatment. Exclude child from school until eyes have been treated and there is no longer any discharge. Strict personal hygiene and careful handwashing.

Disease	Cause	Description/Symptoms	Mode of Transmission	Incubation Period	Period of Communicability	Prevention
Common Cold	Virus	Highly contagious infection of the upper respiratory tract accompanied by slight fever, chills, runny nose, fatigue and muscle aches. Onset may be sudden.	Person to person through direct contact with secretions from the respiratory tract, e.g., coughs, sneezes, eating utensils, etc.	12–72 hours	About 1 day before onset of symptoms to 2–3 days after acute illness.	Prevention through education and good personal hygiene. Avoid exposure.
Dysentery	Bacteria	Sudden onset of vomiting; diarrhea; may be accompanied by high fever, headache, abdominal pain. Stools may contain blood, pus or mucus. Can be fatal in young children.	Fecal-oral transmission. Direct contact with contaminated objects or indirectly through ingestion of contaminated food or water.	1–7 days	Variable; may last up to 4 weeks or longer in the carrier state.	Careful handwashing after bowel movements. Proper disposal of human feces; control of flies. Strict adherence to strict sanitary procedures for food preparation.
Encephalitis	Virus	Sudden onset of headache, high fever, convulsions, vomiting, confusion, neck and back stiffness, tremors and coma.	Spread by bites from disease-carrying mosquitoes; in some areas transmitted by tick bites.	5–15 days	Man is not contagious.	Spraying of mosquito breeding areas and use of insect repellents; public education.
Giardiasis	Parasite (protozoa)	An intestinal parasite infection of the small bowel. Many persons are asymptomatic. Typical symptoms include chronic diarrhea, abdominal cramping, bloating, pale and foul-smelling stools, weight loss and fatigue.	Person to person (fecal to oral route) through direct contact with infected stool (e.g., diaper changes, helping child with soiled underwear; poor handwashing, passed from hands to mouth (toys, food). Also transmitted through contaminated water sources.	1–4 days	As long as parasite is present in the stool.	Infected persons must be treated with medication. Scrupulous handwashing before eating, preparing food, and after using the bathroom. Good sanitary conditions maintained in bathroom areas.

TABLE 9-2   Common Communicable Illnesses (Continued)

COMMUNICABLE ILLNESS	SIGNS AND SYMPTOMS	INFECTIOUS AGENT	METHODS OF SPREAD	INCUBATION PERIOD	LENGTH OF COMMUNICABILITY	CONTROL MEASURES
Hepatitis (Infectious; Type A)	Fever, fatigue, loss of appetite, nausea, abdominal pain (in region of liver). Illness may be accompanied by yellowing of the skin and eyeballs (jaundice) in adults, but not always in children.	Virus	Fecal-oral route; person to person. Spread via contaminated food, milk and water.	10–50 days (average range 30–35 days)	Several days prior to onset of symptoms to not more than 7 days after onset of jaundice.	Exclude from group settings a minimum of 2 weeks following onset. Special attention to careful handwashing after going to bathroom and before eating is critical following an outbreak. Report disease incidences to public health authorities.
Impetigo	Infection of the skin forming crusty, moist lesions usually on the face, ears, and around the nose. Highly contagious. Common among children.	Bacterial	Person to person. Direct contact with discharge from sores; indirect contact with contaminated articles of clothing, tissues, etc.	2–5 days; may be as long as 10 days	Until lesions are healed.	Exclusion from group settings until lesions have been treated with antibiotics for 48–72 hours.
Lice (head)	Lice are seldom visible to the naked eye. White nits (eggs) may be apparent on hair shafts. The most obvious symptom is itching of the scalp, especially behind ears and at the base of the neck.	Head louse	Direct contact with infected persons or with their personal articles, e.g., hats, hair brushes, combs or clothing. Lice can survive for 2–3 weeks on bedding, carpet, furniture, car seats, clothing, etc.	Nits hatch in 1 week and reach maturity within 2 weeks	While lice remain alive on infested persons or clothing; until nits have been destroyed.	Infested children should be excluded from group settings until treated. Nits should first be removed with a fine-tooth comb. Hair should then be washed with a special medicated shampoo. Heat from a hair dryer also helps destroy the eggs. All friends and

Disease	Cause	Symptoms	Transmission	Incubation Period	Period of Communicability	Control
						family members should be carefully checked. The child's environment should be cleaned thoroughly; bedding, clothing, and hair brushes should be washed or dry-cleaned.
Measles (Rubeola)	Virus	Fever, cough, runny nose, eyes sensitive to light. Dark red blotchy rash that often begins on the face and neck then spreads over the entire body. Highly communicable.	Person to person through coughs, sneezes and contact with contaminated articles.	8–13 days; rash develops approximately 14 days after exposure	From beginning of symptoms until 4 days after rash appears.	Most effective control method is immunization. Good personal hygiene, especially handwashing and covering coughs. Exclude child for at least 5 days after rash appears.
Mononucleosis	Virus	Characteristic symptoms include sore throat, intermittent fever, fatigue and enlarged lymph glands in the neck. May also be accompanied by headache and enlarged liver or spleen.	Person to person; often by direct contact with the mouth of an infected person.	10–14 days for children; 30–50 days for adults	Unknown. Organisms may be present in oral secretions for as long as one year following illness.	None known. Child should be kept home until over the acute phase (6–10 days).
Mumps	Virus	Sudden onset of fever with swelling of the salivary glands.	Person to person through coughs and sneezes; direct contact with oral secretions of infected persons.	12–26 days	4–6 days prior to the onset of symptoms until swelling in the salivary glands is gone (7–9 days).	Immunization provides permanent protection. Peak incidence is in winter and spring. Exclude children from school or group settings until all symptoms have disappeared.

TABLE 9-2   Common Communicable Illnesses (Continued)

COMMUNICABLE ILLNESS	SIGNS AND SYMPTOMS	INFECTIOUS AGENT	METHODS OF SPREAD	INCUBATION PERIOD	LENGTH OF COMMUNICABILITY	CONTROL MEASURES
Pinworms	Irritability, and itching of the rectal area. Common among young children.	Parasite; not contagious from animals	Infectious eggs are transferred from person to person by contaminated hands (oral-fecal route). Indirectly spread by contaminated bedding, food, clothing, swimming pool.	Life cycle of the worm is 3–6 weeks; persons can also re-infect themselves	2–8 weeks or as long as a source of infection remains present.	Infected children must be excluded from school until treated with medication; may return after initial dose. All infected and noninfected members of a family must be treated at one time. Frequent handwashing is essential; discourage nail biting or sucking on fingers. Daily baths and change of linen are necessary. Disinfect school toilet seats at least once a day. Vacuum carpeted areas daily. Eggs are also destroyed when exposed to temperatures over 132°F. Education and good personal hygiene are vital to control.
Ringworm	A disease of the scalp, skin or nails. Causes flat, spreading, oval-shaped lesions that may become dry	Fungus	Direct or indirect contact with infected persons, their personal items, showers, swimming pools, theater seats, etc. Dogs and cats may also be infected	1–4 days (unknown for athlete's foot)	As long as lesions are present.	Exclude children from gyms, pools or activities where they are likely to expose others. May return to group care following medical treatment with a fungicidal

Disease	Signs and Symptoms	Cause	Transmission	Incubation	Communicability	Control
	and scaly or moist and crusted. When it is present on the feet it is commonly called athlete's foot. Infected nails may become discolored, brittle, or chalky or they may disintegrate.		and transmit it to children or adults.			ointment. All shared areas such as pools and showers should be thoroughly cleansed with a fungicide.
Rocky Mountain Spotted Fever	Onset usually abrupt; fever (101°–104°F); joint and muscle pain, severe nausea and vomiting, and white coating on tongue. Rash appears on 2nd to 5th day over forehead, wrist and ankles; later covers entire body. Can be fatal if untreated.	Bacteria	Tick bite.	2–14 days; average 7 days	Not contagious from person to person.	Prompt removal of ticks. Administration of antibiotics. Use insect repellent on clothes when outdoors.
Roseola Infantum (6 months to 3 years).	Most common in the spring and fall. Fever rises abruptly (102°–105°F) and lasts 3–4 days; loss of appetite, listlessness, development of rash on trunk, arms and neck lasting 1–2 days.	Virus	Unknown	10–15 days	1–2 days before onset to several days following fading of the rash.	Exclude from school or group care during the acute phase.
Rubella (German Measles)	Mild fever; rash begins on face and neck and rarely lasts more than 3 days. May have arthritislike discomfort and swelling in joints.	Virus	Person to person through direct contact with respiratory secretions, e.g., coughs, sneezes.	14–21 days	From one week prior to 5 days following onset of the rash.	Immunization offers permanent protection. Children must be excluded from school for at least 5 days.

TABLE 9-2 Common Communicable Illnesses (Continued)

COMMUNICABLE ILLNESS	SIGNS AND SYMPTOMS	INFECTIOUS AGENT	METHODS OF SPREAD	INCUBATION PERIOD	LENGTH OF COMMUNICABILITY	CONTROL MEASURES
Scabies	Characteristic burrows or linear tunnels under the skin, especially between the fingers and around the wrists, elbows, waist, thighs and buttocks. Causes intense itching.	Parasite	Direct contact with an infected person.	Several days to 2-3 weeks	Until all mites and eggs are destroyed.	Children should be excluded from school or group care until treated. Affected persons should bathe with prescribed soap and carefully launder all bedding and clothing. All contacts of the infected person should be notified.
Streptococcal Infections (strep throat, fever, scarlatina, rheumatic fever).	High fever accompanied by sore, red throat; may also have nausea, vomiting, headache, and enlarged glands. Development of a rash depends on the infectious organism.	Bacteria	Person to person; direct contact through inhalation of respiratory secretions, e.g., coughs, sneezes. May also be transmitted by food and raw milk.	1-4 days	Throughout the illness and for approximately 10 days afterward unless treated with antibiotics. Medical treatment eliminates communicability within 36 hours. Child may become a carrier if not treated.	Antibiotic treatment is essential. Avoid crowding in classrooms. Practice frequent handwashing, educating children, and careful supervision of food handlers.
Tetanus	Muscular spasms and stiffness, especially in the muscles around the neck and mouth. Can lead to convulsions, inability to breathe, and death.	Bacteria	Organisms enter the body through wounds, especially puncture-type injuries, burns and unnoticed cuts.	4 days to 2 weeks	Not contagious	Immunization every 8-10 years affords complete protection.

SUMMARY

Often preschool teachers and child care providers must contend with outbreaks of communicable illness in their settings. Close contact with others, immature physiological development, and habits typical of particular age groups help to explain the frequency of illness among young children.

A communicable illness is one that is spread or transmitted from one person or animal to another. The infectious process requires the availability of a pathogen, a susceptible host, and a method for transmission. The absence of any one factor will interrupt this process and prevent infection from occurring. An infant or young child who is in good health is more resistant to communicable illness. Most contagious illnesses progress through an incubation, prodromal, acute, and convalescence stage.

Control and management of communicable illness in group settings requires that teachers and child care providers possess some knowledge and understanding of these illnesses. Control measures that preschool teachers and child care providers can implement in their settings include observations, setting policies and guidelines, requiring immunizations, controlling the environment, education, and cooperating with parents.

LEARNING ACTIVITIES

1. Obtain several agar growth medium plates. With sterile cotton applicators, culture one toy and the top of one table in a preschool classroom or child care center. Observe the "growth" after 24 hours and again after 48 hours. Wash the same items with a mild chlorine solution and repeat the experiment. Compare the results.

2. Prepare a memo notifying parents that their child has been exposed to rubella. Be sure to include early symptoms to observe for, the approximate dates when children would be most likely to develop the disease (incubation period), and the name and phone number of a person they can contact to answer questions.

3. Write to the Office of Public Health in your state. Request information on the immunization requirements for preschool children attending child care programs. If possible, obtain data on the percentage of children under 6 years of age that are immunized in your state.

4. Review your own immunization records. Obtain any immunizations necessary to bring it up to date.

UNIT REVIEW

A. Define the following terms.

1. pathogen

2. contagious

3. susceptible

4. incubation period

5. immunity

6. convalescence

7. antibodies

8. communicable illness

B. Match the signs/symptoms in column I with the correct communicable illness in column II.

Column I

1. swelling and redness of white portion of the eye
2. frequent itching of the scalp
3. flat, oval-shaped lesions on the scalp, skin; infected nails become discolored, brittle, chalky, or they may disintegrate
4. high fever; red, sore throat
5. mild fever and rash that lasts approximately three days
6. irritability and itching of the rectal area
7. red rash with blisterlike heads; coldlike symptoms
8. sudden onset of fever; swelling of salivary glands
9. burrows or linear tunnels under the skin; intense itching
10. vomiting, abdominal pain, diarrhea which may be bloody

Column II

a. chickenpox
b. strep throat
c. lice
d. dysentery
e. conjunctivitis
f. ringworm
g. German measles
h. scabies
i. pinworms
j. mumps

C. Briefly answer the following questions.

1. Describe how an illness can be spread by:
   a. direct contact
   b. indirect contact

2. What are some probable causes for the apathy regarding immunization of infants and young children?

3. Where can parents obtain immunizations for their children?

4. Children are contagious during what stages of most communicable diseases?

5. What three factors must be present for an infection to be communicable?

6. Name three early signs of communicable illness that can be observed in young children?

7. Name four control measures that child care facilities can implement to reduce communicable illnesses.

D. Case Study

The teacher has noticed that Kati seems quite restless today and is having difficulty concentrating on any task she starts. She is continuously squirming whether in a chair or sitting on the floor. On a number of occasions throughout the morning, the teacher has observed Kati scratching her bottom.

1. What type of problem might the teacher suspect Kati is having?

2. What control measures should be taken?

3. When can she return to school?

4. For what length of time after an outbreak must the teacher watch for the development of similar problems in other children?

5. What special personal health measures should be emphasized to the other children?

REFERENCES

Center for Disease Control. "Immunization Against Disease 1980." *CDC Monograph,* September 1980.

Highberger, Ruth, and Boynton, Mary. "Preventing Illness In Infant/Toddler Day Care." *Young Children* 38(3), March 1983.

Paskert, Catherine J. "Progress and Focus of the National Childhood Immunization Campaign." *Journal of School Health* 53(6):357–59, August 1983.

Pringle, Sheila, and Ramsey, Brenda. *Promoting the Health of Children.* St. Louis: C. V. Mosby Co., 1982.

Additional Reading

"Childhood Immunization Initiative, U.S. Five Year Follow-up." *Morbidity and Mortality Weekly Report* 31(17):231–32. Atlanta, GA: Center for Disease

Control, May 7, 1982.

"Educators, Health Officials Study Immunization Law Compliance." *Report on Preschool Education,* December 30, 1980.

Hickson, M., and Hinman, A. "A Shot At Success." *Journal of School Health* 51(10):678, 1981.

Mortimer, E. A. "Immunization Against Infectious Disease." *Science,* 200(4344):902–7, May 26, 1978.

O'Brien, M.; Porterfield, J.; Herbert-Jackson, E.; and Risley, T. *The Toddler Center.* Baltimore: University Park Press, 1979.

Pomeranz, Virginia. "Your Child Has Been Exposed (Head Lice, Scabies, Pinworms)." *Parents* 58(3):94, March 1983.

MANAGEMENT OF
ACUTE ILLNESS

Terms to Know

dehydration	*temperature*
listlessness	*fever*
anemia	*disorientation*
hyperventilation	*urinate*
intestinal	*infection*
salmonellosis	*abdomen*
symptom	*Reye's syndrome*

Objectives

After studying this unit, you will be able to:
- *Identify the signs and symptoms of four common illnesses.*
- *Check axillary and oral temperatures with a thermometer.*
- *Describe actions to be taken when a child in a group setting shows signs of illness.*

Children, especially those under three years of age, are very susceptible to illness and infection. Group settings such as preschools, child care centers and elementary schools encourage the rapid transfer of illness among children and adults. Every attempt must be made to establish policies and practices that will protect young children from unnecessary exposure.

IDENTIFYING SICK CHILDREN

Every care provider should know how to identify sick children, Figure 10–1. By learning to recognize the early signs of common illnesses, preschool teachers and child care providers can exclude sick children from group settings. They can also take advantage of these opportunities to promote children's wellness by including educational experiences that teach and strengthen principles of good health.

Guidelines for identifying the early signs of illness help teachers, child care providers and parents work together to control the spread of disease. The following signs and *symptoms* can be incorporated into a center's exclusion policy and serve to determine whether a child should remain in a group care setting or be sent home:

- an oral *temperature* over 99.4°F (37.4°C) or
  axillary temperature over 98°F (36.7°C)
- an upset stomach or vomiting within the past 24 hours
- any intestinal disturbance with diarrhea
- unexplained fatigue, irritability, or loss of appetite
- any undiagnosed rash
- any discharge or drainage from eyes, nose, ears or open sores
- signs of a newly developing cold or severe coughing.

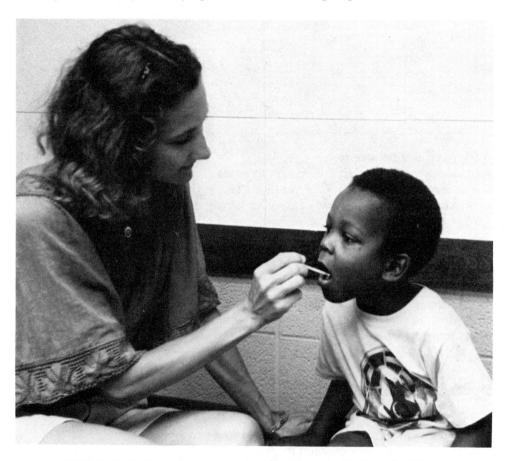

FIGURE 10-1   Every care provider should know how to identify sick children.

Not all of children's acute illnesses are contagious. Persons who work with young children must be able to distinguish conditions that are contagious from those that are limited to an individual child. This information is extremely useful for developing and implementing procedures, such as handwashing, that help limit the spread of illness.

Serious complications can often be avoided if an illness is identified in the early stages. However, teachers and child care providers should never attempt to diagnose children's health problems. Their main responsibility is only to make children comfortable until parents arrive and then to advise the family to contact their physician.

COMMON ILLNESSES

The remaining portions of this unit are devoted to discussions of several illnesses and health complaints commonly experienced by young children.

Colds

Colds are a common ailment of young children (Feinbloom 1978); they may experience as many as three to six colds during a year. Colds are caused by a viral *infection* of the nose and throat. Antibiotics are not effective against most viruses and are of limited value for treating simple colds. However, antibiotics may be prescribed to treat complications or secondary infections that develop.

Teachers and child care providers can recognize the early symptoms of a cold by carefully observing children for:

- a runny nose
- sneezing
- congestion
- "glassy" or watery eyes
- *fever*
- coughing
- a red or sore throat
- red and enlarged tonsils
- white spots on tonsils or throat
- *listlessness,* Figure 10–2

Because colds are highly contagious during the first two or three days, children should be kept home and away from group care settings. Treatment, including bedrest, increased intake of liquids (water, fruit juices, soups), and nonaspirin fever-reducing medication can be provided by the child's parents and is usually adequate for most colds.

Although colds themselves are not serious, complications can sometimes develop. Toddlers and preschool-aged children are often more susceptible to complications such as earaches, bronchitis, croup and pneumonia. Parents can

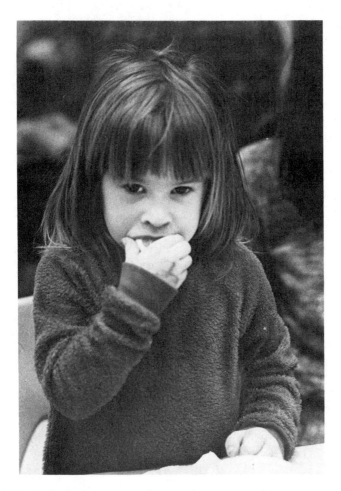

FIGURE 10-2 Listlessness may be an early indication of an oncoming cold.

be cautioned to watch children closely and contact their physician if any complications develop or the child does not improve within four to five days. Parents should also be advised to seek immediate medical attention for children observed to have white spots on their throats or tonsils in order to rule out the possibility of strep throat.

Diaper Rash

Diaper rash is an irritation of the skin in and around the buttocks and genital area. It is caused by prolonged contact with ammonia in urine and organic acids in diarrheal stools. Severe burning leads to affected patches of skin that appear reddened and may be covered with tiny pimples. Diaper rash occurs more often in formula-fed infants than in breast-fed infants (Pringle 1982). Reactions to fabric softeners, soaps, lotions, powders and disposable diapers can also cause diaper rash in infants with sensitive skin.

Prompt changing of wet and soiled diapers followed by a thorough cleansing of the skin is often sufficient prevention and treatment of diaper rash. A thin layer of zinc oxide ointment can also be applied to help protect irritated areas. Allowing the infant to go without diapers and exposing irritated skin to the air also speeds the healing process. Plastic pants and disposable diapers with a plastic outer layer should be avoided because they tend to hold in moisture.

Diarrhea

The term diarrhea refers to frequent watery or very soft bowel movements. They may be foul-smelling and also contain small particles of blood or mucus. Some causes of diarrhea in children include:

- viral, bacterial or parasite infections
- antibiotic therapy
- recent dietary changes
- food allergies
- food poisoning
- illnesses, such as earaches, colds, strep throat or cystic fibrosis

Frequent or prolonged diarrhea can result in *dehydration,* especially in infants and toddlers. Dehydration involves a loss of body water and can occur quickly in young children because of their small body size. Excessive dehydration can be fatal (Chow 1979). For this reason, it is critical that care providers keep exact count of the number and size of bowel movements. It is also important to observe bowel movements for color, consistency, and whether blood, mucus, or pus is present. Medical advice should be sought immediately if diarrhea is severe or the child becomes lethargic or drowsy.

Children who have experienced diarrhea within the past 24 hours should be kept home from preschool or child care settings. Exceptions to this policy would include children whose diarrhea resulted from noncontagious conditions such as food allergies, changes in diet, or recent treatment with antibiotics. However, even these children may not feel well enough to attend school or group care and participate in activities. There is also the problem and inconvenience of frequent accidental soiling.

Most cases of diarrhea can be treated simply by placing the child on a clear liquid diet for a period of 24 hours. Clear broths or soups, flavored gelatin, noncitrus juices, ginger ale, 7-Up, or water can be offered in small amounts. Other liquids and soft foods can gradually be added to the diet. Any complaint of pain that is continuous or located in the lower right side of the *abdomen* should be reported to the child's parents. Parents should, in turn, contact the child's physician.

Dizziness

Occasionally, young children will complain of feeling dizzy, usually after vigorous activity or play. The sensation of spinning or unsteadiness usually lasts only a few seconds. However, repeated complaints of dizziness should be noted and reported to the child's parents. The parents should be advised to contact their physician. Dizziness can be a symptom of other health conditions including:

- ear infections
- fever
- headaches
- head injuries
- *anemia*
- nasal congestion and sinus infections
- brain tumor (rare)

If dizziness is accompanied by any loss of balance or coordination, the child's parents should contact a physician immediately.

Most episodes of dizziness can be treated by having the child lie down or sit in a chair with the child's head resting on or between the knees. The child should be encouraged to remain quiet for a short time after the dizziness has passed. Parents need to be alerted so they can continue to observe the child at home.

Dizziness that occurs because of some underlying health problem will usually not respond to temporary first aid measures. Medical treatment of the problem is necessary before dizziness will disappear entirely.

Earache

Earaches and ear infections occur more frequently during the toddler and preschool years. As children grow older, structures in the nose, ear and throat mature and resistance to infection (antibody formation) increases. As a result, fewer ear infections occur.

Earaches frequently accompany colds and the congestion of allergies. Passageways located between the ear and the nose swell and can lead to a buildup of fluid in the middle ear. This condition is known as otitis media. It is often accompanied by pain and temporary hearing loss (Denk-Glass 1982). Other possible causes of earache can include dental cavities, excess wax, or foreign objects such as stones, pieces of a toy, or food that have been pushed into the ear canal.

Not all children recognize or complain of discomfort due to earaches. This is especially true of children who are too young to talk. Teachers and child care providers can observe children for other signs that may indicate an ear infection, including:

- tugging or rubbing of the affected ear, Figure 10–3.
- refusal to eat or swallow
- redness of the outer ear
- fever
- dizziness

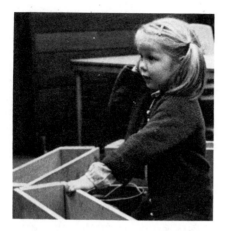

FIGURE 10-3 Tugging on the affected ear may be a sign of earache.

- discharge from the ear canal
- difficulty hearing

Any complaint of ear pain or earache should be checked by the child's physician. Most ear infections must be treated with antibiotics to prevent further complications from developing. Temporary relief from pain can be achieved by having the child rest the affected ear on a warm water bag or blanket while lying down. Care must be used so the child is not accidently burned. Placing a small, dry cotton ball in the opening of the outer ear will sometimes help to lessen the pain of an earache by blocking contact with the air. Excess wax and foreign objects should only be removed by a physician.

Fainting

Fainting, a momentary loss of consciousness, occurs when the blood supply to the brain is temporarily reduced. Possible causes for this condition in young children include:

- anemia
- breathholding
- *hyperventilation*
- extreme excitement or hysteria
- drug reactions
- illness or infection
- poisoning

Initially, children may complain of feeling dizzy or weak. Very quickly the skin becomes pale, cool, and moist, and the child may collapse. Injuries can be avoided by gently lowering the child to the floor.

Immediate care of a child who faints involves lying the child down, and elevating the legs 8 to 10 inches on a pillow. A light blanket can be placed over the child for extra warmth. Breathing is made easier if clothing is loosened from around the neck and waist. No attempt should be made to give the child anything to eat or drink until consciousness is regained. When the child is awake and resting quietly, parents should be notified and encouraged to consult their physician.

Fever

Activity, age, eating, sleeping and the time of day can cause normal fluctuations in children's temperatures. However, an elevated temperature is usually an indication of illness or infection, especially if the child complains of other discomforts such as headache, coughing, nausea or sore throat. Teachers and child care providers may first notice a child's fever by observing:

- flushed or reddened face
- listlessness or desire to sleep
- skin that is warm to the touch
- "glassy" eyes
- loss of appetite
- complaints of not feeling well
- increased perspiration

A child's temperature should be checked if there is any reason to believe that a fever might be present, Table 10–1. Only the oral and axillary methods are recommended for use by teachers and child care providers; only the axillary method should be used with infants. Plastic strip thermometers are not recommended because their readings are not always reliable or accurate. The American Medical Association considers these thermometers "unacceptable substitutes for the standard glass thermometers" (Lewit 1982). Children with an oral temperature over 99.4°F (37.4°C) or axillary temperature over 98°F (36.7°C) should be sent home where they can be monitored and observed by parents. The thermometer should be carefully cleaned after each use, Table 10–2.

Work schedules or prior commitments sometimes make it difficult for parents to come immediately and take a sick child home. When these situations arise, there are measures teachers or care providers can take to make a feverish child more comfortable. The child should be removed from a group setting. If no special sick room is available, the child can be placed in a crib or on a cot in a quiet corner of the room. Other children should be kept away. Cool room temperatures, removing warm clothing and giving extra fluids to drink will help make the child feel more comfortable. Sponging the child with cool water will also help lower a high temperature.

TABLE 10-1   How to Take a Child's Temperature

Oral Method
1. Rinse the thermometer under running water if it has been stored in a chemical solution.
2. Carefully inspect the thermometer for any broken edges, especially around the mercury bulb.
3. Shake the mercury down to the lowest point.
4. Place the thermometer (mercury bulb end) in the child's mouth and under the tongue. Caution children not to bite down on the thermometer, but only to close their lips tightly around it. Continue to hold onto the thermometer as long as it is in the child's mouth. Leave in place 3 minutes.
5. Remove the thermometer. Wipe with a clean tissue. Hold it at eye level and rotate it gently until the mercury level can be read. Normal oral temperature is 98°F–99.4°F (36.7°C–37.4°C).
6. Clean the thermometer thoroughly after each use.

Axillary Method
1. Rinse the thermometer under running water if it has been stored in a chemical solution.
2. Carefully inspect the thermometer for any broken or sharp edges, especially around the bulb.
3. Shake the thermometer down until the mercury is at the lowest point.
4. Place the thermometer against the child's skin under the armpit. Bring the child's arm down and press it gently against the side of the body.
5. Hold the thermometer in place for 5 minutes.
6. Remove and read. Normal axillary temperature is 97°F–98°F (36.1°C–36.7°C).
7. Clean the thermometer thoroughly after each use.

TABLE 10-2   How to Clean a Thermometer

---

1. Wash the thermometer with a soapy cotton ball.
2. Rinse under cool, running water (hot water may cause the thermometer to break).
3. Dry thoroughly.
4. Soak thermometer in an antiseptic solution (isopropyl or rubbing alcohol) for at least 20 minutes.
5. Rinse under running water and store in a clean container.

Headaches

Headaches are not a common complaint of young children. When they do occur, it is usually as a symptom or indication of some other condition, such as:

- bacterial or viral infections
- allergies
- head injuries
- emotional tension or stress
- reaction to medication
- lead poisoning
- hunger
- eye strain

- brain tumor (rare)
- constipation
- carbon monoxide poisoning

In the absence of any fever, rash, vomiting or *disorientation,* children can remain at school and continue to be observed. Frequently, their headaches will disappear with rest and interest in a new activity. Patterns of repeated or intense headaches should be noted and parents encouraged to discuss the problem with the child's physician.

Heat Rash

Heat rash is characterized by fine, red, raised bumps. Generally, it is located around the neck, chest, waistline, cheeks and inner areas of the forearm. Heat rash is caused by a blockage of sweat glands and usually develops suddenly during hot weather or when children are dressed too warmly.

Heat rash is not contagious. However, there are several measures teachers and child care providers can take to make a child more comfortable. Affected areas can be washed with cool water, dried thoroughly and powdered sparingly with baby powder or talc. Overdressing should be avoided, both during summer and winter months. Parents should be encouraged to help children dress in clothing that is lightweight and made of nonsynthetic fabrics.

Sore Throat

Sore throats are a fairly common complaint among young children, especially during the fall and winter seasons. Most sore throats are caused by viral infections that are relatively harmless. Antibiotics are not effective against most viral infections and so are not usually prescribed.

A small percentage of sore throats are caused by streptococcal infection. A throat infection of this type is commonly called strep throat and is highly contagious. Characteristic signs and symptoms of strep throat include:

- sudden onset
- fever
- upset stomach; vomiting
- enlarged lymph glands
- intense redness of the tonsils and throat
- headache
- painful swallowing
- white or yellow patches on the throat or tonsils
- duration of more than three or four days

Children showing any of these signs or symptoms should be sent home and checked by a physician.

It is extremely important not to ignore a child's complaints of sore throat. Strep throat must be identified and treated with antibiotics. A routine throat culture performed by a nurse or doctor can safely determine whether or not a strep infection is present. Left untreated, strep throat can lead to serious complications such as rheumatic fever and rheumatic heart disease (Hamilton 1982).

Stomachaches

Most children experience stomachaches at one time or another. There are many causes for stomachaches in children:

- food allergies or intolerance
- appendicitis
- *intestinal* infections, e.g., parasites, Salmonella
- urinary tract infections
- gas or constipation
- side effect to medication, especially antibiotics
- change in diet
- emotional stress
- need for attention
- hunger
- diarrhea
- vomiting
- strep throat

There are a number of things teachers and child care providers can check to determine whether or not a child's stomach pain is serious. Is the pain continuous, or is it a cramping-type pain that comes and goes? Is there a fever? If no fever is present, the stomachache is probably not serious. Encourage the child to go to the bathroom and see if *urination* or having a bowel movement relieves the pain. Have the child rest quietly to see if the discomfort goes away. Check with the parents to see if the child is taking any medication. Stomach pain or stomachaches should be considered serious if they:

- disrupt a child's activity, e.g., running, playing, eating, sleeping
- cause tenderness of the abdomen
- are accompanied by diarrhea, vomiting or severe cramping
- last longer than 3 to 4 hours
- result in stools that are bloody or contain mucus

If any of these conditions occur while the child is attending preschool or a child care center, parents should be notified and advised to seek prompt medical attention for the child.

Toothache

Tooth decay is the most common cause of toothache. Children may complain of a throbbing pain that sometimes radiates into the ear. Redness and swelling can often be observed around the gumline of the affected tooth. Foods that are hot or very sweet may intensify pain. Similar tooth discomfort may be experienced by older children during the process of losing baby teeth and eruption of permanent teeth.

Toothaches should be checked promptly by the child's dentist. In the meantime, an icepack applied to the cheek on the affected side may make the child more comfortable. Aspirin or aspirin-free products can also be administered by the child's parents for pain relief. Proper brushing after eating will help to eliminate a significant amount of tooth decay, Figure 10–4.

Vomiting

Vomiting is usually a symptom of an illness or other health problem, such as:

- emotional upset
- viral or bacterial infection, e.g., stomach flu, strep throat
- *Reye's syndrome*
- ear infections
- meningitis
- *salmonellosis*

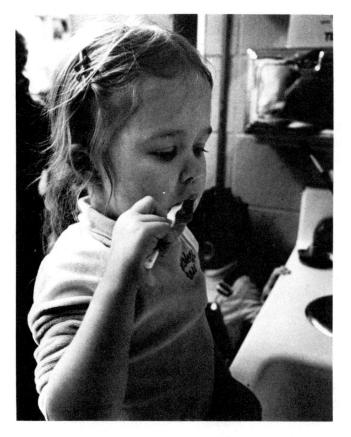

FIGURE 10–4 Brushing the teeth after eating helps to eliminate tooth decay.

- indigestion
- severe coughing
- drug reactions
- head injury
- poisoning

The exact number of times, amount, and composition of vomited material is very important to record. Dehydration and disturbance of the body's chemical balance can occur with prolonged or excessive vomiting. Children should also be observed carefully for:

- high fever
- abdominal pain
- signs of dehydration, e.g., sunken eyes, decreased urination, dryness of the lips and mouth, decreased thirst
- headache
- excessive drowsiness
- difficulty breathing
- sore throat
- exhaustion

Any child who continues to vomit and shows signs of a sore throat, fever or stomach pains should be sent home as soon as possible. The teacher or child care provider should also advise the child's parents to contact their physician for further advice.

In the absence of any other symptoms, a single episode of vomiting may simply be the result of emotional upset, dislike for a particular food, excess mucus, or a reaction to medication. Usually the child feels better immediately after vomiting. These children can remain at the school or child care center and be encouraged to rest until they feel better.

In addition to not feeling well, the act of vomiting itself may be very upsetting and frightening to the young child. Infants should be positioned on their stomachs with their hips and legs raised. This position allows vomited material to flow out of the mouth. Older children should also be watched very closely so they don't choke or inhale vomitus. Extra reassurance and comforting from teachers and child care providers can make the experience less traumatic.

SUMMARY

Illness is a common occurrence whenever groups of children spend time together. Teachers and child care providers must learn to recognize the early signs of illness and exclude sick children in order to protect the entire group.

Exclusion policies serve as guidelines for deciding when a child is too ill to be admitted to preschool or child care programs. Early recognition of noncontagious illnesses can help to avoid serious complications from developing later. Teachers and child care providers can carry out temporary measures to make sick children more comfortable until parents arrive to take them home.

LEARNING ACTIVITIES

1. With a partner, practice taking each other's axillary and oral temperatures. Follow steps for cleaning the thermometer between each use.

2. Divide the class into groups of five to six students. Discuss how each of you feel about caring for children who are ill. Could you hold or cuddle a child with a high fever or diarrhea? What are your feelings about being exposed to children's contagious illnesses? How might you react if an infant just vomited on your new sweater? If you feel uncomfortable around sick children, what steps can you take to better cope with the situation?

3. Select another student as a partner and observe that person carefully for 20 seconds. Write down everything you can remember about this person, such as eye color, hair color, scars or moles, approximate weight, height, color of skin, shape of teeth, clothing, etc. What can you do to improve your observational skills?

UNIT REVIEW

A. Select the best answer from the choices offered.

1. Earaches are often associated with
   a. allergies and stomachaches
   b. colds and allergies
   c. emotional upsets
   d. dizziness

2. Children should be sent home if their oral temperature is over
   a. 36.7°C
   b. 37°C
   c. 98.6°F
   d. 99.4°F

3. Heat rash
   a. can spread rapidly from one child to another
   b. does not usually respond to treatment
   c. is not contagious
   d. requires prompt medical attention

4. Strep throat
   a. can cause headache and vomiting
   b. usually disappears in a few days
   c. is not contagious
   d. is difficult to diagnose

5. Children's toothaches are frequently caused by
   a. pain that radiates from an earache
   b. gum disease
   c. tumors
   d. cavities and decay

B. Describe what you would do in each of the following situations:
1. You have just finished serving lunch to the children, when Mara begins to vomit.

2. The class is involved in a game of Keep-Away. Ted suddenly complains of feeling dizzy.

3. During check in, a parent mentions that his son has been experiencing stomachaches every morning before coming to school.

4. Leandra wakes up from her afternoon nap, crying because her ear hurts.

5. You have just changed a toddler's diaper for the third time in the last hour because of diarrhea.

6. Sami enters the classroom, sneezing and blowing his nose.

7. While you are helping Erin put on her coat to go outdoors, you notice that her skin feels very warm.

8. Richard refuses to eat his lunch because it makes his teeth hurt.

9. While you are cleaning up the blocks, Tommy tells you that his throat is sore and it hurts to swallow.

10. You have just taken Juanita's temperature (orally) and it is 101°F.

REFERENCES

Chow, M.; Durand, B.; Feldman, M.; and Mills, M. *Handbook of Pediatric Primary Care.* New York: John Wiley & Sons, Inc., 1979.

Denk-Glass, Rita; Laber, Susan; and Brewer, Kathryn. "Middle Ear Disease in Young Children." *Young Children* 37(6):51–53, September 1982.

Hamilton, Helen K. (editorial director). *Professional Guide to Diseases.* Springhouse, PA: Intermed Communications, Inc., 1982.

Lewit, E.M. "An Evaluation of Plastic Strip Thermometers." *Journal of the American Medical Association* 247(3):321–25, January 15, 1982.

Pringle, Sheila, and Ramsey, Brenda E. *Promoting the Health of Children.* St. Louis: C.V. Mosby Co., 1982.

Feinbloom, Richard I. *Child Health Encyclopedia.* New York: Dell Publishing Co., 1978.

Additional Reading

Leach, Penelope. *Your Baby and Child: From Birth to Age Five.* New York: Alfred A. Knopf, 1982.

Mother's Encyclopedia and Everyday Guide to Family Health. Edited by Isadore Rossman. New York: Dell Publishing Company, 1981.

Parent's Guide to Baby and Child Medical Care. Edited by Terril H. Hart. Deepha-
ven, MN: Meadowbrook Press, 1982.

Rhodes, Ronald L., et al., *Elementary School Health.* Boston: Allyn and Bacon,
Inc., 1981.

Shiller, Jack G. *Childhood Illness.* New York: Stein and Day Publishers, 1976.

Unit 11
MANAGEMENT OF ACCIDENTS AND INJURIES

Terms to Know

ingested
elevate
resuscitation
paralysis
alkali

submerge
sterile
negligent
reimplant

Objectives

After studying this unit, you will be able to:
- *State the difference between emergency care and first aid.*
- *Identify the ABCs for assessing emergencies.*
- *Name eight life-threatening conditions and state the emergency treatment for each.*
- *Name ten conditions that are nonlifethreatening and state the first aid treatment for each.*
- *Describe the teacher's or child care provider's role and responsibilities as they relate to management of accidental injuries and illness.*

Accident prevention is a major responsibility of preschools and child care centers. This goal is best achieved by providing safe environments, presenting health/safety education, and establishing procedures for handling emergencies.

Unfortunately, many programs overlook the necessity for developing emergency policies and plans until something unexpected happens. To avoid confu-

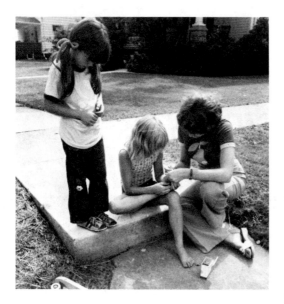

FIGURE 11-1 Every care provider should know the fundamentals of emergency and first aid care (from *Children in Your Life,* Radeloff and Zechman, Delmar Publisher's Inc. 1981).

sion and unfortunate experiences, every early childhood program should establish plans for emergency care. Such plans should include:

- personnel trained in lifesaving and first aid techniques, Figure 11-1.
- staff member(s) assigned to coordinate and direct emergency care
- notarized parental permission forms for each child authorizing emergency medical treatment
- a listing of emergency telephone numbers, including those of parents, hospital, fire department, ambulance, police, poison control
- the availability of a telephone
- arrangements for emergency transportation
- appropriate first aid supplies

These plans should be made available to parents and staff members and reviewed on a regular basis.

Despite careful planning and supervision, accidents, injuries and illness still happen. For this reason, it is very important that preschool teachers and child care providers learn the fundamentals of emergency care and first aid, Table 11-1. Prior training and preparation allow personnel to handle emergencies with skill and confidence (Sousa 1982).

Teachers and care providers are primarily responsible for providing initial and urgent care to young children who are seriously injured or ill. These mea-

TABLE 11-1 Basic First Aid Supplies

adhesive tape—½ and 1 inch widths	scissors—blunt tipped
alcohol	soap—preferably liquid
Band-Aids—assorted sizes	spirits of ammonia
blanket	splints
cotton balls	syrup of ipecac
flashlight	thermometers—2
gauze pads—sterile, 2×2s, 4×4s	tongue blades
hot water bottle	towel—large and small
ice pack	triangular bandages for slings
needle—sewing	tweezers
roller gauze—1- and 2-inch widths	Vaseline
safety pins	

sures are considered to only be temporary and aimed at saving lives, reducing pain and discomfort, and preventing complications and additional injury. Responsibility for obtaining any further treatment or care is then transferred to the child's parents (Sheldon 1983).

EMERGENCY CARE VS. FIRST AID

Emergency care refers to immediate treatment administered for life-threatening conditions. It includes a quick assessment of the emergency ABCs, Table 11-2. The victim is also checked and treated for severe bleeding, shock and signs of poisoning.

TABLE 11-2 The ABCs for Assessing Emergencies

A—Airway	Make sure the air passageway is open and clear. Roll the infant or child onto its back. Support the neck with one hand and gently lift up. Tilt the head back by placing your other hand on the child's forehead. Clear out the mouth with a cloth or your fingers.
B—Breathing	Watch for the child's chest to go up and down. Feel and listen for air to escape from the lungs.
C—Circulation	Check for a pulse. In an infant, feel just below the left nipple. For an older child, the pulse can be felt along the large artery on the side of the neck.

First aid refers to treatment administered for injuries and illnesses that are not considered life-threatening. Emergency care and first aid are based on principles that should be familiar to everyone involved in child care:

1. Stay calm and in control of the situation.

2. Always remain with the child. If necessary, send another adult or child for help.

3. Don't move the child until the extent of injuries or illness can be determined.

4. Quickly evaluate the child's condition, paying special attention to an open airway, breathing and circulation.

5. Carefully plan and administer appropriate emergency care. Improper treatment can lead to other injuries.

6. Don't give any medications unless they are prescribed for certain lifesaving conditions.

7. Don't offer diagnoses or medical advice. Refer the child's parents to health professionals.

8. Summon emergency medical assistance if the injury or illness is too difficult to handle alone.

9. Always inform the child's parents of the injury and first aid care that has been administered.

10. Record all the facts concerning the accident and treatment administered; file in the child's permanent folder.

In most states, legal protection is granted to individuals who administer emergency care, unless their actions are grossly *negligent* or harmful.

LIFE-THREATENING CONDITIONS

Situations that require emergency care to prevent death or serious disability are discussed in this unit. The emergency care techniques and suggestions given are not intended to replace or eliminate the need for teachers and child care providers to complete American Red Cross first aid and cardiopulmonary resuscitation training. Rather, they are included here to enrich basic instruction and to expand the teacher's ability to care for children's emergencies.

Absence of Breathing

Breathing emergencies accompany many life-threatening conditions, e.g., drowning, electric shock, convulsions, poisoning, severe injuries, and choking. Anyone who is involved in the care of young children should complete training in mouth-to-mouth and cardiopulmonary *resuscitation*. This training is available from most local chapters of the American Red Cross.

It is important to remain calm and perform emergency lifesaving procedures quickly and with confidence. Have someone call for an ambulance or emergency medical assistance while you begin mouth-to-mouth breathing. The procedure for mouth-to-mouth breathing follows and is also illustrated in Figure 11–2.

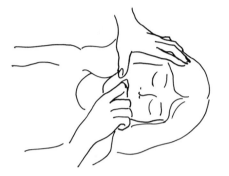

CLEAR CHILD'S MOUTH OF MUCUS OR VOMITUS BY QUICKLY RUNNING YOUR FINGERS AROUND THE INSIDE OF THE CHILD'S MOUTH.

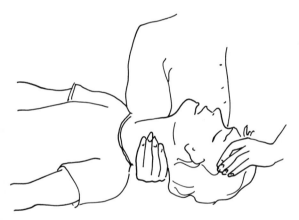

POSITION THE CHILD ON ITS BACK. GENTLY TILT THE HEAD UP AND BACK BY PLACING ONE HAND UNDER THE CHILD'S NECK AND LIFTING UPWARD, AND THE OTHER HAND ON CHILD'S FOREHEAD.

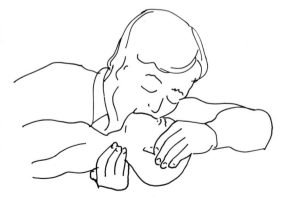

FOR AN INFANT, PLACE YOUR MOUTH OVER THE INFANT'S NOSE AND MOUTH CREATING A TIGHT SEAL. GENTLY GIVE 4 SMALL PUFFS OF AIR INTO THE INFANT'S NOSE AND MOUTH. CHECK FOR BREATHING. CONTINUE BREATHING FOR THE INFANT AT A RATE OF ONE BREATH EVERY 3 SECONDS.

FIGURE 11–2 Emergency breathing techniques for the infant and child.

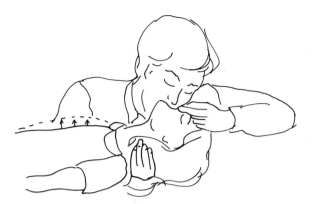

FOR AN OLDER CHILD, PLACE YOUR OPEN MOUTH OVER THE CHILD'S OPEN MOUTH FORMING A TIGHT SEAL. GENTLY PINCH THE CHILD'S NOSTRILS CLOSED. QUICKLY GIVE 4 SMALL BREATHS OF AIR. CHECK FOR BREATHING. CONTINUE BREATHING FOR THE CHILD AT A RATE OF ONE BREATH EVERY 5 SECONDS.

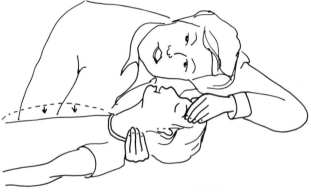

LIFT YOUR HEAD AND TURN IT TO THE SIDE AFTER EACH PUFF. THIS ALLOWS TIME FOR AIR TO ESCAPE FROM THE CHILD'S LUNGS AND ALSO GIVES YOU TIME TO TAKE A BREATH AND TO OBSERVE IF THE CHILD IS BREATHING ON ITS OWN.

FIGURE 11–2 Continued

1. Gently shake the child or infant to determine if the child is conscious or in a deep sleep. Speak the child's name in a loud voice. If the child does not answer, begin emergency breathing procedures immediately.

2. Position the child on its back on a hard surface.

3. Clear the mouth of any mucus or vomitus by quickly running your fingers around the inside of the child's mouth.

4. Gently tilt the child's head up and back by placing one hand under the child's neck and lifting upward and placing the other hand on the child's forehead. **Caution:** Do not tip the head back too far. Tipping the head too far can cause obstruction of the airway in an infant or small child.

5. Carefully listen for any spontaneous breathing by placing your ear next to the child's mouth.

6. **For an infant,** place your mouth over the infant's nose and mouth creating a tight seal. Gently blow 4 small puffs of air into the infant's nose and

mouth. **Caution:** Too much air forced into an infant's lungs may cause the lungs to rupture. Always remember to use small gentle puffs of air from your cheeks.

7. **For an older child,** gently pinch the nostrils closed, place your open mouth over the child's open mouth forming a tight seal. Quickly give 4 small breaths of air in quick succession without pausing between breaths.

8. Observe to see if the chest or abdomen of child is rising to be sure air is entering the lungs.

9. Continue breathing for the child at a rate of one breath every 3 seconds for infants and toddlers, and one breath every 5 seconds for older children and adults.

10. Lift your head and turn it to the side after each puff. This allows time for air to escape from the child's lungs and also gives you time to take a breath and to observe if the child is breathing on its own.

11. Continue breathing procedures until the child breathes alone or emergency medical assistance arrives. DO NOT GIVE UP!

If the entry of air seems blocked or the chest does not rise while administering mouth-to-mouth breathing, check for foreign objects in the airway and remove them if possible. Continue mouth-to-mouth breathing until the child breathes on its own or medical help arrives.

If the child resumes breathing, keep it lying down with its feet slightly elevated. Turn the child's head to one side if vomiting begins. Maintain body temperature by covering with a light blanket. Closely observe the child's breathing until medical help arrives.

Airway Obstruction

Occasionally, infants and young children get food or foreign objects caught in their throats in such a way that the airway is obstructed, Table 11–3. In most

TABLE 11–3 Foods Commonly Linked to Childhood Choking

raw carrots	peanuts and other nuts
hot dogs	cookies
pieces of raw apple	crackers
grapes	potato chips
fruit seeds and pits	pretzels
round and ring-shaped hard candies	popcorn
peanut butter sandwich	gum

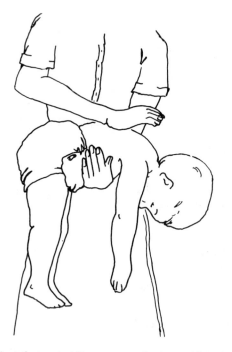

FIGURE 11–3 Position the infant or toddler over your forearm with its head lower than its chest.

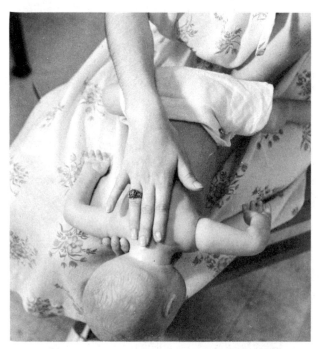

FIGURE 11–4 Position infant face down on your thigh with its head lower than its chest (from *Diversified Health Occupations*, Louise Simmers, Delmar Publishers Inc., 1983).

instances, these objects can be successfully coughed out (Harris 1984). However, emergency lifesaving measures must be started immediately if:

- breathing is labored or absent
- lips and nailbeds turn blue
- cough is weak or ineffective
- the child is unconscious
- there is a high-pitched sound when the child inhales

Emergency first aid techniques used to treat someone who is choking are different for infants and toddlers than they are for older children (Green 1977). Regardless of the child's age first try to remove the object. With the index finger make a sweep of the child's mouth, bringing the finger along one cheek, across the throat from the side, and towards the opposite cheek. Care must be taken not to push straight into the throat as this may push the object further into the airway. If the object cannot be removed easily and the infant or toddler is conscious, do the following:

- Position the infant or toddler face down over the length of your arm with the child's head lower than its chest, Figure 11–3. An alternate approach is to position the child face down on your thigh with the child's head lower than its chest, Figure 11–4. The adult's hand should support the infant's or toddler's head and neck.
- Use the heel of your hand to give 4 quick blows on the child's back between the shoulder blades. **Caution:** Do not use excessive force as this could injure the child.
- Turn the infant or toddler over, face up, with the head held lower than the chest and give 4 quick abdominal thrusts; use 2 or 3 fingers to push upwards on the infant's abdomen, Figure 11–5.
- Repeat the steps (4 back blows, 4 abdominal thrusts) until the object is dislodged or the child loses consciousness.

If the infant or toddler loses consciousness, and is not breathing:

- Have someone call for an ambulance or emergency medical assistance.
- Begin lifesaving breathing procedures.
- Give the infant 4 quick small puffs of air.
- If the infant's lungs inflate, continue giving breathing assistance only. If the lungs cannot be inflated, give 4 puffs of air, 4 back blows, 4 abdominal thrusts, then check the mouth for the object. Repeat these steps until help arrives or the object is dislodged.

Note: This procedure is currently recommended by the American Red Cross. However, the use of the abdominal thrust in infants is not promoted by some major health organizations who are responsible for establishing emergency procedures. **Caution:** It is imperative that teachers and child care providers check with local emergency authorities to be sure they learn and understand the application of approved methods in emergency situations.

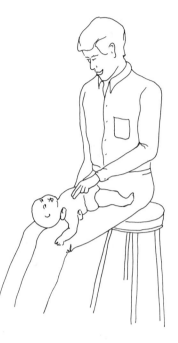

FIGURE 11–5 With the infant face up and its head lower than its chest, give four quick abdominal thrusts using two or three fingers to push upwards on the infant's abdomen.

To give emergency aid to the older child who is choking, first try to remove the object from the blocked airway. If this is not successful, support the child and give 4 rapid blows to the back between the shoulder blades. If the object is still not dislodged, proceed with the Heimlich maneuver, Figure 11–6.

1. Stand or kneel behind the child with your arms around the child's waist.

2. Make a fist with one hand, thumbs tucked in.

3. Place the fisted hand against the child's abdomen immediately below the tip of the rib cage and slightly above the navel.

4. Grasp your fisted hand with your other hand.

5. Press your fisted hand into the child's abdomen with a quick upward thrust.

6. Repeat the procedure until the object is dislodged.

7. If the child stops breathing, administer mouth-to-mouth breathing until medical help arrives.

8. After the object is dislodged and breathing is restored, be sure the child receives medical attention.

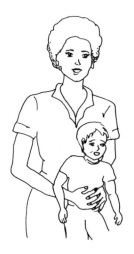

STAND OR KNEEL BEHIND THE CHILD WITH YOUR ARMS AROUND THE CHILD'S WAIST.

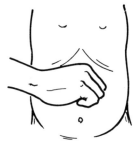

MAKE A FIST WITH ONE HAND. PLACE THE FISTED HAND AGAINST THE CHILD'S ABDOMEN BELOW THE TIP OF THE RIB CAGE, SLIGHTLY ABOVE THE NAVEL.

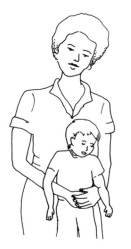

GRASP THE FISTED HAND WITH YOUR OTHER HAND. PRESS YOUR FISTS INTO THE CHILD'S ABDOMEN WITH A QUICK UPWARD THRUST.

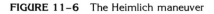

FIGURE 11-6   The Heimlich maneuver

Shock

Shock frequently accompanies injuries especially those that are severe and, therefore, it should be anticipated. Shock can also result from extreme emotional upset, bleeding, pain, heat exhaustion, poisoning, burns, and fractures. It is a serious emergency and requires immediate first aid treatment in order to prevent death. The signs of shock include:

- skin that is pale, cool, and clammy
- bluish discoloration around lips, nails, and ear lobes
- increased perspiration
- weakness
- rapid, weak pulse
- dilated pupils, blurred vision
- rapid, shallow breathing
- extreme thirst
- nausea and vomiting
- confusion, anxiety, restlessness

Teachers and child care providers can carry out the following emergency first aid measures to treat the child in shock:

1. Have someone call for emergency medical assistance.

2. Quickly try to identify the main cause of shock and treat the cause first, e.g., bleeding, poisoning.

3. Keep the child lying down.

4. Elevate the child's feet 8 to 10 inches, if there is no indication of fractures or head or back injuries.

5. Maintain body heat by placing one blanket under the child and covering the child lightly with another blanket.

6. If the child complains of thirst, moisten a clean cloth and use it to wet the child's lips, tongue, and inside of mouth.

7. Stay calm and reassure the child until medical help arrives.

8. Observe the child's breathing closely; give mouth-to-mouth resuscitation if necessary.

Asthma

Asthma is a disorder of the respiratory system characterized by periods of wheezing, gasping and difficult breathing. Acute asthma attacks are thought to be triggered by allergic reactions, infections and emotional upsets or stress. An infant's or child's life is placed in grave danger during an attack because of the intense struggle to breathe (Feinbloom 1978).

Remaining calm and confident during a child's asthmatic attack is one of the most important first aid measures. At the same time, teachers and child care providers can also:

1. Reassure the child.

2. If the child has medication at the center that is to be given in the event of an acute asthmatic attack, administer it immediately.

3. Encourage the child to relax and breathe slowly and deeply (anxiety makes breathing more difficult).

4. Have the child assume a position that is most comfortable (breathing is usually easier when sitting or standing up).

5. Offer small sips of water or juice to offset fluid loss due to rapid breathing; use care so that the child does not accidently choke.

6. Summon emergency medical help immediately if the child shows signs of extreme fatigue, loss of consciousness or blue discoloration of the nail-beds and lips.

7. Have someone call the child's parents.

Bleeding

Occasionally, young children receive injuries such as a deep gash or jagged laceration that bleed profusely. Severe bleeding requires prompt emergency first aid treatment. Again, it is extremely important that the teacher or child care provider act quickly, yet remain calm. To stop bleeding:

1. Place a pad of *sterile* gauze or clean material over the wound.

2. Apply firm pressure directly over the site of bleeding, using the flat parts of the fingers.

3. Maintain pressure for approximately 5 to 10 minutes before letting up.

4. *Elevate* the bleeding part on a pillow if there is no sign of a fracture.

5. If blood soaks through the bandage, place another pad over the original bandage; bleeding may restart if the pad next to the skin is disturbed.

6. When bleeding is stopped, secure the pad in place.

7. If bleeding cannot be stopped by direct pressure, locate the nearest pressure point above the injury and apply pressure, Figure 11–7.

8. Summon emergency medical assistance if bleeding comes in spurts or cannot be stopped.

9. Use a tourniquet **only** if a body part has been amputated. If bleeding cannot be stopped with any other method, apply a tourniquet with the understanding that amputation afterward is a possible risk.

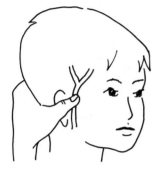

PRESS THUMB AGAINST THE BONE SLIGHTLY IN FRONT OF THE EAR.

PRESS FINGERS AGAINST THE HOLLOW SPOT IN THE JAW.

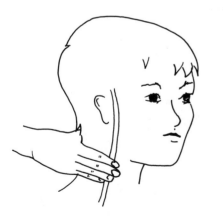

PLACE THUMB AGAINST THE BACK OF THE NECK. FINGERS SHOULD BE PLACED ON THE SIDE OF THE NECK CLOSE TO THE WINDPIPE; PRESS TOWARD THE THUMB. **CAUTION:**   DO NOT PLACE FINGERS OVER THE WINDPIPE.

FIGURE 11-7   Pressure points used to control bleeding

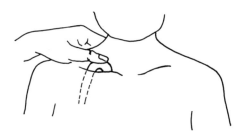

PRESS THUMB IN THE GROOVE
BEHIND THE COLLARBONE.

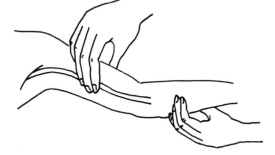

PLACE FINGERS ON THE INNER
ARM AT THE EDGE OF THE BICEP
MUSCLE HALFWAY DOWN THE ARM.
KEEP THUMB ON OUTER ARM AND
PRESS TOWARD THE BONE.

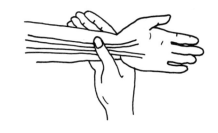

PLACE THUMB ON INNER WRIST
AND PRESS TOWARD THE BONE.

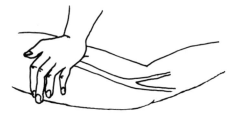

PLACE HEEL OF HAND ON INNER
THIGH AT THE CREASE OF THE
GROIN AND PRESS AGAINST THE
BONE.

FIGURE 11–7 Continued

Save all blood-soaked dressings. Doctors will need them to estimate the
amount of blood loss. Contact the child's parents when bleeding is under control
and advise them to seek medical attention for the child.

TABLE 11-4   Signs and Symptoms of Hypoglycemia and Hyperglycemia

HYPERGLYCEMIA (diabetic coma)
Causes
 High blood sugar caused by too little available insulin, improper diet, illness, stress, or omitted dose of insulin.

Symptoms
 • Slow, gradual onset
 • Respirations slow and deep
 • Increased thirst
 • Skin flushed and dry
 • Confusion
 • Staggering; appears as if drunk
 • Drowsiness
 • Sweet smelling, winelike breath odor

Treatment
 Call the child's doctor immediately. Keep the child quiet and warm.

HYPOGLYCEMIA (insulin shock)
Causes
 Low blood sugar caused by too much insulin, insufficient amounts of carbohydrates, increased activity, decreased food intake, and illness.

Symptoms
 • Sudden onset
 • Skin cool and clammy
 • Faintness
 • Shakiness
 • Nausea
 • Headache
 • Hunger
 • Respirations rapid and shallow
 • Convulsions
 • Unconsciousness

Treatment
 If conscious, quickly administer a sugar substance, e.g., orange juice, hard candy, or sugar cube. Call the child's doctor.

 If unconscious, rush the child to a hospital.

Diabetes

Two major medical emergencies associated with diabetes are hypoglycemia and hyperglycemia. Emergency first aid treatment requires that the teacher or child care provider quickly distinguish between the two conditions. The causes and symptoms of these complications are, in many respects, opposites of each other, Table 11-4.

Hypoglycemia, or insulin shock, is caused by low levels of sugar in the blood. It can occur whenever a diabetic child receives either an excess amount of insulin or an insufficient amount of food. Other causes may include illness, delayed eating times, or increased activity. Similar symptoms are experienced by nondiabetic children when they become excessively hungry. Hypoglycemia can be reversed very quickly by administering a sugar substance. Orange juice is ideal for this purpose because it is absorbed rapidly by the body. Sugar cubes and hard candies such as lollipops or Life-Savers are also good sources of quick sugar.

Hyperglycemia, or diabetic coma, results when there is too much sugar circulating in the blood stream. This condition is a potential problem for every diabetic child. Illness, infection, emotional stress, poor dietary control, fever, or a dose of insulin that is forgotten or too small can lead to hyperglycemia. Any time a teacher or care provider recognizes the symptoms of hyperglycemia in a diabetic child, the parents should be notified immediately so they can consult with the child's physician. Emergency treatment usually requires the administration of insulin by medical personnel.

Drowning

Drowning is a frequent cause of accidental death among young children. Mouth-to-mouth resuscitation is necessary to restart breathing and can be started while the child is being taken out of the water. The Heimlich maneuver has recently been suggested as a method for emptying water from the lungs, thus allowing more space for air to be introduced during mouth-to-mouth resuscitation.

The child who has been rescued from drowning is likely to vomit during resuscitation attempts because large amounts of water are often swallowed. Therefore, the child's head should be turned to one side to decrease the possibility of choking. Also, observe closely for signs of shock.

Even if a child appears to have fully recovered from a near drowning incident, medical care should be obtained immediately. Complications such as pneumonia can develop from water remaining in the lungs.

Electric Shock

Although it is a natural reaction, never touch the child until the source of electricity can be turned off or disconnected. Quickly unplug the cord, or remove the appropriate fuse from the fusebox, or turn off the main breaker switch. A dry nonconductive object such as a piece of wood, folded newspaper or magazine, or rope can be used to push or pull the child away from the source of current. Be sure to stand on something dry such as a board or cardboard while you attempt to rescue the child.

Severe electric shock can cause breathing to stop, severe burns, symptoms of shock, and the heart to stop beating. To treat the infant or young child who has received an electrical shock do the following:

1. Have someone call for emergency medical assistance while you remove the child from the source of electric current.

2. Begin mouth-to-mouth breathing if the child is not breathing.

3. Observe for and treat signs of shock and burns.

4. Rush the child to a medical facility as quickly as possible.

Head Injuries

The greatest danger of severe head injuries is internal bleeding (Meier 1983). Signs of bleeding may develop within hours following the injury or perhaps not until several days after the injury. During this time, the infant or young child should be observed carefully for:

- weakness or *paralysis*
- repeated or forceful vomiting
- severe headache
- drowsiness
- unequal size of the pupils of the eye
- bleeding or clear fluid coming from the nose or ears
- speech disturbances
- poor coordination or balance
- disorientation
- double vision
- seizures
- any area of increased swelling beneath the scalp

If any of these signs develop, call the child's parents and have them contact the child's physician immediately.

Children who receive even a minor blow or bump to the head should not be moved until it can be determined that there are no fractures or additional injuries. If the injury does not appear to be serious, the child should be encouraged to rest or play quietly for the next few hours. Always report to parents any blow or injury to a child's head regardless of how insignificant it may seem at the time. Several days of careful observations for changes in the child's behavior or physical status are very important.

Scalp wounds have a tendency to bleed profusely causing even minor injuries to appear more serious than they actually are. Therefore, when a child receives an injury to the scalp, it is important not to become overly alarmed at the sight of profuse bleeding. Pressure applied directly over the wound with a clean cloth or gauze dressing is usually sufficient to stop most bleeding. An ice pack can also be applied to the area to decrease swelling and pain. The child's parents should be advised of the injury so they can monitor its progress.

Poisoning

Poisoning in preschools and child care centers can result from a variety of materials including plants and berries, cleaning products, chemicals or insecticides. However, the possibility that a small child may have *ingested* something on the way to school, such as berries, aspirin, medication or perfume from a mother's purse also cannot be overlooked. The signs of poisoning appear suddenly and include:

TABLE 11-5 Poisonous Substances

Strong Acid and Alkalis	Petroleum Products	All Others
bathroom, drain and oven cleaners	charcoal lighter	medicines
battery acid	cigarette lighter fluid	plants
dishwasher soaps	furniture polish and wax	berries
lye	gasoline	cosmetics
wart and corn remover	kerosene	fingernail polish
	naphtha	remover
	turpentine	insecticides
		mothballs
		weed killers

- nausea or vomiting
- abdominal cramps or diarrhea
- skin that feels cold and clammy
- burns visible around the mouth, lips and tongue
- restlessness
- convulsions
- confusion or disorientation
- loss of consciousness

Emergency treatment of accidental poisoning is determined by the type of poison the young child has ingested (Keim 1983). Poisons are categorized into three basic types: strong acids and *alkalis,* petroleum products, all others. Some examples of each type are shown in Table 11-5.

The first step in treating any case of accidental poisoning is always the same—*call the nearest hospital or Poison Control Center for instructions!* Before calling, quickly try to identify what the child has swallowed and, if possible, the approximate amount. If the container cannot be located, do not delay calling.

If the poison is a strong acid or alkali, redness and burns may be visible around the child's mouth, lips and tongue. Do not induce vomiting as vomiting can cause additional burning when the poison comes back up. If the child is conscious, have the child drink one or two glasses of milk to dilute the poison. Follow the instructions received from the Poison Control Center or rush the child to the nearest hospital.

If the poison is a petroleum product the odor of gasoline or kerosene may be detected on a child's breath. The child should be rushed to the nearest hospital. Again, do not induce vomiting. Petroleum products can cause a special form of pneumonia if any of the vomited material is inhaled into the lungs.

For all other types of poisons, call the Poison Control Center for instructions. If the child is conscious, give it one to two glasses of milk to drink in order to dilute the poison. In most cases, you will be advised to make the child vomit. This can be achieved by either giving syrup of ipecac according to directions, or causing the child to gag by touching the back of the throat with a finger, spoon handle or other blunt object.

Continually observe the child for signs of shock while administering other first aid measures. Never attempt to make an unconscious child vomit or drink any type of liquid. If the unconscious child begins to vomit, turn its head to one side to prevent aspiration of vomited material. Contact the child's parents as soon as possible.

CONDITIONS THAT ARE NOT LIFE THREATENING

Most of children's injuries and illnesses are not life threatening but they do require first aid. Teachers and child care providers are not qualified nor expected to provide comprehensive medical treatment. However, they can perform temporary first aid to limit complications and make children more comfortable until parents arrive and assume responsibility for the child's care. The remainder of this unit describes conditions typically encountered with young children that require first aid care.

Abrasions, Cuts and Other Minor Skin Wounds

Simple cuts, scrapes and abrasions are among the most common types of injury young children experience. First aid care is concerned primarily with the control of bleeding and the prevention of infection. To care for the child who has received a simple skin wound do the following:

1. Wash your hands thoroughly before caring for the wound.

2. If the wound is bleeding, apply direct pressure on the wound with a clean or sterile pad.

3. When bleeding has been stopped clean the wound carefully with soap and water or hydrogen peroxide. Begin at the center of the wound and cleanse in a circular motion toward the outer edges. This method reduces the amount of bacteria and foreign matter that is carried across the wound.

4. Cover the wound with a sterile bandage, Figure 11–8.

5. Inform parents of the wound and remind them to check if the child's tetanus immunization is up to date.

Bites

Human and animal bites are painful and can lead to serious infection. The possibility of rabies should be considered with any animal bite that is unpro-

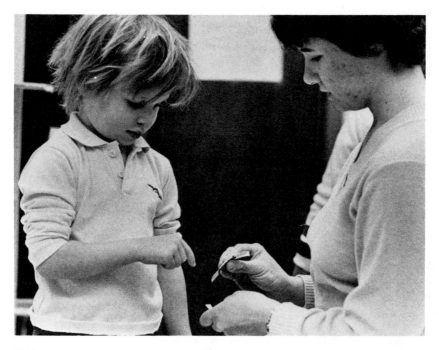

FIGURE 11-8 A bandage helps to protect cuts and skin abrasions against infection.

voked, unless the animal is known to be free of the rabies virus. A suspected animal should be confined and observed by a veterinarian for a period of ten days. In cases where the bite was provoked, the animal is not as likely to be rabid. First aid care for human and animal bites includes the following:

1. If possible, let the wound bleed for a short time to help remove the animal's saliva.

2. Cleanse the wound thoroughly with soap and water or hydrogen peroxide.

3. Cover the wound with a dressing.

4. Notify the child's parents and advise them to have the wound checked by the child's physician.

Most insect bites cause little more than local skin irritations. However, some children are extremely sensitive to certain insects, especially bees, hornets, wasps and spiders. When stung or bitten, these children may experience severe allergic reactions, including:

- difficulty breathing
- joint pain
- abdominal cramps

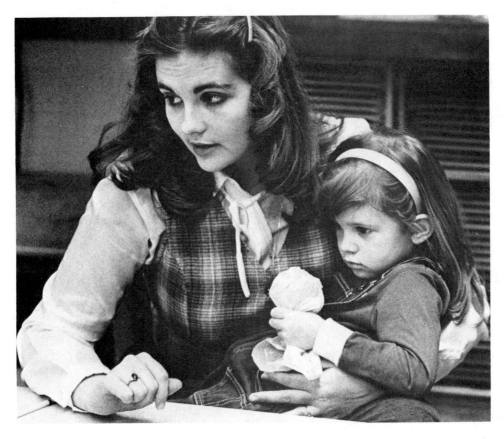

FIGURE 11-9 Having the child hold a bag of ice can help reduce the swelling and pain from an insect bite to the finger.

- vomiting
- fever
- red, swollen eyes
- hives or generalized itching

Allergic reactions to insect bites can be life threatening. If a child experiences any of these reactions, immediately do the following:

1. Keep the child quiet.

2. If the child has medication for this type of allergic reaction at school, administer it immediately.

3. Place an ice pack on the bite and position the affected body part so that it is lower than the heart.

4. Call for emergency medical assistance, especially if the child has never experienced this type of reaction before.

Most first aid measures for insect bites are temporary and aimed at relieving discomfort and preventing infection. If a stinger remains in the skin after a bee, wasp or hornet bite, it can be carefully removed with a tweezers or by scraping the skin with a dull knife. A paste of baking soda and water applied to the area relieves some discomfort. An ice pack can also be used to decrease swelling and pain, Figure 11–9.

Blisters

A blister is a collection of fluid that builds up beneath the outer layer of skin. Blisters most commonly develop from rubbing or friction, burns, or allergic reactions.

First aid care of blisters is aimed at protecting the irritated skin from infection. If at all possible, blisters should not be broken. However, if they do break, wash the area with soap and water and cover with a bandage.

Bruises

Bruises result from the rupture of small blood vessels beneath the skin. They are often caused by falls, bumps and blows. Fair-skinned children tend to bruise more easily. First aid care is aimed at controlling subsurface bleeding and swelling. Apply ice or cold packs to the bruised area for 15 to 30 minutes and repeat 3 to 4 times during the next 24 hours. Later, warm moist packs can be applied to improve healing. Alert parents to watch for signs of infection and unusual bleeding if the bruising is extensive or severe.

Burns

Burns are classified according to how deeply the skin is burned:

- first degree—surface skin is red
- second degree—surface skin is red and blistered
- third degree—burn is deep; skin and underlying tissues are brown or white and charred

Immediate first aid care of burns includes the following:

1. Quickly *submerge* the burned part in cold water for 15 to 30 minutes. Cool water temperatures lessen the depth of burn as well as decrease swelling and pain.

2. Elevate the burned part to relieve discomfort.

3. Cover the burn with a sterile gauze dressing and tape in place. *Do not* use greasy ointments or creams. Dirt and bacteria can collect in the ointments and creams increasing the risk of infection. If the burn covers a large area

or causes blistering, notify the child's parents immediately and advise them to contact the child's physician.

Chemical burns should be rinsed for 10 to 15 minutes under cool running water. Remove any clothing that might have some of the chemical on it. Call the nearest Poison Control Center for further instructions. Also, check the label on the chemical container for any additional first aid measures. The child's parents should be contacted and advised to check with their physician.

Eye Injuries

Children's curiosity and active play can lead to a variety of eye injuries. Most injuries are simple and can be treated by the teacher or child care provider (Green 1977). It is very important to inform parents of any eye injury so they can continue to observe the child and consult the child's physician if necessary.

A sudden blow to the eye from a snowball, wooden block or other hard object is usually quite painful. First aid treatment includes the following:

1. Keep the child quiet.

2. Apply an ice pack to the eye for 15 minutes if there is no bleeding.

3. Use direct pressure to control any bleeding around the eye; cleanse and cover wounds with a sterile gauze pad.

4. Report any complaint of inability to see or of seeing spots to the child's parents so they can immediately contact the child's physician.

Foreign particles such as sand, cornmeal or specks of dust frequently find their way into children's eyes. Although it is very natural for children to want to rub their eyes, this must be discouraged to prevent further injury to the eyeball. Often spontaneous tearing will be sufficient to wash the object out of the eye. If the particle is visible, it can also be removed with the corner of a clean cloth or flushed out using an eye syringe and warm water. If the particle cannot be removed easily, the eye should be covered and medical attention sought.

An object that penetrates the eyeball must not be removed. Place a paper cup, funnel or small cardboard box over *both* the object and the eye. Place a gauze pad over the unaffected eye and secure both dressings in place by wrapping a bandage around the head. Movement of the injured eyeball should be kept to a minimum and can be achieved by covering both eyes. Seek immediate medical treatment.

A thin cut on the eye's surface can result from a piece of paper, toy, or child's fingernail. Injuries of this type cause severe pain and tearing. The teacher should cover *both* of the child's eyes with a gauze dressing. Notify the parents and advise them to take the child for immediate medical treatment.

Chemical burns to a child's eye are very serious. Quickly tip the child's head toward the affected eye. Gently pour large amounts of warm water over the eyeball for at least 15 minutes. Meanwhile, have someone contact the parents or make arrangements to have the child transported to a medical facility.

Fractures

A fracture is a break or crack in a bone. A teacher or child care provider can check for possible fractures by observing the child for:

- particular areas of extreme pain or tenderness
- an unusual shape or deformity of a bone
- a break in the skin with visible bone edges protruding
- swelling
- a change in skin color around the injury site

A child who complains of pain after falling should not be moved, especially if a back or neck injury is possible. Have someone call for an ambulance or emergency medical assistance. Keep the chid warm and observe carefully for signs of shock. Avoid giving the child anything to eat or drink in case surgery is necessary.

Fractures should be splinted and firmly supported before the child is moved. Splints can be purchased from medical supply stores or improvised from items such as a rolled-up magazine or blanket, a ruler, a piece of board or a tissue box. Never try to straighten a fractured bone. Cover open skin wounds with a sterile pad but do not attempt to clean the wound. Elevate the splinted part on a pillow and apply an ice pack to reduce swelling and pain. Watch the child closely for signs of shock. Contact the child's parents immediately and have them contact the child's physician.

Frostbite

Infants and young children should be watched very closely during extremely cold weather so they don't remove hats, boots or mittens. Frostbite occurs within minutes and most commonly affects the nose, ears, cheeks, fingers and toes. Frostbite results when body tissue is frozen. The skin takes on a waxy, white appearance and may be blistered. The child with frostbite often suffers from extreme pain or feels none at all. First aid treatment for frostbite consists of the following:

- Rewarm the affected part by immersing it in lukewarm, then warm water. **Caution:** Never use hot water.
- Handle the frostbitten part with care; avoid rubbing or massaging the part as this could further damage frozen tissue.
- Cover the frostbitten area with sterile gauze.

- Wrap the child in a blanket for extra warmth.
- Contact the parents so they can take the child for medical treatment.

Heat Exhaustion and Heat Stroke

First aid treatment of heat related illness depends on distinguishing heat exhaustion from heat stroke. The following symptoms can be observed in a child who is suffering from heat exhaustion:

- skin is pale, cool and moist with perspiration
- weakness or fainting
- thirst
- nausea
- abdominal cramps
- headache
- normal body temperature

Heat exhaustion is not a life-threatening condition. It usually occurs when a child has been playing vigorously in extreme heat or too much sunshine. First aid treatment for heat exhaustion is similar to that of shock:

1. Have the child lie down.

2. Elevate the child's feet 8 to 10 inches.

3. Sponge the child's face and body with cool water.

4. Offer sips of cool water, about one-half glass every 15 minutes for one hour.

Heat stroke or "sunstroke" is a life-threatening condition that requires immediate treatment. Failure of the body's temperature-regulating mechanism during extremely hot weather allows a child's temperature to rise rapidly and dangerously. Symptoms of heat stroke include:

- high body temperature (102°F–106°F)
- dry, flushed skin
- headache
- convulsions
- vomiting
- diarrhea, abdominal cramps
- unconsciousness
- shock

Emergency treatment for heat stroke is aimed at cooling the child as quickly as possible:

1. Remove the child's outer clothing.

2. Sponge the child's body with cool water or rubbing alcohol. The child can also be placed in a cool tub of water or gently sprayed with a garden hose.

3. Elevate the child's legs to decrease the possibility of going into shock.

4. If the child is conscious, offer sips of cool water.

5. Have someone notify the child's parents and advise them to contact the child's physician immediately.

Nosebleeds

Accidental bumps, allergies, nose picking or sinus congestion can all cause a child's nose to bleed. Most nosebleeds are not serious and can be stopped quickly. If a nosebleed continues more than 30 minutes, get medical help. To stop a nosebleed, do the following:

1. Place the child in a sitting position.

2. Firmly grasp the child's nostrils and squeeze together for at least five minutes before releasing the pressure.

3. If bleeding continues, place a small roll of cotton in each nostril; pinch the nostrils together for approximately ten minutes. Gently remove the cotton when bleeding stops.

4. Apply an ice pack to the bridge of the nose to slow down bleeding.

5. Encourage parents to discuss the problem with the child's physician if nosebleeds occur repeatedly.

Seizures

Seizures occur in infants and young children for a variety of reasons. Simple precautionary measures can be taken during and immediately after a seizure to protect a child from additional injury and include the following:

1. Encourage everyone to remain calm.

2. Carefully lower the child to the floor.

3. Move furniture and other objects out of the way.

4. Do not hold the child down.

5. Do not attempt to force any protective device into the child's mouth.

6. Loosen tight clothing around the child's neck and waist to make breathing easier.

7. Watch carefully to make sure the child is breathing.

8. Call for emergency assistance if the seizure lasts longer than 15 minutes.

9. Turn the child to one side after the seizure to prevent choking.

Following the seizure, the child can be moved to a quiet area and encouraged to rest or sleep. Always be sure to notify the child's parents of the seizure.

Splinters

Most splinters under the skin's surface can be easily removed with a steril- ized needle and tweezers. Sterilize the instruments by soaking them in alcohol or holding them in an open flame. Clean the skin around the splinter with soap and water or alcohol before starting and after it is removed. Cover the area with a bandage. If the splinter is very deep, do not attempt to remove it. Inform the child's parents to seek medical attention.

Sprains

A sprain is caused by an injury to the tissues around a joint. It is usually very difficult to distinguish a sprain from a fracture without seeing an X ray. If there is any question, it is always best to splint the injury and treat it as if it were broken. Elevate the injured part and apply ice packs for several hours. Notify the child's parents and encourage them to have the child checked by a physician.

Tick Bites

Ticks are small, oval-shaped insects that generally live in wooded areas and on dogs. On humans, ticks frequently attach themselves to the scalp or base of the neck. The child is seldom aware of the tick's presence. Rocky Mountain Spotted Fever is a rare complication of the tick bite. If a child develops chills and fever following a known tick bite, medical treatment should be sought at once.

Ticks should be removed carefully so that all parts are removed. Cover the tick with mineral oil or Vaseline and leave on for at least one-half hour. This closes off the tick's breathing pores. Then, carefully lift the tick off with tweezers, being sure to get all parts. Wash the area thoroughly with soap and water. Watch the site for signs of infection.

Tooth Emergencies

The most common type of tooth injury is teeth that are chipped or loosened. A tooth that is loosened will often tighten itself back up after a few days.

If a tooth is completely dislodged, the child should be seen by a dentist. If the lost tooth is a deciduous or baby tooth, the dentist will usually not attempt to replace it. If the tooth is a permanent tooth, it should be kept wet by immediately wrapping it in a damp cloth or placing it in a cup of water to which a small amount of salt has been added. Often, the tooth can be *reimplanted* if it is done within an hour of the injury.

SUMMARY

Emergency care is the immediate care given for life-threatening conditions. First aid is treatment given for conditions that do not endanger life.

Plans and procedures established ahead of time allow preschool teachers and child care providers to respond efficiently and effectively during times of emergency. These plans include having trained personnel on hand, a coordinator of emergency care, notarized permissions for treatment, a telephone and listings of emergency telephone numbers, transportation, and adequate first aid supplies.

Training in lifesaving and first aid techniques is essential. These skills allow teachers and child care providers to fulfill their responsibility to save lives, relieve pain, and prevent complications. However, teachers do not diagnose or offer medical advice; they are only required to provide temporary care. Any additional treatment that is necessary is the responsibility of the child's parents.

LEARNING ACTIVITIES

1. Complete a Red Cross basic first aid course.

2. Design a poster or bulletin board illustrating emergency first aid for a young child who is choking. Offer your project to a local preschool or child care center where it can be displayed for parents to see.

3. Divide the class into small groups of students. Discuss and demonstrate the emergency first aid care for each of the following situations. A child:

   - burned several fingers on a hot plate

   - ate de-icing pellets

   - splashed turpentine in the eyes

   - fell from a climbing gym

   - is choking on popcorn

   - slammed fingers in a door

   - is found chewing on an extension cord

4. As a class project, prepare listings of emergency services and telephone numbers in your community. Distribute them to local early childhood centers.

UNIT REVIEW

A. Complete each of the given statements with a word selected from the following list. Take the first letter of each answer and place it in the appropriate
   space following question 10 to spell out one of the basic principles of first aid.

airway	evaluate
breathing	plans
diagnose	pressure
elevate	responsible
emergency	resuscitation

   1. Always check to be sure the child is _____.

   2. The immediate care given for life-threatening conditions is
      _____ care.

   3. Early childhood programs should develop _____ for handling
      emergencies.

   4. If an infant is found unconscious and not breathing, begin mouth-to-
      nose/mouth _____ immediately.

   5. The first step in providing emergency care is to quickly _____
      the child's condition.

   6. Bleeding can be stopped by applying direct _____.

   7. When evaluating a child for life-threatening injuries, be sure to check for
      a clear _____, breathing and circulation.

   8. Parents are _____ for any additional medical treatment of a
      child's injuries.

   9. Treatment of shock includes _____ the child's legs 8 to 10
      inches.

   10. Teachers never _____ or give medical advice.

   A basic principle of first aid is   __ __   __ __ __ __ __ __ __ __

B. Select the best answer from the choices offered to complete each statement.

   1. In a case of sunstroke, you would expect the child's temperature to be
      a. normal
      b. elevated
      c. below normal
      d. unstable

2. Emergency treatment of accidental poisoning
   a. includes making the child vomit
   b. is always the same
   c. depends on the type of poison ingested
   d. is based on the child's age and body weight

3. Signs of head injuries
   a. may not show up for several days
   b. are always immediately visible
   c. are nothing to worry about if the child can get up and walk away
   d. are usually not serious

4. Bleeding can be stopped by
   a. elevating the injured part
   b. applying direct pressure
   c. placing an ice pack on the site
   d. all of these

5. A chemical burn to the eye should be treated *immediately* by
   a. bandaging the eye and rushing the child to a medical facility
   b. flushing the eye with warm water for 15 minutes
   c. calling the child's parents
   d. left alone so that the child's excess tears can wash the chemical out

6. Immediate treatment of burns includes
   a. submerging the burned part in cold water
   b. applying warm packs to the burned area to aid healing
   c. covering the burned area with an ointment
   d. all of these

7. A diabetic child with symptoms of hypoglycemia should be given
   a. insulin
   b. dry toast
   c. nothing to eat or drink
   d. a glass of orange juice

8. In mouth-to-mouth resuscitation, the rate of breathing for a 7-year-old child is
   a. once every 3 seconds
   b. 30 times per minute
   c. once every 5 seconds
   d. 5 times per minute

9. The Heimlich maneuver is used to treat a child who is
   a. overweight
   b. in shock
   c. asthmatic
   d. choking

10. Frostbitten fingers should be
    a. massaged briskly to increase circulation
    b. quickly placed in water as hot as the child can tolerate
    c. rewarmed quickly in lukewarm water
    d. elevated to reduce pain and swelling

REFERENCES

Feinbloom, R.I. *Child Health Encyclopedia.* New York: Dell Publishing Co., 1978.

Green, Martin I. *A Sigh of Relief.* New York: Bantam Books, 1977.

Harris, C.; Baker, S.; Smith, G.; and Harris, R. "Childhood Asphyxiation by Food." *Journal of the American Medical Association.* 251(7):2231–35, May 4, 1984.

Keim, Katherine A. "Preventing and Treating Plant Poisonings in Young Children." *Journal of Maternal Child Health* 8(4):287–89, July/August 1983.

Meier, Ellen M. "Evaluating Head Trauma in Infants and Children." *Journal of Maternal Child Health* 8(1):54–57, January/February 1983.

Multimedia First Aid. The American Red Cross, 1981.

Additional Reading

First Things First. Upjohn Laboratories, 99 Park Avenue, 3rd Floor, New York, New York 10016. (A children's first aid booklet)

Hunt, W. Thomas. *Elements of Emergency Health Care and Principles of Tort Liability for Educators.* Dubuque, IA: Kendall/Hunt Publishing Co., 1973.

Rhodes, R.; Hafner, K.; Larren, K.; and Rollins, L.M. *Elementary School Health.* Boston: Allyn and Bacon, Inc., 1981.

VanBiervliet, A., and Sheldon-Wildgen, J. *Liability Issues In Community-based Programs.* Baltimore: Brookes Publishing Co., 1981.

Sheldon, Jan B. "Protecting the Preschooler and the Practitioner: Legal Issues in Early Childhood Programs." In *Early Childhood Education: Special Environmental, Policy and Legal Considerations,* edited by E. Goetz and K. E. Allen. Rockville, MD: Aspen Publications, 1983.

Sousa, Barbara. "School Emergencies—Preparation Not Panic." *Journal of School Health* 52(7):437–40, September 1982.

CHILD ABUSE AND NEGLECT

Terms to Know

abuse	intentionally
neglect	verbal assault
discipline	failure to thrive
punishment	mandatory
reprimand	expectations
innocent	precipitating

Objectives

After studying this unit, you will be able to:
- *Distinguish between abuse and neglect.*
- *Identify three types of abuse and two types of neglect.*
- *State four ways that teachers can help abused or neglected children.*
- *Describe characteristics of abusive adults and abused children.*
- *Identify six sources of support and assistance for abusive and neglectful parents.*
- *Describe actions the teacher should take in a case of suspected child abuse.*

There is no completely accurate way to determine the number of *abuse* and *neglect* incidences in this country. However, it is estimated that roughly one million cases of child abuse occur in the United States each year (Gibson 1984). Many times that number probably go unreported. In addition, two to three thousand children die every year as a result of inhumane treatment. Many more are severely injured, suffer permanent physical and mental damage or develop serious emotional problems.

Although child abuse and neglect have occurred throughout history, it is only in the last fifteen to twenty years that public attention has been drawn to the problem. Only now are professionals and lay persons beginning to realize the magnitude of child abuse and neglect as they occur in our society.

Accounts of child abuse date from ancient times to the present. Throughout history children have been abused in every imaginable way, including physical, mental, verbal and sexual abuse. Understandably, the most vulnerable victims of abusive practices have always been handicapped and very young children. In many societies, children had no rights or privileges whatsoever including the right to live.

Perhaps one of the first child abuse cases in this country to attract widespread public attention involved a young girl named Mary Ellen. Friends and neighbors were concerned about the regular beatings Mary Ellen received from her adoptive parents. However, in 1874 there were no organizations responsible for dealing with the problems of child abuse and neglect. Consequently, Mary Ellen's friends contacted the New York Society for the Prevention of Cruelty to Animals on the basis that she was a human being and, therefore, also a member of the animal kingdom. Her parents were found guilty of cruelty to animals and eventually Mary Ellen was removed from their home. This incident brought gradual recognition of the fact that some form of care and protection was needed for the many maltreated, abandoned and handicapped children in this country.

Although child abuse continued to be a major problem, it wasn't until 1961 that the subject once again received national attention. For a period of years, Dr. C. Henry Kempe studied various aspects of child abuse. He was greatly concerned about children whose lives were endangered. He first introduced the phrase "battered child syndrome" in 1961 during a national conference that he organized to discuss the problems related to harsh treatment of children (Kempe 1980).

Nearly twelve years later, on January 31, 1974, the Child Abuse Prevention and Treatment Act (Public Law 93–247) was signed into law creating the National Center on Child Abuse and Neglect. The law also required states, for the first time, to establish definitions, policies, procedures and laws regarding child abuse and neglect. As a result, there are many variations in definitions and reporting procedures.

The passage of Public Law 93–247 marked a turning point in the history of child abuse and neglect. For the first time, each state was to appoint an agency vested with the legal authority to investigate and prosecute incidences of maltreatment.

DISCIPLINE VS. PUNISHMENT

Concern over the maltreatment of children came about because of major changes in public attitude toward the rights of families to *discipline* their children and the invasion of family privacy. For decades, the right to punish or discipline children as families saw fit was considered a parental privilege. Consequently, outsiders often overlooked or ignored incidences of cruelty to children so as not to interfere in a family's personal affairs. Eventually, however, educators, professionals, neighbors and concerned friends realized that maltreatment of young children should no longer be tolerated. It became apparent that someone had to speak out against brutality and represent the innocent children who were being victimized by their families and caretakers.

One of the most difficult aspects of this problem is deciding at what point discipline or *punishment* becomes abuse or neglect. For example, when does a spanking or verbal *reprimand* constitute abuse? In an attempt to establish some guidelines, the federal government passed legislation forcing states to define abuse and neglect and to establish policies and procedures for handling individual cases.

ABUSE AND NEGLECT

Abuse and neglect are generally defined as any situation or environment in which a child is not considered safe because of inadequate protection that may expose the child to hazardous conditions, or because of caretakers who mistreat or *intentionally* inflict injury on the child. For legal purposes, a child is defined as an individual under 18 years of age, Figure 12–1. As further insight is gained into the problem, specific categories of abuse and neglect have been identified:

- physical abuse
- emotional or verbal abuse
- sexual abuse
- physical neglect
- emotional or psychological neglect

Of all the types, physical abuse is the easiest to recognize because the signs are usually quite visible. Physical injuries may include cuts, burns, bruises, bites, welts, fractures, and missing teeth or hair; often there is a combination of old and untreated injuries present.

Incidences of physical abuse frequently begin as an *innocent* means of punishment; in other words, most parents do not set out to intentionally harm their child. However, during the process of disciplining the child, quick tempers and uncontrollable anger lead to punishment that is severe and sufficiently violent to cause injuries and sometimes death. It is often difficult to predict when and if incidences of physical abuse will be repeated as it is more likely to occur during times when the abuser has lost control. Consequently, days, weeks and even months may pass between attacks.

Emotional or verbal abuse is very difficult to detect and prove. Unrealistic parental demands and expectations not based on the child's age and abilities are generally to blame for this form of abuse. Children subjected to this type of abuse live in an environment that is often unpredictable. Consequently, they are *verbally assaulted* and repeatedly criticized, harrassed and belittled for both their behavior and achievements. Understandably, preschool and school-aged children are the most likely victims of emotional abuse. One of the first indications that a child has suffered from verbal abuse is changed or disturbed behavior. Unfortunately, the effects of verbal abuse are often delayed and cumulative, developing gradu-

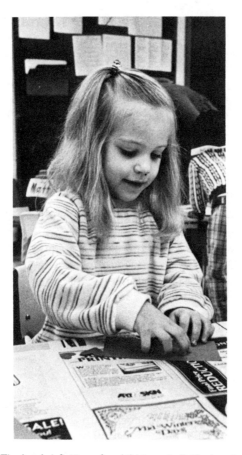

FIGURE 12-1   The legal definition of a child is an individual under 18 years of age.

ally over a period of time. This fact makes it difficult to identify and correct the situation before it leaves permanent scars on a child's personality or development.

Sexual abuse includes any sexual involvement between an adult and a child, including fondling, exhibitionism, rape, and incest. Such acts are considered abuse regardless of whether or not the child agreed to participate (Schultz 1982). It is felt that children are not capable of making rational decisions in these situations or that often they are not free of adult pressure to make the decision they would like to make. Each year there are an estimated 100,000 cases of sexual abuse in the United States (Thomas 1980). Far more cases go unreported than with other forms of abuse. Many times sexual abuse is discovered indirectly or not until years later. Baby-sitters, relatives, caretakers, teachers, and parents have all sexually abused children.

Failure of a parent or legal caretaker to provide for a child's basic needs and care is considered physical neglect. Children may be denied adequate or appropriate food, shelter, clothing, personal cleanliness or medical and dental care. In many states, parents who fail to send their children to school or encourage regular attendance are also guilty of neglect. Grounds for physical neglect can also result from leaving children unsupervised.

Emotional or psychological neglect is perhaps the most difficult of all types to identify and document. For this reason, many states do not include it in their reporting laws. Emotional neglect reflects a basic lack of parental interest or responsiveness to a child's psychological needs and development. Parents fail to see the need to show affection or converse with their infant or child. The absence of emotional stimulation, such as hugging, kissing, touching, conversation, or indications of pleasure or displeasure, can lead to developmental delays and stunted physical growth. The term *failure to thrive* is used to describe this condition when it occurs in infants and young children. Absence of measurable gains in either weight or height is often one of the first indications of psychological neglect.

REPORTING LAWS

Reporting laws support the philosophy that parenthood carries with it certain obligations and responsibilities toward children, Figure 12–2. Punishment of abusive adults is not the primary concern. Instead, the purpose of these laws is to protect children who are not of legal age from maltreatment and exploitation. Every attempt is made to maintain family unity by helping families find solutions to problems that may contribute to child abuse. Criminal action against parents is reserved for only those cases where the parents are not willing or able to cooperate with treatment programs.

Each case of child abuse and/or neglect involves a unique and complex set of conditions (O'Brien 1980). Home environments, work stresses, personalities, temperaments and other factors vary. For this reason, most child abuse laws and definitions are purposefully written in general terms. This practice allows the legal system and social agencies greater flexibility in determining whether or not a parent has acted irresponsibly.

Nearly every state requires physicians to report all cases of suspected abuse and neglect. Reporting is also *mandatory* for additional groups of professionals, including:

- teachers
- nurses
- day care providers
- dentists
- psychologists
- law enforcement personnel
- social workers

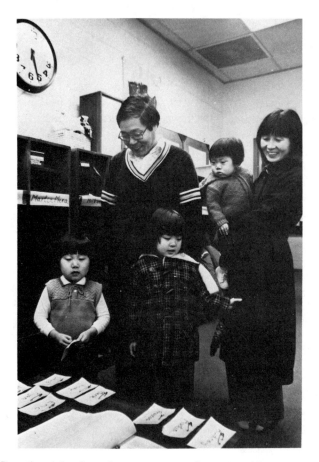

FIGURE 12–2 Parenthood involves the acceptance of certain obligations and responsibilties toward children.

However, it is important that anyone who suspects a child is being abused or neglected contact the nearest child protection authorities. Failure to report prolongs a potentially harmful situation for the child, and can result in criminal prosecution and fines.

Initial reports can be made by telephone. A written report is usually requested within several days, Table 12–1. All information is kept strictly confidential, including the identity of the person making the report. Protection against liability and criminal charges is extended in most reporting laws to anyone who reports abuse or neglect without intent to harm another person.

Suspicions of abuse and neglect do not have to be proven before they are reported. If teachers or child care staff have reason to believe that a child is being mistreated or inadequately cared for, child protective services should be contacted immediately. Trained personnel will meet with the family and evaluate the situation. Also, when an abuse or neglect report is filed by a teacher or child care provider, it is not necessary to inform the parents.

TABLE 12-1   Items to Include in a Written Child Abuse/Neglect Report

---

1. The name and address of the child and the parents or caretakers (if known).
2. The child's age.
3. The nature and extent of the child's injuries or description of neglect including any evidence of previous injuries or deprivation.
4. The identity of the offending adult (if known).
5. Other information that the reporting person believes may be helpful in establishing the cause of injuries or neglect.

FACTORS CONTRIBUTING TO ABUSE AND NEGLECT

Abusive adults come from all levels of social, economic, educational, racial, religious and occupational backgrounds (Pelton 1978). They live in rural areas as well as small towns and large cities. It is a common misconception that child abuse and neglect are committed by people who are uneducated, alcoholics, or have low income. While it is true that the incidence of abuse and neglect is higher among this group, like most assumptions about complex social and economic issues generalizations often are too simple.

Perhaps one reason why individuals from disadvantaged families are reported more often is because of their greater use of, and dependency on, public and social services. Furthermore, daily living is often more stressful for low income families. Simply finding adequate food, clothing, housing and transportation can be an overwhelming task.

On the other hand, persons from upper socioeconomic levels generally can afford private medical care and the services of multiple doctors in nearby cities. These factors may make it easier to cover up abuse or neglect and avoid being caught.

To help understand the complex nature of child abuse and neglect, three risk factors have been identified:

- characteristics of abusing adults
- presence of a child who is different
- environmental stresses

It is usually thought that for abuse and neglect to take place, all three risk factors are present at the same time.

Characteristics of Abusive Adults

More is known about the personalities and traits of the abusive adult than perhaps any other aspect of child abuse and neglect. Certain behaviors and predispositions are known to be consistent from one case to another. Although not every abusive adult fits the description, likewise not all persons who fit the pattern are necessarily abusive.

Many abusive adults have been abused as children. Consequently, they believe that harsh punishment is the only way to discipline children because this is the method with which they are most familiar. Repeated anger, rejection and fear have filled their lives. They often turn to early marriage and children to satisfy the need to be wanted and loved. Only a small percentage of abusive parents have drug or alcohol-related problems.

Feelings of inadequacy and poor self-image are also typical. As if to reinforce these feelings, they often seek jobs that they see as having little importance and status, such as factory work, waitressing and cleaning. Their relationships with people, including spouses, are often unstable. A lack of trust makes it difficult for them to get along with others. The inability to form supportive friendships gradually leads to social isolation and feelings of helplessness.

An absence of good parenting skills is also common among many abusive adults. Inadequate knowledge often gives the impression that a parent does not care about their child. However, in many instances, it is simply that parents do not know how to provide proper care and protection for their children. Consequently, their expectations for children are unrealistic and developmentally inappropriate based on the child's age. For example, a parent may become angry and abusive because a fifteen-month-old child wets the bed, a toddler spills milk, or a seven year old loses a mitten.

Many abusive adults also have a low tolerance for stress or have a great deal of stress in their lives. They are easily frustrated, impulsive and impatient with children. Eventually, anger provokes abuse.

Presence of a Child Who Is Different

Often an abusive parent or adult singles out one child whom they consider to be different in some way from their *expectations*. These differences may be real or only imagined, but the adult is convinced they exist. Qualities that are frequently cited by abusive adults include a child who is:

- handicapped
- disobedient or uncooperative
- physically unattractive
- unintelligent
- hyperactive
- fussy
- clumsy
- frequently ill
- very timid or weak
- similar in appearance to someone the adult dislikes

Children under three years of age and handicapped children are the most frequent victims of abuse. However, abuse incidents are also very high among children born out of wedlock or from unwanted or unplanned pregnancies, and among stepchildren. Neglect is more commonly reported among infants and children over six years of age. Both sexes are abused and neglected almost equally.

Environmental Stresses

All families face conflict and crises from time to time. However, some families are able to cope with stressful events better than others. In the case of abusive or neglectful families, environmental stresses are usually the *precipitating* factor. That is, a conflict is sufficient to push them to action (abuse) or withdrawal (neglect) as a caretaker.

The abusive or neglectful adult often reacts to stressful events without distinguishing the true magnitude of the conflict. Instead, they find all crises overwhelming and difficult to deal with. The following examples illustrate the wide range of physical and environmental stresses that can lead to loss of control when they occur in combination with other factors:

- flat tire
- clogged sink
- broken window
- lost keys
- loss of a job
- illness, injury or death
- financial pressures
- divorce or other marital problems
- moving
- birth of another child

Some of these events may seem trivial in comparison to others. Yet, they may become the "straw that breaks the camel's back" and may be responsible for triggering abusive behavior when they occur in conjunction with other stressful events. A parent or caretaker frequently responds by losing control and reacting inappropriately regardless of the seriousness of the actual event. In turn, anger and frustration are taken out on the child.

THE ROLE OF THE TEACHER

Teachers and child care providers are in an ideal position to help identify children who are abused and neglected. Close daily contact with children makes it possible to observe unusual behaviors and changes in physical appearance, Table 12–2. Also, a teacher may be the only person a child trusts enough to discuss abusive treatment.

For these reasons, teachers in most states are required by law to report suspected cases of abuse and neglect. (Department of Health, Education and Welfare 1975). They are not required to prove their beliefs as long as the report is

TABLE 12-2 Observation List for Recognizing Abused and Neglected Children

Physical Abuse
- repeated or unexplained injuries, e.g., burns, fractures, bruises, bites, eye or head injuries
- frequently complains of pain
- wears clothing to hide injuries; may be inappropriate for weather conditions
- reports harsh treatment
- frequently late or absent; arrives too early or stays after dismissal from school
- unusually fearful of adults, especially parents
- appears malnourished or dehydrated
- avoids logical explanations for injuries
- withdrawn, anxious or uncommunicative or may be outspoken and disruptive
- lacks affection, both giving and seeking
- may be given inappropriate food, beverage or drugs

Emotional Abuse
- generally unhappy; seldom smiles or laughs
- aggressive and disruptive or unusually shy and withdrawn
- reacts without emotion to unpleasant statements and actions
- displays behaviors that are unusually adult or childlike
- delayed growth and/or emotional and intellectual development

Sexual Abuse
- underclothing torn, stained or bloody
- complains of pain or itching in the genital area
- has venereal disease
- has difficulty getting along with other children, e.g., withdrawn, babylike, anxious
- rapid weight loss or gain
- sudden failure in school performance
- involved in delinquency, including prostitution, running away, alcoholism or drug abuse
- fascination with body parts; talks about sexual activities

Physical Neglect
- repeatedly arrives unclean; may have a bad odor from dirty clothing or hair
- is in need of medical or dental care; may have untreated injuries or illness
- frequently hungry; begs or steals food while at school
- dresses inappropriately for weather conditions; shoes and clothing often sized too small or too large
- is chronically tired; falls asleep at school, lacks the energy to play with other children
- has difficulty getting along with other children; spends much time alone

Emotional Neglect
- poor academic performance
- appears apathetic, withdrawn and inattentive
- frequently absent or late to school
- uses any means to gain teacher's attention and approval
- seldom participates in extracurricular activities
- engages in delinquent behaviors, e.g., stealing, vandalism, sexual misconduct, abuse of drugs or alcohol

Source: Adapted from *New Light on an Old Problem*. U.S. Department of Health, Education and Welfare, (DHEW Publication No. 70-31108), Washington, DC, 1978.

made in good faith. By making a report, the teacher is merely indicating that a family or individual may be in need of help.

Child abuse and neglect is often exhibited as a pattern of behavior. Therefore, it is important that teachers document each incidence. Written reports should be precise and include the following information:

- the type, location, size and severity of any injury
- the child's explanation of how the injury occurred
- any explanation provided by the parents or caretakers of how the injury happened
- obvious signs of neglect, e.g., malnutrition, uncleanliness, inappropriate dress, excessive fatigue, lack of medical or dental care
- recent or drastic changes in the child's behavior
- quality of parent/child interactions.

Such information is useful for deciding on appropriate services and rehabilitative treatment programs for individuals and families. A teacher's written observations can also be extremely valuable to child protective agencies as evidence should the need arise.

Helping Abused or Neglected Children

As educators, preschool teachers and child care providers also play an important role in helping maltreated children deal with the effects of abuse and neglect. As a positive role model, the teacher can accept children for what they are, listen to their problems, encourage their efforts and praise their successes (Evans 1980). For many children it may be the first time any adult has shown a sincere interest in them as a person without threatening or causing them harm.

As a trusting relationship is established, children can gradually be encouraged to verbalize their feelings. Play therapy is especially useful with young children. It can help them act out anger, fears, and anxieties related to abusive incidents. Housekeeping activities and doll play are ideal activities for this purpose. Talking about how the doll (child) feels when it is mistreated can help to bring out a child's real feelings about their own treatment. At the same time, teachers can demonstrate good parenting skills, such as appropriate ways to treat and care for the dolls.

Artwork can also be an effective means for helping young children express their feelings and concerns. For example, self-portraits may reveal an exaggeration of certain body parts or how children actually feel about themselves. Pictures may also depict unusual practices that children have been subjected to, such as being tied up or locked in a closet or dark room.

Extreme caution must be exercised in any attempt to interpret children's artwork. A child's immature drawing skills and lack of special training can easily lead an inexperienced observer to misinterpretation and false conclusions. Therefore, it is best to view unusual items in children's drawings as additional clues, rather than absolute indications of abuse or neglect.

Annoying or irritating behaviors used by some children to gain attention can sometimes trigger an adult's abusive actions. Teachers can help children with such behaviors by teaching them how to express their feelings in ways that are both appropriate and socially acceptable. For example, a teacher might say, "Rosa, if you want another cracker, you need to use your words to ask for it. No one can understand you when you whine or cry." They can also do much to build and strengthen trusting relationships with these children. Gradually, the abused or neglected child's self-concept will also improve as teachers:

- respond to children in a loving and accepting manner
- set aside a private space that children can call their own
- establish gradual limits for acceptable behavior; set routines and schedules that provide order in children's lives that often have been dominated by turmoil
- let children know they are available whenever they need someone, whether it be for companionship, extra attention, or reassurance, Figure 12–3.
- take time to prepare children for new experiences; knowing what is expected enhances the "safeness" of the child's environment
- encourage children to talk about their feelings, fears and concerns.

Little attention has been paid to helping children recognize when they are being severely mistreated. Unless children are informed otherwise, it is difficult

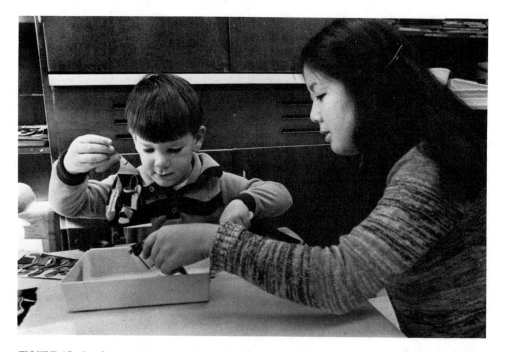

FIGURE 12–3 Caring adults can provide extra companionship, reassurance and individualized attention.

for them to realize that being beaten, forced to engage in sexual activity, or left alone for days is not normal or the type of treatment they deserve. Materials are slowly being developed for children, especially in the area of sexual abuse, Table 12–3. A variety of professionals, including nurses, doctors, mental health personnel, social workers and psychologists also can be called upon to aid in the development and presentation of such programs. Even when children do not fully understand the problems involved with something as complex as abuse and neglect, it is useful for them to know when and where to go for help.

TABLE 12–3   Sexual Abuse Resources for Children

"My Body: A Book to Teach Young Children How to Resist Uncomfortable Touch." Send $2.95 to:
Planned Parenthood of Snohomish County
Book Order
2730 Hoyt
Everett, WA 98201
(206) 259–0096
A resource book is also available for parents and teachers to use in conjunction with the above booklet. To order, send $5.00 ($1.25 postage and handling) to the same address and request "A Parent's Resource Booklet."

"Private Zone" by Frances S. Dayee. To order, send $2.00 ($.75 postage and handling) to:
The Charles Franklin Press
Department FW, 18409
90th Avenue W.
Edmonds, WA 98020

"Red Flag, Green Flag People" by Joy Williams. Send $4.00 to:
Rape and Abuse Crisis Center of Fargo-Moorhead
317 8th Street North
Fargo, ND 58102
(701) 293–7273

"No More Secrets" by Caren Adams and Jennifer Fay. Order from:
Impact Publishers
P.O. Box 1094
San Luis Obispo, CA 93406

"He Told Me Not To Tell." To Order, send $2.95 to:
Network Publications
ETR Associates
1700 Mission St., Suite 203
P.O. Box 8506
Santa Cruz, CA 95061–8506

"Ice Cream Isn't Always Good." To order, send $1.00 to:
Project Two
P.O. Box 5092–FD
F.D.R. Station
New York, NY 10150

Helping Parents

Parenting is a demanding task (Gibson 1984). Many parents today have not had the same opportunities to learn parenting skills that past generations once had. Without sound knowledge and adequate resources, everyday stresses can lead to abusive and neglectful treatment of children.

There are many ways teachers can help parents. Contacts with parents provide opportunities for recognizing families in crises and helping them find solutions to their problems. Teachers can share valuable skills and a wealth of knowledge with parents to improve their child-rearing practices and strengthen family unity. Supportive relationships can also be established through parent-teacher interactions. These are important as early intervention and prevention measures.

On a more structured basis, teachers can get involved in presenting a series of discussions or workshops that would be useful to parents. These could be sponsored by a school, child development center or in cooperation with other community agencies. Topics most parents will find of interest include:

- information on child growth and development
- identification and management of behavior problems
- principles of good nutrition
- how to meet children's social and emotional needs at different stages
- preventive health care for preschool and school-aged children
- locating and utilizing community resources
- stress and tension relievers for parents
- financial planning
- organizing a parent self-help group

Participation in community organizations and public awareness programs is another valuable contribution teachers can make. With knowledge of community resources and services available to children and parents, teachers and child care providers can direct families to appropriate sources of help. This can be one of the most important steps in avoiding abusive and neglectful situations. A wide range of services is offered in most communities, including:

- protective services
- day care and "crisis" nurseries
- mental health counseling for parents, children and families
- help or "hot lines"
- temporary foster homes
- homemaker services
- transportation
- financial assistance
- parenting classes
- employment assistance
- home visitors
- self-help or support groups

Inservice Training

Teachers and child care providers are morally and legally responsible for recognizing the early signs of child abuse and neglect. However, to be effective, they need to be well informed. Through inservice training sessions, teachers can gain the basic knowledge and understanding necessary to carry out this function. Suggested topics for inservice programs might include:

- an explanation of relevant state laws
- teachers' rights and responsibilities
- how to identify child abuse and neglect
- development of a school policy and procedures for handling suspected cases
- exploration of teachers' and staff reactions to abuse and neglect
- identifying community resources and services
- ways to help abused and neglected children in the classroom.

SUMMARY

Child abuse and neglect are not new problems. However, passage of the Child Abuse Prevention and Treatment Act (Public Law 93–247) has gradually brought about increased public awareness of the problem, along with legal protection for the children involved.

Each state has had to develop its own legal definition of what constitutes abuse and neglect. In general, resulting laws are designed to encompass any situation in which a child is not likely to be safe from abuse and neglect. For legal purposes, five categories of abuse and neglect have been identified: physical abuse, emotional or verbal abuse, sexual abuse, physical neglect, emotional or psychological neglect.

The major purpose of child abuse laws is to protect children and strengthen the family as a unit. Most states require teachers and child care personnel to report suspected incidences of child abuse or neglect to a designated agency.

The probability for abuse and neglect is thought to be greatest when a combination of three factors occur simultaneously: characteristics of abusing adults, the presence of a child who is different, environmental stresses.

Frequently, abusive adults were themselves abused or neglected as children. As a group, abusive adults tend to exhibit feelings of inadequacy, poor self-image, isolation, loneliness and difficulty handling stressful situations. They often lack good parenting skills and proper knowledge of child growth and development. They commonly believe that harsh forms of punishment are necessary to discipline children.

The risk and incidence of abuse and neglect are known to be greater for certain groups of children. Those who are handicapped, under three years of age, viewed as being different by parents, born out of wedlock or are stepchildren run the highest risk for being abused and neglected.

A crisis or series of crises is often the factor that triggers explosive or inattentive behaviors on the part of the adult caretaker. Low tolerances for stress and limited ability to deal with it make every crisis seem overwhelming.

Teachers perform many valuable roles in the prevention and treatment of child abuse and neglect through:

- identification and documentation of suspected cases
- emotional support for abused or neglected children
- helping children learn socially acceptable behaviors
- alerting children to situations involving maltreatment in the home and community
- parent education
- participation in community programs
- inservice training

These many contributions are essential to lowering the incidence of child abuse and neglect.

LEARNING ACTIVITIES

1. Gather statistics on the incidence of child abuse and neglect for your city, county and state. Compare them to the national rates.

2. Write a two-minute public service announcement for radio and television alerting the community to the problems of child abuse and neglect.

3. Locate at least five agencies or services in your community that provide assistance to abusive or neglectful families. Collect materials from these agencies describing their services.

4. Prepare a pamphlet to help young children recognize abusive and neglectful situations and how to protect themselves.

UNIT REVIEW

A. Briefly define each of the following terms:

1. child

2. abuse

3. neglect

4. reporting laws

5. environmental stresses

B. Complete the given statements by selecting the correct answer from the following list.

teachers	sexual
trust	childhood
physical	definition
psychological	expectations
neglect	identify
confidential	reported

1. A child's fascination with body parts and talk about sexual activities may be an indication of _____ abuse.

2. Public Law 93–247 requires states to write a legal _____ of child abuse and neglect.

3. Injury that is intentionally inflicted on a child is called _____ abuse.

4. Malnutrition, lack of proper clothing or inadequate adult supervision are examples of physical _____.

5. Verbal abuse sometimes results because of unrealistic parent demands and _____.

6. Emotional or _____ neglect is one of the most difficult forms of neglect to identify.

7. Reporting laws usually require _____ to report suspected cases of child abuse and neglect.

8. Information contained in reports of child abuse or neglect is kept _____.

9. Many abusive adults were abused during their own _____.

10. Lack of _____ makes it difficult for many abusive and neglectful adults to form friendships.

11. Daily contact with children helps teachers to _____ children who are abused or neglected.

12. Abuse or neglect does not have to be proven before it should be _____.

C. Briefly answer each of the following questions.

1. List five clues that would help teachers recognize a child who is being physically abused.

2. What should teachers do if they suspect that a child is being abused or neglected?

3. What information should be included in both an oral and written report?

4. State four ways that teachers and child care providers can help abused and neglected children in the classroom.

5. List six types of services that are available in many communities to help abusive or neglectful families.

6. Why does the incidence of child abuse and neglect appear to be higher among disadvantaged families?

D. Case Study

When it was time for snacks, four-year-old Jimmy said he wasn't hungry and refused to come over and sit down. At the teacher's gentle insistence, Jimmy reluctantly joined the other children at the table. Tears began to roll down his cheeks as he tried to sit in his chair. Jimmy's teacher watched for a few moments and then walked over to talk with him. Initially, he denied that anything was wrong, but later told the teacher that he "had fallen the night before and hurt his leg."

The teacher took Jimmy aside and comforted him. She asked Jimmy if he would show her where he had been hurt. When Jimmy loosened his jeans, the teacher observed what appeared to be a large burn with some blistering approximately two inches in length by one inch in width on his left buttock. Several small bruises were also evident along one side of the burn. Again, the teacher asked Jimmy how he had been hurt and again he replied that "he had fallen."

1. What actions should Jimmy's teacher take? Should she tell anyone else?

2. Would you recommend that Jimmy's teacher report the incidence right away or wait until she has gathered more evidence? Why?

3. To whom should the teacher report what she observed?

4. Using the information provided, write up a complete description of Jimmy's injury.

5. If you were Jimmy's teacher, would your feelings and responses be any different if this was a first-time versus a repeated occurrence?

6. Is it necessary for the teacher to notify Jimmy's parents before making a report?

7. In what ways can the teacher be of immediate help to Jimmy?

8. What should the teacher do if this happens again?

REFERENCES

Child Abuse and Neglect: The Problem and Its Management. Vol. 1. Washington, DC: Department of Health, Education and Welfare. Publication No. (OHD) 75–30073, 1975.

Evans, Marilyn, and Hansen, Beverly. *Guide To Pediatric Nursing.* New York: Appleton-Century-Crofts, 1980.

Gibson, Janice. "The Specter of Child Abuse." *Parents* 59(3):128, March 1984.

Helberg, June L. "Documentation In Child Abuse." *American Journal of Nursing* 83(2):234–39, February 1983.

Kempe, C. Henry, and Helfer, Ray. *The Battered Child.* Chicago: University of Chicago Press, 1980.

O'Brien, Shirley. *A Crying Shame.* Provo, UT: Brigham Young University Press, 1980.

Pelton, Leroy H. "Child Abuse and Neglect: The Myths of Classlessness." *American Journal of Orthopsychiatry* 48:608–16, October 1978.

Schultz, Leroy. "Child Sexual Abuse In Historical Perspective." *Social Work and Child Sexual Abuse,* Fall/Winter 1982.

Thomas, Joyce N. "Yes, You Can Help A Sexually Abused Child." *RN* 43(8):23–29, August 1980.

Additional Reading

Children's Defense Budget: An Analysis of the President's F.Y. 1984 Budget and Children. Washington, D.C.: Children's Defense Fund, 1983.

Child Abuse and Neglect: A Training Guide for Treating the Child and Family. Edited by N.B. Ebeling and D.A. Hill. Littleton, MA: John-Wright-PSG, Inc., 1983.

Ellerstein, Norman S. *Child Abuse and Neglect.* New York: John Wiley and Sons, 1981.

National Center on Child Abuse and Neglect: Sexual Abuse of Children (Selected Readings). U.S. Department of Health and Human Services, 1980.

Rose, Barbara C. "Child Abuse and the Educator." *Focus on Exceptional Children* 16(9):1–13, May 1980.

Tschirhart-Sanford, Linda. *The Silent Children: A Parent's Guide to the Prevention of Child Abuse.* New York: McGraw-Hill Book Co., 1980.

Young, L. *Wednesday's Children.* New York: McGraw-Hill, 1964.

SIX

FOODS AND NUTRIENTS: BASIC CONCEPTS

Unit 13
NUTRITIONAL GUIDELINES

Terms to Know

essential   nutrient-density
nutrient strength   overnutrition
nutrient weakness   Index of Nutrient Quality

Objectives

After studying this unit you will be able to:
- Classify foods according to the Basic Four Food Groups.
- State nutrient strengths and nutrient weaknesses for each of the Basic Four Food Groups.
- State the differences between the Recommended Daily Dietary Allowances and the United States Recommended Daily Allowances.
- Explain nutrient density.
- Determine the relative nutrient contribution of foods using the Index of Nutrient Quality formula.

Good nutrition affects the health and well-being of individuals of all ages. It is important to note that all persons throughout life need the same nutrients, but in varying amounts. Small children need nutrients for growth and energy; adults need nutrients to maintain or repair body tissue and to provide energy.

To teach good food habits, the care provider or parent must first set a good example. Children frequently model behaviors they see in people they love and admire, such as parents and teachers. To set a good example, the care provider must possess the knowledge to maintain good personal nutrition. A good basic understanding of one's own nutrient needs is essential for good personal dietary practices. The ability to apply nutrition knowledge to the care of children will hopefully follow.

Nutrition is the study of food and how it is used by the body. Nutritionists study foods because foods contain nutrients, which are chemical substances with specific uses in the body. The body has three basic uses for nutrients:

- sources of energy
- materials for growth and maintenance of body tissue
- regulation of body processes

Table 13–1 shows the relationship between nutrients, their food sources and functions.

TABLE 13–1   Nutrients: Their Food Sources and Functions

FOOD SOURCE	NUTRIENT	FUNCTION
Dairy	Carbohydrates	
Protein	Fats	Energy
Fruits and Vegetables	Proteins	
Grains	Minerals	Growth
	Water	
	Vitamins	Regulation

Nutrients are needed in adequate amounts for normal body function to take place. An inadequate supply of nutrients or poor utilization of nutrients lead to abnormal body function which is detrimental to overall good health.

Approximately fifty nutrients are known to be *essential* for humans. An essential nutrient is one which must be provided by food substances as the body is unable to manufacture it in adequate amounts. Scientists have been able to determine the approximate amounts of many nutrients needed by the body. Information is also available listing the amounts of many nutrients found in specific foods.

Good nutrition is dependent upon combinations of foods which provide nutritious meals on a daily basis. In the interest of simplifying this process, a number of meal plans or guidelines have been developed. Any of the guidelines discussed will promote healthful eating habits; the choice lies with the individual and may depend on time available, ease of use, and interest.

Regardless of the guideline selected, the common factor necessary for good nutrition is the inclusion of a wide variety of foods. A variety of foods is most likely to supply the greatest number of nutrients. Some foods contain many nutrients while others contain only a few nutrients. No single food contains enough of all nutrients to support life. The only exception is breast milk, which contains all the nutrients known to be needed by an infant until about three months of age. If a person consumes adequate amounts of the following "leader" nutrients, other nutrients will, theoretically, be consumed in large enough amounts to meet body needs.

Protein	Vitamin C	Niacin
Carbohydrate	Thiamin	Calcium
Fat	Riboflavin	Iron
Vitamin A		

A pattern of consuming the same food over time provides the same nutrient strengths and also the same nutrient weaknesses.

THE BASIC FOUR FOOD GROUPS

The simplest and easiest plan for good nutrition is the Basic Four Food Groups (Guthrie 1983). This plan is made up of four groups of foods:

- The Dairy Group
- The High Protein Group
- The Fruit and Vegetable Group
- The Grain Group

The foods within each group provide similar amounts of leader nutrients. Each group is marked by *nutrient strengths* and *nutrient weaknesses.* Nutrient strengths are nutrients which occur in relatively large amounts in the foods within a group. Nutrient weaknesses are those nutrients which are found in small amounts or not at all within a food group. The Basic Four Food Group plan is easy to follow because the units used are foods rather than nutrients. (It is easier to plan 2 to 3 servings of milk than it is to plan 800 milligrams of calcium.) Numbers of servings from each group are the basis for planning daily intakes when following the Basic Four Food Groups. The number of servings are listed for each group; the small child's serving is approximately half that suggested for adults. A good rule of thumb when planning food for children is "one tablespoon of food per each year of age."

The Dairy Group

The Dairy Group includes milk and dairy products. Children should have a total of three cups of milk or the equivalent from this group daily. The servings may be divided into one-half cup portions in consideration of children's smaller appetites and capacity. Adults need two cups of milk or the equivalent daily. Equivalent foods include cheeses, yogurt, ice cream, custards and puddings. Equivalent amounts of foods may vary due to the addition of other ingredients such as fruit or sugar. Foods which provide calcium equal to that in one cup of milk are:

$1\frac{1}{2}$ ounces cheddar cheese
1 cup pudding
$1\frac{3}{4}$ cup ice cream
1 cup plain yogurt

Nutrient Summary: Dairy Group

Nutrient Strengths	Nutrient Weaknesses
Calcium	Vitamin C
Protein	Iron
Riboflavin	

The High Protein Group

The recommended daily amount from the High Protein Group is two or more servings. The amount of food in a serving varies with the age of the individual. Small children need and often will eat only 1 to 1½ ounces in a serving, while the adult serving consists of 2 to 3 ounces of meat or equivalent. Beef, veal, pork, lamb, fish and poultry are included in the High Protein Group. Other foods included in this group are eggs, legumes such as dry peas and beans, nuts and nut butters, Figure 13–1. Cheese may also be substituted for meats; however, it should be remembered that cheeses do not contain iron which is a nutrient strength of the High Protein Group. The following foods contain protein equal to that in one ounce of meat:

> 1 egg
> 1 ounce of cheese
> ¼ cup cottage cheese
> ½ cup dried peas or beans
> 2 tablespoons peanut butter

Nutrient Summary: High Protein Group

Nutrient Strengths	Nutrient Weaknesses
Protein	Calcium
Thiamin	Vitamin C
Niacin	Vitamin A
Iron	

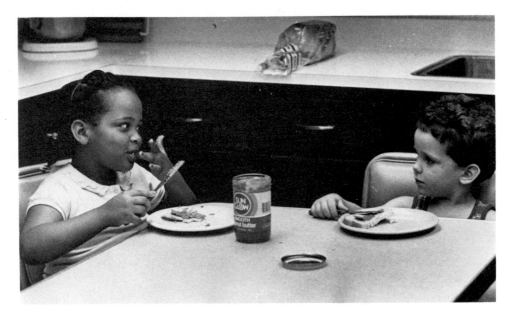

FIGURE 13–1 Peanut butter is a popular food from the High Protein Food Group.

TABLE 13-2   Good to Excellent Sources of Vitamin C

Orange*	Tomatoes*
Orange Juice*	Grapefruit*
Strawberries*	Mustard greens
Cauliflower	Spinach
Broccoli	Cabbage
Sweet Peppers, red or green	Tangerine*

*May cause allergic reactions

Fruit and Vegetable Group

The Fruit and Vegetable Group consists of a large number of fruits and vegetables. Fruits and vegetables contribute a great variety of nutrients. The following rules are helpful in choosing wisely from this group.

1 serving daily—citrus fruit or juice, or other fruit or vegetable rich in Vitamin C, Table 13-2.

1 serving every other day—dark green vegetable or deep orange vegetable or fruit, or other fruit or vegetable rich in Vitamin A, Table 13-3.

2 servings daily—choose a variety from the remaining foods from this group.

The daily total should include four or more servings from the Fruit and Vegetable Group. An adult serving is ½ cup canned fruit, vegetable or juice, or one medium-sized piece of raw fruit. The child's serving is about half that of the adult serving.

Nutrient Summary: Fruit and Vegetable Group

Nutrient Strengths	Nutrient Weaknesses
Vitamin A	Good Quality Protein
Vitamin C	Fat
Fiber	Vitamin B_{12}

TABLE 13-3   Good to Excellent Sources of Vitamin A

Liver	Winter Squash
Carrots	Greens
Pumpkin	Apricots
Sweet Potatoes	Watermelon*
Spinach	Broccoli

*May cause allergic reactions

The Grain Group

Such foods as breads, breakfast cereals, pastas and flour make up the Grain Group. Food choices from this group should be whole grain or enriched products. Whole grain products retain all of the grain. Enriched breads and cereals are products that have been processed and specified amounts of nutrients have been added. The nutrients which are added are iron, thiamin, riboflavin, and niacin. The amounts of these added nutrients are equal to those found in the whole grain.

A serving from this group consists of one slice of bread, one cup of dry, ready-to-eat cereal or ½ cup of cooked cereal or pasta. As with the other groups, the child's serving is one-half the adult serving. Four or more servings daily are recommended.

Nutrient Summary: The Grain Group

Nutrient Strengths	*Nutrient Weaknesses*
Iron	Calcium
Thiamin	Vitamin A
Niacin	Vitamin C
Riboflavin	
Complex Carbohydrates	

OTHER FOODS

Many foods commonly eaten do not fit precisely into one of the Basic Four Food Groups. Refined sugars, oils and fats, and alcohol are not included in the Basic Four but make contributions to the average person's diet. These foods are often listed under a grouping called Other Foods. In general, the nutrient content of this group is low and the calorie content is high. The addition to the diet of large amounts of foods from the Other Foods group can dilute the nutrient content of foods from the Basic Four Food Groups. Table 13–4 illustrates the dilution of the Vitamin C in an apple by the addition of sugar and fat. Calorie content increases, with the addition of sugar. Further increases in calories occur with the addition of fat and flour in making apple pie. At the same time the calories are increasing the amount of Vitamin C present decreases.

TABLE 13–4   Comparison of Caloric Increase and Nutrient Decrease
When Sugar and Fats Are Added to the Diet

	CALORIES	VITAMIN C
Apple, raw, 3/ #	80	6 mg
Applesauce, sweetened, 1 cup	230	3 mg
Apple pie, ¹/₇ pie	342	2 mg
Pie a la Mode, ¹/₇ pie plus ½ cup ice cream	480	2 mg

Source: Home and Garden Bulletin No. 72.

RECOMMENDED DAILY DIETARY ALLOWANCES

Recommended Daily Dietary Allowances (RDA) are guidelines published by the National Academy of Sciences for the amounts of nutrients needed by most healthy people, categorized according to age and sex. These guidelines are up-dated about every five years in an effort to reflect the most up-to-date knowledge about nutrient needs. The latest revision was done in 1980, Table 13–5.

In order for the Recommended Daily Dietary Allowances guidelines to be meaningful, nutrient content of foods must be known (check the references at the end of this unit). Evaluation of a diet by means of the Recommended Daily Dietary Allowances guidelines requires the following steps:

1. List the amounts of all foods and beverages consumed during the day.

2. Using a nutrient table, determine the nutrient content of each food and beverage consumed.

3. Total the amount of each nutrient consumed during the day.

4. Determine if nutrients consumed are in sufficient amounts by comparing the total amount of each nutrient consumed with the Recommended Daily Dietary Allowances for the appropriate age and sex group.

UNITED STATES RECOMMENDED DAILY ALLOWANCES (U.S. RDA)

The United States Recommended Daily Allowances are adapted by the Food and Drug Administration from the National Academy of Sciences Recommended Daily Dietary Allowances. The U.S. RDA differ from the Recommended Daily Dietary Allowances in the following ways:

- The U.S. RDA groups all persons over four years of age in one group.
- U.S. RDA levels are usually equal to the highest Recommended Daily Dietary Allowances for a specific nutrient, Table 13–6.

U.S. RDA are a means of helping the consumer determine which foods are good sources of nutrients, Table 13–7. Nutrient information is found on food labels in terms of percentages of U.S. RDA, Figure 13–2.

U.S. DIETARY GUIDELINES

U.S. Dietary Guidelines are a proposal of the U.S. Senate Select Committee on Nutrition (Dietary Guidelines 1979). They are based on many hours of testimony and opinions and knowledge of numerous experts in nutrition. The Guidelines were proposed as a result of great concern about possible relationships

TABLE 13–5 Recommended Daily Dietary Allowances,[a] Revised 1980.
Designed for the maintenance of good nutrition of practically all healthy people in the U.S.A.

	Age (years)	Weight (kg)	Weight (lbs)	Height (cm)	Height (in)	Protein (g)	Vitamin A (µg R.E.)[b]	Vitamin D (µg)[c]	Vitamin E (mg α T.E.)[d]	Vitamin C (mg)	Thiamin (mg)	Riboflavin (mg)	Niacin (mg N.E.)[e]	Vitamin B6 (mg)	Folacin (µg)[f]	Vitamin B12 (µg)	Calcium (mg)	Phosphorus (mg)	Magnesium (mg)	Iron (mg)	Zinc (mg)	Iodine (µg)
Infants	0.0–0.5	6	13	60	24	kg × 2.2	420	10	3	35	0.3	0.4	6	0.3	30	0.5[g]	360	240	50	10	3	40
	0.5–1.0	9	20	71	28	kg × 2.0	400	10	4	35	0.5	0.6	8	0.6	45	1.5	540	360	70	15	5	50
Children	1–3	13	29	90	35	23	400	10	5	45	0.7	0.8	9	0.9	100	2.0	800	800	150	15	10	70
	4–6	20	44	112	44	30	500	10	6	45	0.9	1.0	11	1.3	200	2.5	800	800	200	10	10	90
	7–10	28	62	132	52	34	700	10	7	45	1.2	1.4	16	1.6	300	3.0	800	800	250	10	10	120
Males	11–14	45	99	157	62	45	1000	10	8	50	1.4	1.6	18	1.8	400	3.0	1200	1200	350	18	15	150
	15–18	66	145	176	69	56	1000	10	10	60	1.4	1.7	18	2.0	400	3.0	1200	1200	400	18	15	150
	19–22	70	154	177	70	56	1000	7.5	10	60	1.5	1.7	19	2.2	400	3.0	800	800	350	10	15	150
	23–50	70	154	178	70	56	1000	5	10	60	1.4	1.6	18	2.2	400	3.0	800	800	350	10	15	150
	51+	70	154	178	70	56	1000	5	10	60	1.2	1.4	16	2.2	400	3.0	800	800	350	10	15	150
Females	11–14	46	101	157	62	46	800	10	8	50	1.1	1.3	15	1.8	400	3.0	1200	1200	300	18	15	150
	15–18	55	120	163	64	46	800	10	8	60	1.1	1.3	14	2.0	400	3.0	1200	1200	300	18	15	150
	19–22	55	120	163	64	44	800	7.5	8	60	1.1	1.3	14	2.0	400	3.0	800	800	300	18	15	150
	23–50	55	120	163	64	44	800	5	8	60	1.0	1.2	13	2.0	400	3.0	800	800	300	18	15	150
	51+	55	120	163	64	44	800	5	8	60	1.0	1.2	13	2.0	400	3.0	800	800	300	10	15	150
Pregnant						+30	+200	+5	+2	+20	+0.4	+0.3	+2	+0.6	+400	+1.0	+400	+400	+150	h	+5	+25
Lactating						+20	+400	+5	+3	+40	+0.5	+0.5	+5	+0.5	+100	+1.0	+400	+400	+150	h	+10	+50

[a] The allowances are intended to provide for individual variations among most normal persons as they live in the United States under usual environmental stresses. Diets should be based on a variety of common foods in order to provide other nutrients for which human requirements have been less well defined.

[b] Retinol equivalents. 1 retinol equivalent = 1 µg retinol or 6 µg β-carotene.

[c] As cholecalciferol. 10 µg cholecalciferol = 400 I.U. vitamin D.

[d] α tocopherol equivalents. 1 mg d-α-tocopherol = 1 α T.E.

[e] 1 N.E. (niacin equivalent) is equal to 1 mg of niacin or 60 mg of dietary tryptophan.

[f] The folacin allowances refer to dietary sources as determined by Lactobacillus casei assay after treatment with enzymes ("conjugases") to make polyglutamyl forms of the vitamin available to the test organism.

[g] The RDA for vitamin B12 in infants is based on average concentration of the vitamin in human milk. The allowances after weaning are based on energy intake (as recommended by the American Academy of Pediatrics) and consideration of other factors such as intestinal absorption.

[h] The increased requirement during pregnancy cannot be met by the iron content of habitual American diets nor by the existing iron stores of many women; therefore the use of 30–60 mg of supplemental iron is recommended. Iron needs during lactation are not substantially different from those of nonpregnant women, but continued supplementation of the mother for 2–3 months after parturition is advisable in order to replenish stores depleted by pregnancy.

Source: Food and Nutrition Board, National Academy of Sciences, National Research Council, Washington, DC, 1980.

TABLE 13-6   Comparison of U.S. RDA for Adults and Children

NUTRIENT	ADULT	CHILDREN UNDER 4	% OF ADULT USRDA
Vitamin A	5000 I.U.	2500 I.U.	50
Vitamin C	60 mg	40 mg	67*
Thiamin	1.5 mg	0.7 mg	47
Riboflavin	1.7 mg	0.8 mg	47
Niacin	20 mg	9 mg	45
Calcium	1.0 mg	0.8 mg	80**
Iron	18 mg	10 mg	56

Note: A child serving is one-half of an adult serving. Half servings provide a similar percent of U.S. RDA for a child for all nutrients except Vitamin C and calcium.

*Four servings of fruits and vegetables including one rich source of Vitamin C are recommended to ensure enough Vitamin C.

**A total of 3 cups of milk (½ cup servings) is recommended in order to meet calcium needs.

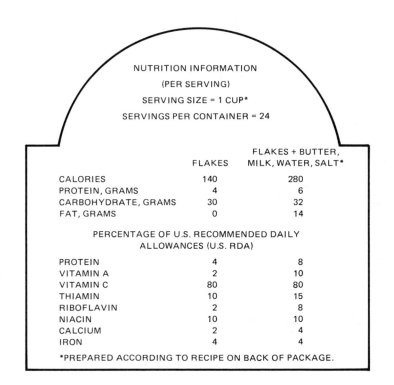

NUTRITION INFORMATION

(PER SERVING)

SERVING SIZE = 1 CUP*

SERVINGS PER CONTAINER = 24

	FLAKES	FLAKES + BUTTER, MILK, WATER, SALT*
CALORIES	140	280
PROTEIN, GRAMS	4	6
CARBOHYDRATE, GRAMS	30	32
FAT, GRAMS	0	14

PERCENTAGE OF U.S. RECOMMENDED DAILY ALLOWANCES (U.S. RDA)

PROTEIN	4	8
VITAMIN A	2	10
VITAMIN C	80	80
THIAMIN	10	15
RIBOFLAVIN	2	8
NIACIN	10	10
CALCIUM	2	4
IRON	4	4

*PREPARED ACCORDING TO RECIPE ON BACK OF PACKAGE.

FIGURE 13-2   Percentages of U.S. Recommended Daily Allowances are shown on some food labels.

TABLE 13-7   United States Recommended Daily Allowances (U.S. RDA)

	ADULTS AND CHILDREN 4 OR MORE YEARS OF AGE (For use in labeling conventional foods and also for "special dietary foods")	INFANTS	CHILDREN UNDER 4 YEARS OF AGE	PREGNANT OR LACTATING WOMEN
			(For use only with "special dietary foods")	
Nutrients which **must** *be declared on the label (in the order below)*				
Protein	45 g "high quality protein" 65 g "proteins in general"		—	—
Vitamin A	5000 IU	1500 IU	2500 IU	8000 IU
Vitamin C (or ascorbic acid)	60 mg	35 mg	40 mg	60 mg
Thiamin (or vitamin B_1)	1.5 mg	0.5 mg	0.7 mg	1.7 mg
Riboflavin (or vitamin B_2)	1.7 mg	0.6 mg	0.8 mg	2.0 mg
Niacin	20 mg	8 mg	9 mg	20 mg
Calcium	1.0 g	0.6 g	0.8 g	1.3 g
Iron	18 mg	15 mg	10 mg	18 mg
Nutrients which **may** *be declared on the label (in the order below)*				
Vitamin D	400 IU	400 IU	400 IU	400 IU
Vitamin E	30 IU	5 IU	10 IU	30 IU
Vitamin B_6	2.0 mg	0.4 mg	0.7 mg	2.5 mg
Folic acid (or folacin)	0.4 mg	0.1 mg	0.2 mg	0.8 mg
Vitamin B_{12}	6 μg	2 μg	3 μg	8 μg
Phosphorus	1.0 g	0.5 g	0.8 g	1.3 g
Iodine	150 μg	45 μg	70 μg	150 μg
Magnesium	400 mg	70 mg	200 mg	450 mg
Zinc	15 mg	5 mg	8 mg	15 mg
Copper	2 mg	0.5 mg	1 mg	2 mg
Biotin	0.3 mg	0.15 mg	0.15 mg	0.3 mg
Pantothenic acid	10 mg	3 mg	5 mg	10 mg

Courtesy of the U.S. Food and Drug Administration.

between *overnutrition* and some degenerative diseases. They are presented here in summary.

Eat a Variety of Foods. A variety of foods should be eaten daily, including fruits, vegetables, whole grain and enriched grain products, dairy foods, meats, poultry and legumes (dry beans and peas).

Maintain Ideal Weight. Body weight remains steady when calories taken in equal calories expended. When more calories are taken in than are expended, weight gain occurs. Loss of weight results from taking in less calories than are expended. Programs for weight loss must recognize that weight loss results from reduced calorie intake or increased activity or a combination of both. Adequate nutrients must be provided even when calories are reduced. A steady loss of 1 to 2 pounds per week is safest.

Avoid Too Much Fat, Saturated Fat, and Cholesterol. This guideline is the most controversial of those proposed. Fats are found in such foods as butter, eggs, salad dressing, meats, and some dairy products. Saturated fats and cholesterol are found in animal foods such as meats, eggs, butter and whole milk.

Eat Food With Adequate Starch and Fiber. Starchy foods include fruits, vegetables, beans, peas, and whole grains. Vegetables, fruits, whole grains and legumes are also excellent sources of fiber (a source of bulk in the diet).

Avoid Too Much Sugar. Refined sugar provides calories but no other nutrients. Tooth decay has been associated with sugar consumption. Other health problems such as obesity may result when refined sugar contributes to excess calories.

Avoid Too Much Sodium. Sodium is found in salt and occurs naturally in foods such as milk, meats, eggs, and some vegetables. Many food additives in addition to salt contain sodium. Americans consume more than adequate amounts of sodium. The guidelines suggest reducing or omitting the salt added to foods and avoiding salty foods such as pickled or cured meats, catsup, mustard, chips, pretzels, and salted nuts.

If You Drink Alcohol, Do So in Moderation. Alcohol contributes many calories and few nutrients. Its use is associated with numerous health and social problems.

NUTRIENT DENSITY

Adequate nutrients are more easily obtained with high calorie intakes. However, in recent years, actual caloric requirements have decreased as a result of reduced physical activity. Therefore, the required nutrients must now be obtained from foods which contain fewer calories. This is very difficult if food choices are calorie-dense. The *nutrient density* of a food indicates the amount of nutrients relative to calories contributed. *Index of Nutrient Quality* (INQ) is one means of determining nutrient-density or *calorie-density,* Table 13–8.

The formula for determining the Index of Nutrient Quality is:

$$INQ = \frac{\% \text{ of U.S. RDA of nutrient/serving}}{\% \text{ of total daily energy requirement/serving}}$$

TABLE 13-8   Index of Nutrient Quality (INQ)

	CHILD 4-6	WOMAN	MAN
Suggested daily caloric need	1800	2000	2500
Calories per serving (from label)	120*	240	240
% of daily calories per serving (calculated)	7	12	10
% of U.S. RDA (from label)	40*	80	80
INQ	40/7 = 5.7	80/12 = 6.6	80/10 = 8.0

*half servings

The information necessary to determine the Index of Nutrient Quality may be easily obtained from the labels of many packaged foods. Two steps are necessary:

1. Calculate the percentage of the calorie intake represented by a serving of a food (calories per serving divided by daily caloric requirement).

2. Find the ratio between the percentage of the U.S. RDA of a nutrient in a serving of food and the percentage of caloric intake per serving (percent of U.S. RDA divided by percent of daily calories).

$$\frac{\% \text{ U.S. RDA}}{\% \text{ daily calories}}$$

An INQ of 1.0 indicates that a food contains calories and nutrients in the same proportions. An INQ of less than 1.0 indicates more calories than nutrients (calorie-dense). INQ may be used in the following rule of thumb to determine nutritious foods:

4 leader nutrients with INQ of 1
or
2 leader nutrients with INQ of 2

SUMMARY

Nutrition is the study of nutrients and how the human body uses them. Foods serve as sources of nutrients; the body uses the nutrients from foods.

Various food guidelines ease the problem of knowing which foods and how much of them to select to provide adequate amounts of essential nutrients.

The Basic Four Food Groups divide foods into groups which contain similar kinds and amounts of nutrients. The Basic Four is easily understood by most people and therefore is widely used.

Recommended Daily Dietary Allowances are guidelines for the amounts of nutrients needed by most healthy persons, divided according to age and sex groups.

United States Recommended Daily Allowances (U.S. RDA) help the consumer to determine if a food is a good or poor source of nutrients. Many packaged foods are labeled to show percentages of U.S. RDA contained in a serving. Amounts of nutrients suggested by the U.S. RDA tend to be higher than the Recommended Daily Dietary Allowances for individuals.

The U.S. Dietary Guidelines and the Index of Nutrient Quality (INQ) are suggestions to help people eat nutritiously and yet deal with the harmful effects of overnutrition.

The major factor to remember in the use of any guideline is the selection of as wide a variety of foods as possible.

LEARNING ACTIVITIES

1. Using the following format, summarize each of the Basic Four Food Groups:
   a. Recommended number of servings
      • child
      • adult (where different)
   b. Recommended size of serving
      • child
      • adult
   c. Nutrient strengths
   d. Nutrient weaknesses

2. Plan a day's diet for a 4-year-old child. Include the recommended number of servings and the appropriate serving sizes from the Basic Four Food Groups.

3. Assume that a child is allergic to citrus fruit and strawberries (common food allergies). What fruit and/or vegetable choices could be substituted to provide adequate Vitamin C? Use the nutrient content table in Appendix A to determine if the substitution meets the Recommended Daily Dietary Requirements (45 mg).

4. Visit a child care center. Analyze the posted menus according to Basic Four Food Groups. Identify nutrient strengths of each food served. How many leader nutrients are represented?

UNIT REVIEW

A. CROSSWORD PUZZLE

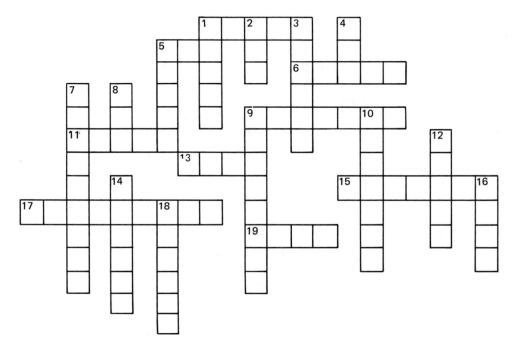

ACROSS

1. Calcium is a major nutrient strength of this group.

5. Federal agency which devised U.S. RDA.

6. Breads, cereal and pastas are examples.

9. Important factor in good nutrition.

11. Refined carbohydrate associated with tooth decay.

13. A food from the High Protein Group.

15. A mineral found in large amounts in the Dairy Group.

17. Substances found in food; they perform specific functions in the body.

19. Mineral found in the Grain and High Protein Groups.

DOWN

1. Recommended _____ Dietary Allowances

2. Nutrient density

3. A food from the Dairy Group.

4. Recommendations for most healthy people.

5. Adds bulk to the diet.

7. Nutrients which must come from foods.

8. Meat alternate; a food in the High Protein Group.

9. Vitamin A and _____ are nutrient strengths of the Fruit and Vegetable Group.

10. Vitamin strength of Grain and High Protein Group.

12. Plans for eating wisely are called _____ lines.

14. An excellent source of Vitamin C is _____ fruits.

16. A beverage from the Dairy Group.

18. A vitamin used to enrich bread.

B. Multiple Choice. Select the best answer.

1. The Recommended Daily Dietary Allowances are
   a. recommended amounts of food
   b. required amounts of food
   c. recommended amounts of nutrients
   d. minimum amounts of nutrients

2. The Recommended Daily Dietary Allowances are for
   a. children only
   b. adults only
   c. individuals 4 years of age or older
   d. nearly all healthy people

3. In comparison to the Recommended Daily Dietary Allowances, the United States Recommended Daily Allowances are:
   a. higher
   b. lower
   c. the same
   d. varied by age/sex group

4. The United States Recommended Daily Allowances are devised to be used
   a. to analyze diets
   b. on food labels
   c. by the Food and Drug Administration
   d. in planning special diets

5. The Basic Four Food Groups are
   a. Dairy, Grains, High Protein, Fruit and Vegetable
   b. Fruit and Vegetable, Fats, Dairy, High Protein
   c. Grains, Sugar and Sweets, High Protein, Dairy
   d. Dairy, High Protein, Water, Fruit and Vegetable

6. The nutrient strengths of the Fruit and Vegetable Group are
   a. calcium and protein
   b. thiamin and niacin
   c. vitamin C and vitamin A
   d. vitamin B_{12}

7. The food group which is the major contributor of calcium to the diet is
   a. Fruit and Vegetable Group
   b. Dairy Group
   c. High Protein Group
   d. Bread and Cereal Group

8. Nutrient density refers to the
   a. nutrient-calorie ratio of a food
   b. recommended numbers of servings of food
   c. nutrients lacking in a food substance
   d. none of these

9. A food furnishes 10 percent of the daily need for energy and 25 percent of U.S. RDA for thiamin. INQ for that food for thiamin is
   a. 0.4
   b. 10
   c. 2.5
   d. 25

10. U.S. Dietary Guidelines are
    a. federal regulations
    b. dietary changes which may be desirable for health
    c. a means of ensuring adequate food supply
    d. dietary changes which authorities agree must be made in the American diet

C. Briefly answer the following questions.

1. Betsy, age 3½ years, drinks milk to the exclusion of adequate amounts of food from other food groups. What nutrient is Betsy receiving in excess? What two nutrients are most likely to be deficient?

2. Jason, age 4 years, refuses to eat vegetables. He will occasionally accept a small serving of applesauce but no other fruits. What two nutrients are probably deficient in Jason's diet?

3. Jeremy, age 3 years, is allergic to milk and dairy products. What nutrient is deficient in Jeremy's diet?

D. Match the foods in column I to the appropriate food group in column II. Some foods may include more than one food group.

Column I
1. navy beans
2. rice
3. spaghetti
4. hamburger pizza
5. macaroni and cheese
6. peanut butter sandwich
7. french fries
8. ice cream
9. popcorn
10. carbonated beverages

Column II
a. Dairy Group
b. High Protein Group
c. Grain Group
d. Fruit and Vegetable Group
e. Other Foods

REFERENCES

Dietary Goals for the United States. 2d ed. Washington, DC: Senate Select Committee on Nutrition and Human Needs, 1979.

Guthrie, H.A. *Introductory Nutrition.* 5th ed. St. Louis: The C.V. Mosby Company, 1983.

Nutrition Labeling: Tools for Its Use. Agriculture Information Bulletin No. 382. Washington, DC: U.S. Department of Agriculture, 1975.

Nutritive Value of Foods. Home and Garden Bulletin No. 72. Washington, DC: U.S. Department of Agriculture.

Composition of Foods. Agriculture Handbook No. 8. Washington, DC: U.S. Department of Agriculture.

Nutrition and Your Health: Dietary Guidelines for Americans. Washington, DC: United States Department of Agriculture.

Unit 14
NUTRIENTS THAT PROVIDE ENERGY

Terms to Know

basal metabolic rate	absorption
energy	metabolism
calories	PUFA
gram	linoleic acid
digestion	enzyme

Objectives

After studying this unit, you will be able to:
- Identify the three classes of nutrients which supply energy.
- State the amount of energy supplied by each class of nutrients.
- List three factors which determine individual energy requirements.
- Identify foods containing good sources of energy-supplying nutrients.
- Calculate daily caloric requirements of a child based on the child's weight.
- Plan a day's diet eliminating refined sucrose.

Energy is generally defined as the ability to do work. Examples of work done by the body are (1) moving the body, (2) building new tissues, (3) maintaining body temperature, and (4) digesting, absorbing and metabolizing food. Energy is required for all body functions. In terms of survival, the need for energy is second only to the need for oxygen and water.

The amount of potential energy in a food is expressed in *calories,* e.g., a one-cup serving of ice cream supplies 185 calories. The energy cost of a given activity is also measured and expressed in calories, e.g., swimming for 30 minutes expends about 150 calories.

Carbohydrates, fats, and proteins found in foods supply energy for the body's activities. Vitamins, minerals and water are necessary for the release of potential energy stored in carbohydrates, fats, and proteins. Vitamins, minerals, and water do not themselves supply any calories. The relative numbers of calories contained in carbohydrates, fats, and proteins are:

- carbohydrates—4 calories per gram
- fat—9 calories per gram
- proteins—4 calories per gram

A *gram* is a metric unit of measurement for weight. There are 28 grams in one ounce, and 454 grams in one pound. A metal paper clip weighs about one gram.

Every individual has different energy requirements; these requirements vary slightly on a day-to-day basis. Individual energy requirements are determined by:

- basal metabolic rate (BMR)
- physical activity
- energy spent to release energy from food (dietary thermogenesis)

The *basal metabolic rate* (BMR) is a term used to describe the energy needed just to carry on vital involuntary body processes. A BMR test is conducted when the body is completely at rest—at least 12 hours after eating, after a restful sleep, in comfortable room temperature, with no exercise, activity, or emotional excitement preceding the test. The BMR measures the energy required for blood circulation, breathing, cell activity, body temperature maintenance, heartbeat, and other involuntary activities. It does not measure voluntary activity.

Physical activity is the aspect of energy need that is subject to the greatest conscious control. For instance, participation in tennis or swimming as a recreational activity requires far more energy than reading or watching television, Figure 14–1. Children should be encouraged to participate in physical activity. The benefits of physical activity include motor development, the opportunity for socialization, a sense of accomplishment, and increased fitness. The additional calories required by increased physical activity provide the opportunity for the intake of additional nutrients.

Dietary thermogenesis refers to the energy required to *digest, absorb,* transport, and *metabolize* nutrients in food. This factor accounts for approximately 10 percent of the total energy requirement.

Growing children need more energy per unit of body weight than adults, Figure 14–2. Growth requires energy for division and/or enlargement of existing cells (Alford and Bogle 1983). Rates of growth, physical activity and body size cause variations in the amount of energy needed by individual children. The number of calories needed daily is calculated on the basis of normal body weight. A four-year-old child needs approximately 40 calories per pound of body weight. (The energy needs of infants are detailed in Table 14–1.) For comparison, a moderately active adult female requires only approximately 18 calories per pound; a moderately active adult male needs approximately 21 calories per pound. (Moderately active has been described as equal time "on the feet and on the seat.")

Balancing the number of calories eaten with the number of calories expended results in stable body weight. Eating fewer calories than are needed leads to weight loss. The result of eating too few calories is more serious in growing children than in adults. Too few calories can result in slowed growth as a result of burning body tissue to provide needed energy for body function. Children need

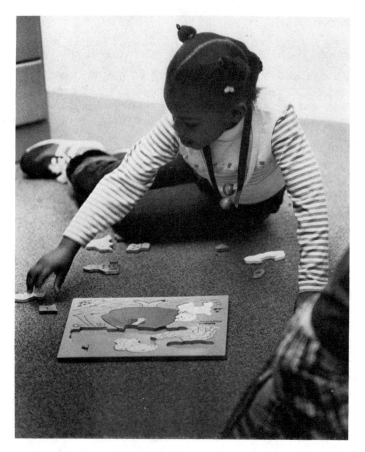

FIGURE 14–1   Quiet activities require lesser amounts of energy.

sufficient calories from carbohydrates and fat to spare protein which is needed for growth.

Too many calories consumed over a period of time may lead to obesity. Obese children are often less active than their slimmer playmates, and may

TABLE 14–1   The Energy Needs of Infants

AGE (years)	WEIGHT (pounds)	LENGTH (inches)	ENERGY NEEDS (calories)
0.0–0.5	13	24	lb × 53 Calories
0.5–1.0	20	28	lb × 48 Calories

Source: Adapted from Recommended Dietary Allowances, 1980.

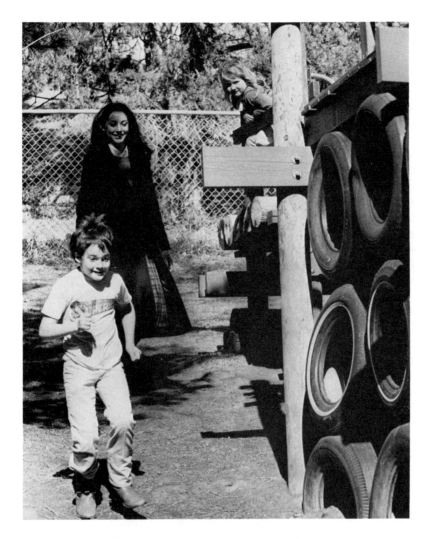

FIGURE 14-2 The energy needs of active growing children are relatively greater than those of an adult.

require fewer calories due to their lower activity level. The obese child's bulkier body can lead to less coordinated movements and greater danger of accidents. Obese children are often teased by their playmates and excluded from play activities. Exclusion from play groups often adds to problems encountered by the obese child, such as poor self-image, decreased fitness level, and fewer opportunities for socialization. The child with a weight problem should be encouraged to exercise and offered adequate amounts of nutrient-dense foods. Calories should not be drastically reduced, as reduction of calories may result in reduction of essential nutrients (Brody 1982).

CARBOHYDRATES AS ENERGY SOURCES

Carbohydrates should be primary sources of energy for children. At least half the energy required by a child should be derived from carbohydrates. A child requiring 1600 calories should derive at least 800 calories from carbohydrates; eight hundred calories are supplied by 200 grams of carbohydrates. Many experts recommend a minimum intake for adults of 125 grams (500 calories) of carbohydrates daily. Children need more, but the exact minimum amount needed is not known. The main portion of carbohydrates should be complex with no more than 10 percent of calories coming from refined sugar.

Foods which contain complex and unprocessed carbohydrates are wise choices for children's snacks. Fresh fruits and vegetables, fruit and vegetable juices, and whole grain products such as breads, cereals, and crackers are nutritious and readily accepted snack foods for growing children. Carbohydrates are present in foods in simple, refined, and complex forms.

Consumption of refined sugar has increased since 1900; the use of complex carbohydrates such as starches has dropped during that same period. Current nutrition recommendations suggest increased amounts of complex carbohydrates and decreased amounts of refined sugars. This simply means less sugar and more starch and fiber from the Grain and the Fruit and Vegetable Food Groups. Three general types of carbohydrates are found in foods: monosaccharides, disaccharides, and polysaccharides.

Monosaccharides

Monosaccharides (simple sugars) consist of one simple sugar unit that needs no further digestion prior to absorption. This makes monosaccharides sources of quick energy. Examples of monosaccharides are:

- glucose
- fructose
- galactose

Glucose is the form in which sugar is normally carried in the blood and which is required for use by body cells. Glucose occurs in such foods as honey, some fruits and vegetables, and corn syrup. However, most glucose in the blood is a result of digestion of compound sugars and polysaccharides.

Fructose is present in honey and in fruits, and is sweeter than either glucose or sucrose (table sugar). In some cases, smaller amounts of fructose may be used to give a desired degree of sweetness.

Galactose is not found free in foods. It results from the digestion of lactose.

Disaccharides

Disaccharides (compound sugars) are made up of two simple sugars joined together. Compound sugars must be digested to their component simple sugars before they can be absorbed and utilized by the body. Two important examples of disaccharides are:

- sucrose
- lactose

In its refined form, sucrose is commonly known as table sugar. Sucrose is found in sugar beets and sugar cane and in fruits, vegetables, and honey. When sucrose occurs in fruits and vegetables it is accompanied by other essential nutrients such as vitamins, minerals and water, Figure 14–3. Refined sucrose, or table sugar, is the cause of concern in several aspects of health. Refined table sugar contributes no nutrients—only calories. For this reason, calories from table sugar are frequently called "empty calories." Eating too many empty calories can lead to obesity accompanied by a deficiency of some essential nutrients. Children who are allowed to eat too many foods containing refined sugar may not be hungry for more healthful foods containing the nutrients they need.

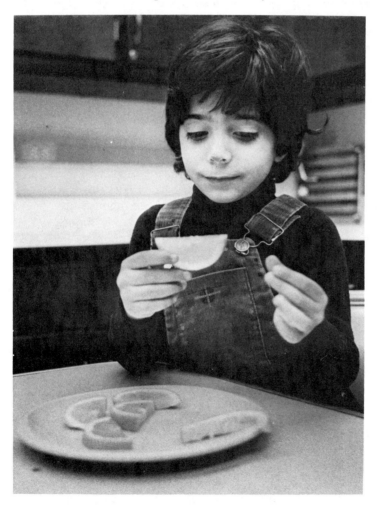

FIGURE 14–3   Sugar in fruits is accompanied by other essential nutrients.

Refined sucrose has also been linked to tooth decay in children. Other important factors contributing to tooth decay are the stickiness of the food containing the sugar, the frequency of eating, the frequency of toothbrushing, whether the sugar is contained in a meal with other foods or in a snack, and whether the sugar-containing food is accompanied by a beverage.

Lactose is found in milk and is referred to as "milk sugar." It is the only carbohydrate found in an animal-source food. Lactose occurs in milk of mammals, including breast milk. It has advantages over other sugars in that lactose aids in establishing and maintaining beneficial intestinal bacteria. Calcium is more efficiently used by the body if lactose is also present. Fortunately, calcium and lactose occur in the same food—milk.

While usually a beneficial sugar, lactose can present problems to some individuals. Some persons of non-Northern European descent do not produce the *enzyme* to break lactose down to its component simple sugars which can be absorbed (Alford and Bogle 1982). This lactose intolerance may cause intestinal discomfort, cramping, gas, and diarrhea. Often small amounts of milk (1–2 cups a day in small feedings) are tolerated. Dairy products such as yogurt and buttermilk are tolerated better than milk. Adults tend to display more severe lactose intolerance than do children.

Polysaccharides

Polysaccharides (complex carbohydrates) are composed of many units of simple sugar joined together. Complex carbohydrates must be broken down to their component simple sugars before the body can absorb and use them. Digestion of only one complex carbohydrate can result in thousands of simple sugars. Polysaccharides which are important to human nutrition are:

- starch
- cellulose
- glycogen

Starches are digestible complex carbohydrates. They are found in large amounts in grains, legumes, and root vegetables such as potatoes and carrots. When contained in these foods, starches are accompanied by vitamins and minerals which the body needs. Starches are desirable components of a healthful diet.

Cellulose is an indigestible complex carbohydrate. Humans cannot digest cellulose; therefore, it cannot be absorbed and used by body cells. Cellulose is thus an important source of bulk or fiber in the diet. Cellulose is found in whole grains, nuts, legumes, and fruits and vegetables. It is also thought to provide some detergent effect to teeth thus aiding good dental health.

Another complex carbohydrate of importance is glycogen. Glycogen is often referred to as animal starch. It is the form in which carbohydrate is stored in the body for future conversion into sugar and subsequent use for performing body activity. There is no food source for glycogen. It is formed from blood glucose and is converted when needed by the body back into glucose.

FATS AS ENERGY SOURCES

Fats are the richest food source of energy, supplying nine calories per gram consumed. Foods in which fats are readily identified are butter, margarine, shortening, oils, and salad dressings. Less obvious sources of fats are meats, whole milk, egg yolks, nuts, and nut butters. Fruits and vegetables contain little fat; with the exception of the avocado which is quite rich in fat. Grains and cereal products are naturally low in fat. However, the many baked goods such as cakes, pies, doughnuts, and cookies that use grain products are high in added fat. Some dietary fat is required for good health. However, no minimum amount of dietary fat has been recommended. On the contrary, recommendations have been made to reduce average fat intake to about 30 percent of total calories. For a child requiring 1600 calories, this means 480 calories or 50–55 grams of fat in the diet.

Although they provide more than twice as much energy per gram than carbohydrates, fats are a less desirable energy source for children. Fats are harder to digest than carbohydrates and are accompanied by fewer essential nutrients. However, fats should not be totally eliminated from the diet since they furnish the essential fatty acid, serve as carriers of fat-soluble vitamins, and give a feeling of satiety or fullness. The practice of lowering a very young child's fat intake through the use of skim milk is questionable. Most authorities believe that this practice may lead to insufficient calorie intake and *linoleic acid* deficiency. In addition, skim milk may provide excessive intakes of protein and minerals, resulting in difficulty in excreting minerals or urea (Williams and Caliendo 1984). Children under two years of age should not be given skim milk in an effort to lower fat. Beyond 2 years of age, low fat (2%) milk may be given.

Fats in foods are present in the form of triglycerides. Before fats present in foods can provide energy they must undergo digestion and absorption into the body. Digestion of dietary fats produces:

- fatty acids
- glycerol

The resulting fatty acids and glycerol can be absorbed for use by the body. Fatty acids in foods are either saturated or unsaturated.

Saturated fatty acids are those which are saturated with hydrogen. Fats found in animal-source foods such as meat, milk, and eggs contain fatty acids which are saturated. Fats containing predominantly saturated fatty acids are solid at room temperature, and are often accompanied by cholesterol. Cholesterol and saturated fats have been extensively investigated as undesirable dietary components. However, after years of study, few definite conclusions have been reached regarding the role of dietary cholesterol in disease or the advisability of lowering the fat and cholesterol intake of children.

A fatty acid which is not completely saturated with hydrogen is said to be an unsaturated fatty acid. Unsaturated fats are usually soft at room temperature or are in oil form.

Fats found in plant-source foods such as corn oil or sunflower oil contain mostly unsaturated fatty acids. Many plant oils are polyunsaturated, which means the fatty acids contain numerous unfilled attachment sites. Polyunsaturated fatty acids are often called PUFAs. Linoleic acid is the one polyunsaturated fatty acid that is essential for all humans, but is needed in greater amounts for infants and children than is needed for adults. Linoleic acid cannot be produced by the body and so must be obtained from food sources. Plant-source foods are better sources of this essential fatty acid than animal-source foods.

Glycerol is a three-carbon alcohol. It is utilized as an energy source.

PROTEINS AS ENERGY SOURCES

Proteins are the third class of nutrients which the body can use as an energy source. Proteins supply four calories per gram; the same amount of energy as that derived from carbohydrates. "Eating protein to meet energy needs . . . represents a waste like burning furniture for heat when firewood is available" (Longacre 1976). Proteins must be digested to their component amino acids prior to absorption and utilization by the body.

Each protein is unique in the number, arrangement, and specific amino acids from which it is built. Since proteins (amino acids) function as materials to build body tissues and as regulators of body functions they will be discussed in detail in subsequent sections.

SUMMARY

Energy is defined as the ability to do work. Carbohydrates, proteins, and fats in foods are sources of energy for the body, Table 14–2. Energy needs vary from individual to individual; children need more energy per pound of body weight than adults. Individual energy needs are based on (1) basal metabolic rate, (2) physical activity, and (3) energy spent to get energy from food (dietary thermogenesis).

Carbohydrates supply four calories per gram. Carbohydrates occur in several forms: monosaccharides (simple sugars), disaccharides (compound sugars) and polysaccharides (complex carbohydrates). Sugars, starches and cellulose are carbohydrates which are important in foods.

Fats supply nine calories per gram. Fatty acids are either saturated or unsaturated, depending on the amount of hydrogen contained. Oils, dairy products, eggs, and meats are sources of fat.

Proteins supply four calories per gram. Proteins are composed of amino acids and are found in meats, eggs, legumes and dairy products.

TABLE 14–2 Summary of Energy-supplying Nutrients

NUTRIENT	CALORIES PER GRAM	CONVERSION NEEDED FOR USE IN BODY	FOOD SOURCES
Carbohydrate	4		
Monosaccharides (simple sugars)		none needed	
glucose			honey, some fruits and vegetables, corn syrup
fructose			honey and fruits
galactose			none
Disaccharides (compound sugars)		simple sugars	
sucrose			sugar beets, sugar cane, honey, fruits, vegetables
lactose			milk
Polysaccharides (complex carbohydrates)		simple sugars	
starch			grains, legumes, root vegetables
cellulose		nondigestible	whole grains, nuts, legumes, fruits, vegetables
glycogen			none
Fat	9	fatty acids and glycerol	
saturated			meats, eggs, milk and dairy products
unsaturated			plant-source foods, corn oil, vegetable oils
Protein	4	amino acids	meats, eggs, legumes, dairy products

LEARNING ACTIVITIES

1. Using the mock cereal label given in Figure 14–4, determine the following:
   a. the number of calories derived from carbohydrate
   b. the approximate percentage of total calories derived from:
      (1) starches and related carbohydrates
      (2) sucrose and other sugars

MUNCHIE CRUNCHIES

Nutrition Information Per Serving

Serving Size	1 oz (¾ c)	With ½ c Vitamin D Milk
Servings per package	13	
Calories	110	190
Protein	2 g	6 g
Carbohydrate	25 g	31 g
Fat	0 g	4 g

Ingredients: Corn, Sugar, Salt, Malted Cereal Syrup, Leavening, Vitamin C, Niacin, Thiamin, Iron

Made by

Cruncho Inc.
123 Main Street
Anywhere, USA 00000

Carbohydrate Information

Starch and related carbohydrates	23 g	23 g
Sucrose and other sugars	2 g	8 g

FIGURE 14-4 Mock cereal label

Is this cereal predominantly starch or sucrose? Why is the amount of sucrose and related sugars increased with the addition of milk? Do starches and complex carbohydrates increase with the addition of milk?

2. Using the mock cereal label given in Figure 14–4, determine those ingredients which contribute to total carbohydrate. Further classify those ingredients which contribute to sucrose or compound sugars. Hint: Dextrose, corn syrup, malt syrup, and corn sugar are all forms of simple or compound sugars.

3. Calculate the caloric requirement of a 4-year-old child who weighs 42 pounds.

4. Determine the number of calories in a serving of food which contributes the following:
carbohydrate—12 grams
protein—8 grams
fat—10 grams

UNIT REVIEW

A. Multiple Choice. Select the best answer.

1. Energy is defined as
   a. running and playing
   b. activity
   c. physical activity
   d. the ability to do work

2. Nutrients which supply energy are
   a. carbohydrates, proteins, and water
   b. carbohydrates, fats, and vitamins
   c. carbohydrates, fats, and proteins
   d. carbohydrates, proteins, and vitamins

3. A food which has 20 grams of carbohydrates and 2 grams of protein yields how many calories?
   a. 198 calories
   b. 188 calories
   c. 88 calories
   d. 98 calories

4. The factor affecting energy requirements which may be consciously controlled by the individual is
   a. basal metabolic rate
   b. physical activity
   c. energy spent to get energy from food
   d. none of the above

5. A four-year-old child weighing 40 pounds needs approximately
   a. 1200 calories daily
   b. 1900 calories daily
   c. 800 calories daily
   d. 1600 calories daily

6. Energy cannot be derived from energy-supplying nutrients without the help of
   a. vitamins
   b. minerals
   c. water
   d. all of these

7. The food combination that contains the most *carbohydrates* is
   a. butter, milk, corn oil
   b. meat, milk, eggs
   c. bread, fruits, vegetables, meat
   d. bread, fruits, vegetables, milk

8. The food combination that contains the most *protein* is
   a. vegetables, milk, eggs
   b. meat, milk, eggs
   c. bread, fruits, vegetables, meat
   d. bread, fruits, vegetables, milk

9. The food combination that contains the most *fat* is
   a. butter, milk, corn oil
   b. meat, milk, eggs
   c. bread, fruits, vegetables, meat
   d. bread, fruits, vegetables, milk

10. At least half of the calories in a child's diet should be derived from
    a. protein
    b. carbohydrate
    c. fat
    d. minerals

11. The nutrient that provides the greatest amount of energy per gram is
    a. protein
    b. carbohydrate
    c. fat
    d. vitamins

12. The nutrient which can perform functions other than supplying energy is
    a. protein
    b. carbohydrate
    c. fat
    d. none of these

13. Fats found in beef, lamb, and butter contain more
    a. polyunsaturated fatty acids
    b. unsaturated fatty acids
    c. saturated fatty acids
    d. linoleic acid

14. Fatty acids found in vegetable oils such as corn oil are predominantly
    a. polyunsaturated
    b. saturated
    c. solid at room temperature
    d. none of these

15. Cholesterol is found in
    a. eggs
    b. butter
    c. foods of animal origin
    d. all of these

16. Proteins are composed of
  a. polyunsaturated fatty acids
  b. unsaturated fatty acids
  c. amino acids
  d. simple sugars

17. Proteins can be used to
  a. supply energy
  b. build body tissue
  c. regulate body functions
  d. all of these

18. Cellulose adds bulk to the diet because it
  a. is indigestible
  b. contains saturated fatty acids
  c. is composed of amino acids
  d. is easily digested

B. Match the terms in column II to the correct phrase in column I.

Column I	Column II
1. a simple sugar	a. amino acids
2. digestible complex carbohydrate	b. cellulose
3. found in meats, dairy products, legumes, and eggs	c. protein
	d. carbohydrate
4. building blocks of proteins	e. glucose
5. found in grains, fruits, vegetables, and dairy products	f. fats
	g. starch
6. richest source of energy	h. sucrose
7. indigestible complex carbohydrate	
8. table sugar	

C. Case Study

Terry, age 5, has several decayed teeth. His dentist has suggested a program of good dental hygiene plus limiting his intake of refined sucrose.

1. Plan a day's diet for Terry which contains at least 200 grams of carbohydrates without any refined sucrose (table sugar). Use the following *average* amounts of carbohydrates:

bread, cereals, pastas	15 grams/serving
fruits and juices	10 grams/serving
starchy vegetables	7 grams/serving
milk	12 grams/serving

REFERENCES

Alford, B., and Bogle, M.L. *Nutrition During the Life Cycle.* Englewood Cliffs, NJ: Prentice-Hall, Inc. 1982.

Brody, J. *Jane Brody's Nutrition Book.* New York: Bantam Books, Inc., 1982.

Longacre, D. J. *More-with-Less Cookbook,* Scottsdale, PA: Herald Press, 1976.

Williams, E. R., and Caliendo, M.A. *Nutrition: Principles, Issues and Applications.* New York: McGraw Hill Book Company, 1984.

Unit 15
NUTRIENTS THAT PROMOTE GROWTH OF BODY TISSUES

Terms to Know

amino acids
incomplete protein
complete protein
minerals

complementary proteins
collagen
hemoglobin
iron deficiency anemia

Objectives

After studying this unit, you will be able to:
- State how growth occurs.
- Name three classes of nutrients that promote growth of body tissue and list food sources for each.
- Describe the role that proteins, minerals, and water play in body growth.
- Differentiate between nonessential and essential amino acids.
- Identify food sources for complete protein and for incomplete protein.
- Identify examples of complementary incomplete proteins.

Growth may be defined as an increase in physical size of either the entire body or of any body part. Growth may occur by (1) an increase in the number of cells, or by (2) an increase in the size of individual cells. At various stages of the child's life, either or both types of growth may be occurring.

Infancy and early childhood are periods of rapid growth, Figure 15–1. During the first six months of life, infants can be expected to approximately double their birth weight. By the end of the first year, their birth length should have increased by 50 percent. Birth weight and length are the baselines for evaluating infant growth. The preschool child normally more than doubles birth length and increases birth weight five to six times.

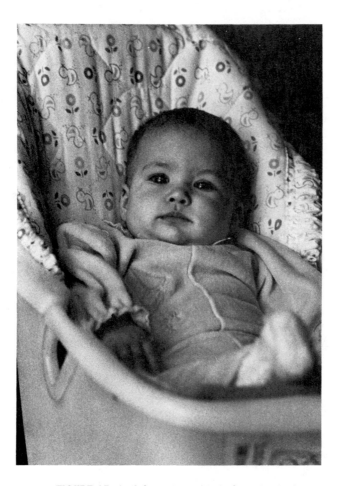

FIGURE 15-1 Infancy is a period of rapid growth.

PROTEINS FOR GROWTH

Proteins play an important role in growth. Protein is the material from which all body cells are built. Approximately 15 percent of body weight is protein. Examples of types of body tissues which consist of large amounts of protein are muscles, glands, organs, bones, blood and skin.

Proteins are composed of hundreds of individual units called *amino acids.* The human body is able to manufacture some of the amino acids it needs to build proteins; these amino acids are termed nonessential amino acids. Amino acids which the body cannot manufacture in needed amounts must be provided by proteins in foods; these amino acids are termed essential amino acids. The amino acids which are essential for humans are:

- histidine
- isoleucine
- leucine
- lysine
- methionine
- phenylalanine
- threonine
- tryptophan
- valine
- arginine (currently under investigation as essential)

When all essential amino acids occur in adequate amounts in food protein, that protein is said to be a *complete protein*. Complete proteins occur in animal-source foods such as meats, milk, eggs and cheese. Soybeans are a plant source of complete protein.

Incomplete proteins are those which lack adequate amounts of one or more essential amino acids. Proteins from plant sources such as grains, legumes other than soybeans, and vegetables are incomplete proteins. Gelatin, an animal-source food, is also an incomplete protein.

Complete protein intake may also be achieved by combining two or more *complementary* incomplete proteins. A food that supplies an amino acid that is absent or in low quantities in another food is said to complement that food. For example, wheat, which is deficient in lysine, may be combined with peanuts, which contain adequate amounts of lysine but lack another essential amino acid provided by wheat (Vyhmeister 1984). The resulting combination of wheat and peanuts contains all the essential amino acids and is equivalent to a complete protein. The wheat-peanut combination could be served as a peanut butter sandwich. Plant proteins tend to be less costly than complete animal proteins.

Rapidly growing children need some complete protein or equivalent combinations daily to support that growth. A greater amount of incomplete protein is needed to achieve the equivalent of a complete protein (Lappe 1975). For instance, 1 cup of beans is required to complement 2²/₃ cups of rice (Longacre 1976).

Small children may not have enough stomach capacity to hold the larger amounts of food they must eat to meet their protein needs solely from incomplete protein. Free amino acids resulting from digestion of food protein must be used within a short time as they are not stored for future use. Therefore, the more efficient complete proteins are better able to support rapid growth.

Many favorite dishes are good examples of combinations of proteins which result in the equivalent of a complete protein. Foods may be combined in either of two ways to obtain adequate protein for less money than by using the more costly complete protein sources:

- complementary proteins—incomplete protein combined with another incomplete protein to equal complete protein.

TABLE 15-1 Nutrient Requirements of Infants

AGE (yr)	WEIGHT (lb)	PROTEIN (gm/#)	CALCIUM (mg)	IRON (mg)
0.0–0.5	13	1	360	10
0.5–1.0	20	0.9	540	15

> *Examples:* peanut butter sandwich, beans and rice, chili, peas and rice, macaroni salad with peas, lentil soup with crackers, navy beans with cornbread, baked beans and brown bread

- supplementary proteins—incomplete protein combined with a small amount of complete protein to equal complete protein.

> *Examples:* macaroni and cheese, rice pudding, cheese sandwich, cheese pizza, cereal and milk

Protein Requirements

The total amount of protein needed daily is based on desirable body weight. An infant's requirements for protein and other nutrients are shown in Table 15-1. Due to the infant's extremely rapid rate of growth, nutrient needs are greater in relation to size during infancy than at any other period of life.

Growing children need more protein per pound than adults. Approximately $2/3$ gram of protein for each pound of body weight is recommended for a child weighing 45 pounds; this child needs approximately 30 grams of protein a day. To be meaningful, these figures must be considered in terms of amounts of food. The following selection of foods provides slightly more than the 30 grams of protein recommended for a 4-year-old child.

Food	*Protein*
2 cups milk	16 grams
1½ slices bread	3 grams
2 ounces meat or meat alternate	14 grams
	TOTAL 33 grams

Table 15-2 shows a menu that would provide the daily recommended amount of protein for a child.

MINERALS FOR GROWTH

Minerals are inorganic elements that help to regulate body functions, and also help to build body tissue. This unit deals with minerals that help to build body tissue. The regulatory functions performed by minerals will be covered in the succeeding unit.

TABLE 15-2 Menu Supplying Recommended Daily Allowances of Protein for 4- to 6-Year-Old Children

Breakfast	Grams of Protein
½ c fruit juice	trace
½ c dry oat cereal	1
½ c milk*	4
½ banana	trace
Midmorning Snack	
½ c milk*	4
½ slice buttered toast	1
Lunch	
½ peanut butter and jelly sandwich (1 slice bread, ½ tablespoon peanut butter, ½ tablespoon jelly)+	4
carrot sticks	1
½ apple	trace
½ c milk*	4
Midafternoon Snack	
½ c fruit juice	trace
Dinner	
1 chicken leg (1 oz)*	6
¼ c rice	1
¼ c broccoli	trace
¼ c strawberries	trace
½ c milk*	4
TOTAL	30 grams of protein

* Complete protein
+ Complementary proteins

Minerals provide no energy. They are required in far smaller amounts than are energy-producing nutrients. For example, RDA for protein is 30 grams for a 4-year-old child; this amount is slightly more than one ounce. In contrast, the RDA for calcium for that same child is 0.8 grams. Other minerals are required in even smaller amounts.

Growth involves creating increased amounts of body tissue, which requires attention to receiving adequate amounts of specific minerals. Two types of body tissues most dependent on minerals for growth are bones and teeth, and blood.

Building Bones and Teeth

Calcium and phosphorus are the major minerals found in bones and teeth, Figure 15-2. Bones are formed by the deposition of phosphorus and calcium

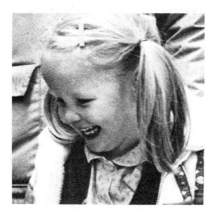

FIGURE 15–2   Calcium and phosphorus are needed for strong teeth and bones.

crystals on a flexible protein base composed of *collagen.* Young childrens' bones are soft and pliable; as growth occurs the amount of calcium and phosphorus deposited in their bones increases, resulting in larger, harder bones. While bones appear to be solid and unchanging, calcium, phosphorus and other minerals are replaced on a regular basis. The calcium content of bone is thought to be replaced every five years. Children need calcium not only for bone growth, but also for replacement of existing bone.

Sources of Calcium.   Dairy foods are the major food source of calcium. With the exception of a few vegetables, calcium is not found in large amounts in any other food source. Milk, cheese and yogurt are excellent sources of calcium. Custards, puddings, and ice cream provide calcium, but they also contain varying amounts of added sugar and fat which reduces their nutrient density relative to calcium.

The calcium content of many dishes may be increased by the addition of nonfat dry milk. The addition of nonfat dry milk to casseroles, cooked cereals, breads, and ground meat dishes not only increases the amount of calcium and protein in those dishes, but also improves the quality of the incomplete proteins in pastas, cereals, or flours.

Sources of Phosphorus.   Phosphorus is also found in dairy foods as well as other high protein foods. Good sources of phosphorus are milk, meats, fish, eggs, and grain products. Calcium and phosphorus occur in approximately equal amounts in milk. Ideally, calcium and phosphorus should be obtained in about equal amounts; the recommended daily amount for both minerals is 0.8 gram for children. It is easier to obtain phosphorus than calcium since it occurs in more kinds of foods. The balance between calcium and phosphorus may be upset if a child is permitted to drink large amounts of carbonated beverages which contain phosphorus in the form of phosphoric acid (Cross 1984). If the child drinks more carbonated beverages than milk, phosphorus in the diet outweighs calcium and calcium absorption may be impaired. This could result in reduced deposition of calcium in the bones and, in extreme cases, withdrawal of calcium from the bones.

The Role of Fluoride. Fluoride should be considered in connection with bone and tooth formation. Many communities add fluoride to the community water supply in an effort to reduce tooth decay in children. Fluoride-containing tooth-pastes are also recommended for use by children. Fluoride incorporated into a growing tooth from drinking water makes the tooth harder and more resistant to decay. Fluoride applied to the exterior surface of the tooth is also thought to reduce the incidence of decay. Excess amounts of fluoride may cause mottling and brown-staining of the teeth. Children who are drinking fluoridated water should be taught not to swallow toothpaste after brushing in order to prevent possible excess consumption.

The most consistent source of fluoride is the local water supply; either as naturally-occurring fluorine or as fluoride added to a level of 1 p.p.m. (1 part fluoride per million parts of water). Food sources of fluoride are variable and depend on the fluorine content of the soil where grown.

Building Blood

Iron is a mineral that is essential to the formation of hemoglobin. *Hemoglobin* is the iron-containing protein in red blood cells that carries oxygen to the cells and removes waste (carbon dioxide) from the cells. Normal growth depends on a healthy blood supply to nourish an increasing number of cells. Iron plays an important role in the formation of healthy blood.

Iron-deficiency anemia is often found in children 2 to 3 years of age. Iron-deficiency anemia is characterized by low levels of hemoglobin in red blood cells, which results in the cells' reduced ability to carry oxygen to tissues. The end result is reduced growth rate, fatigue, lack of energy, possible reduction in learning ability, and reduced resistance to infections.

Sources of Iron. The High Protein Food Group and the Grain Food Group are the best sources of iron. Liver is an especially rich source of iron. Milk, which is usually a major part of the diet of young children, contains very little iron. A child who drinks large amounts of milk to the exclusion of iron-containing foods may not receive enough iron to support a growing blood supply.

Studies of the nutritional status of preschool children have repeatedly indicated that neither calcium nor iron is received in adequate amounts. There may be several reasons for this. One reason may be that neither calcium nor iron are widely distributed in foods. Also, many factors affect the absorption of calcium and iron. Therefore, the presence of either mineral in foods does not always assure that the mineral will be absorbed for use by body cells. Another factor may be that many foods containing calcium or iron are expensive.

Factors Which Affect Absorption of Calcium and Iron

Calcium	Factor	Iron
↑	Adequate Vitamin C	↑
↑	Increased Need	↑
↓	Large Dose	↓
↓	Fiber (bulk) in Diet	↓
↓	High Protein Level	↑

Factors which *increase* the absorption of calcium and iron:

- Vitamin C aids in keeping calcium and iron more soluble and, therefore, more readily absorbed by the body.
- Vitamin C maximizes the absorption of iron in foods in the same meal.
- In cases where need is increased, inadequate intake or rapid growth-absorption of calcium and iron is increased.

Factors which *decrease* the absorption of calcium and iron:
- Large single doses of calcium and iron are not as well-absorbed as several smaller doses.
- Large amounts of fiber in the diet speed intestinal movement, decreasing the time calcium and iron are in contact with absorption surfaces.

Proteins aid the overall absorption of iron; the iron in meats (known as heme iron) is more readily absorbed than the iron in grains and other nonmeat foods. Protein has the opposite effect on calcium in that high intakes of protein may increase the need for calcium.

THE ROLE OF WATER

Water is an important constituent of all body tissues. Approximately 60 percent of normal adult body weight is water; an infant's body weight is nearly 75 percent water. A gradual decline in water content occurs throughout the life cycle. Need for water is affected by body surface area, environmental temperature, and activity. Water is essential for survival; humans can survive much longer without food than they can without water. Water is supplied to the body through drinking water and other beverages, solid foods, and water that results from energy metabolism.

Vomiting and diarrhea cause excess loss of water which can very rapidly cause dehydration. This is especially threatening to infants, toddlers, and small children, since the amount of water loss necessary to produce dehydration is small in comparison to that of an adult.

Children experience more rapid loss of water through evaporation and dehydration than do adults. Since children are busily involved in other activities, they may need reminders to drink fluids, Figure 15–3. This is important at any time but especially in hot weather. Both children and adults should be encouraged to

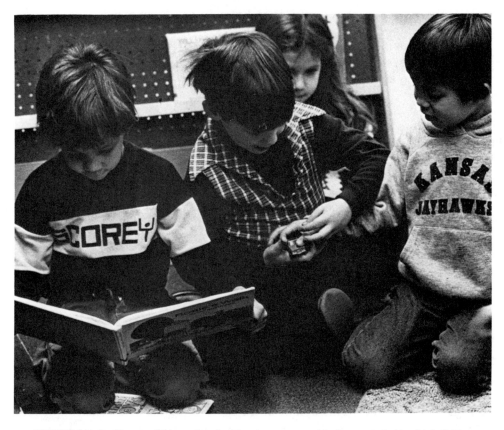

FIGURE 15-3 Young children absorbed in play may need to be reminded to drink fluids.

drink water rather than sugared beverages since the presence of sugar is known to slow the absorption of water (DeVries 1980).

SUMMARY

Growth is an increase in the physical size of either the entire body or any part of the body. Growth occurs both by increasing the number of cells and increasing the size of the cells.

Nutrients most necessary to build body tissue are proteins, minerals, and water. Proteins are components of every living cell and are composed of individual units called amino acids. Essential amino acids must be provided in food proteins since the body cannot manufacture them in needed amounts. Proteins which contain all the essential amino acids in adequate amounts for growth are said to be complete proteins. Meats, fish, poultry, soybeans, eggs and dairy products contain complete proteins. Proteins which lack one or more essential amino acids in adequate amounts are said to be incomplete proteins; examples are grains, most legumes, and vegetables.

Complementary incomplete proteins may be combined to make up the equivalent of a complete protein at a lower cost.

Calcium and phosphorus are the major constituents of bone and teeth. Crystals of calcium and phosphorus are deposited on a flexible protein base composed of collagen. As increasing amounts of calcium and phosphorus are deposited, bones become harder.

The major food source of calcium is the Dairy Food Group. Milk, cheese, and yogurt are excellent sources of calcium. Phosphorus is more widely distributed in foods, since it is found in the Dairy Food Group, High Protein Food Group, and Grain Food Group.

Blood cell formation depends on the presence of adequate amounts of iron. Iron is the mineral component of hemoglobin, a protein found in red blood cells. Food sources of iron are the High Protein Food Group and the Grain Food Group. Liver is the richest food source of iron; some green vegetables such as spinach contain iron, but much of it is in an insoluble form.

Many factors can interfere with the absorption of both calcium and iron.

Water is a constituent of all body tissues, making up 60–75 percent of body weight. Sources of water are beverages, solid foods and water derived from metabolism for release of energy.

LEARNING ACTIVITIES

1. Compare nutrition information labels from prepared cereals. Common iron content levels are 100% USRDA, 45% USRDA and 25% USRDA. After reviewing the "Factors that Affect Absorption of Calcium and Iron," discuss which cereal(s) would be the wisest choice in terms of iron absorption. What other step(s) could be taken to increase the absorption of the iron available in the cereal?

2. Explain why early childhood is a time of risk for iron-deficiency anemia. Consider factors such as food groups in which iron occurs, typical food preferences, and relative ease of eating various foods.

3. Determine the amount of protein recommended for a child who weighs 42 pounds.

UNIT REVIEW

A. Match the terms in column II with the definition in column I. Use each term in column II only once.

Column I	Column II
1. an essential amino acid	a. calcium
2. a nutrient class which functions both to build tissues and provide energy	b. Dairy Food Group
	c. iron

3. the mineral component of hemoglobin
4. the mineral which is a major component of bones and teeth
5. the food group which provides the
   greatest amounts of calcium
6. the food group which provides the
   greatest amounts of iron
7. a nutrient class which helps to regulate body processes and also helps to
   build body tissue
8. comprises approximately 60 percent
   of normal adult body weight

d. High Protein Food
   Group
e. lysine
f. minerals
g. protein
h. water

B. Multiple Choice. Select the correct choice.

1. The two major *mineral* components of bones and teeth are
   a. protein and calcium
   b. phosphorus and iron
   c. calcium and phosphorus
   d. protein and water

2. Proteins are composed of
   a. amino acids
   b. fatty acids
   c. simple sugars
   d. carbon, hydrogen, and oxygen

3. Collagen forms the flexible protein matrix upon which bone is built. Collagen is composed of
   a. fatty acids
   b. amino acids
   c. calcium
   d. phosphorus

4. Amino acids which cannot be manufactured within the body are termed
   a. nonessential
   b. essential
   c. complete
   d. incomplete

5. Essential amino acids must be derived from
   a. within the body
   b. food sources
   c. other amino acids
   d. all of these

6. Proteins from animal sources are
   a. complete
   b. incomplete
   c. complementary
   d. saturated

7. Sources of complete protein are
   a. meat, eggs, milk
   b. cereals, pastas, legumes
   c. fruits, vegetables, grains
   d. butter, cream, salad dressings

8. Examples of incomplete complementary proteins are
   a. macaroni and cheese
   b. tuna and noodles
   c. cornflakes and milk
   d. rice and peas

9. A factor that helps iron and calcium absorption is
   a. adequate Vitamin C
   b. a large amount of fiber
   c. a large single dose
   d. all of these

10. Dairy products are excellent sources of the *mineral*
    a. iron
    b. calcium
    c. protein
    d. none of these

11. The mineral that is usually consumed in less than adequate quantities by preschoolers is
    a. calcium
    b. iron
    c. protein
    d. none of these

12. The nutrient which makes up the greatest percentage of body weight is
    a. protein
    b. water
    c. calcium
    d. iron

13. The means by which growth occurs is
    a. increase in cell size
    b. increase in total body size
    c. increase in number of cells
    d. both a and c

14. Which of the following would provide water for the body?
    a. lettuce
    b. milk
    c. metabolism for release of energy
    d. all of these

C. Case Study

The following chart shows a fairly typical daily intake for Timothy, age 4½. Consider this daily pattern in terms of balance between calcium and phosphorus.

> Breakfast:
>   1 slice of toast
>   1 scrambled egg
>   ½ cup orange juice
> Midmorning Snack:
>   2 graham crackers (milk offered but refused)
> Lunch:
>   2 fish sticks
>   ¼ cup peas
>   ½ slice bread
>   water (milk offered but refused)
> Midafternoon Snack:
>   1 small soft drink
> Dinner:
>   hamburger
>   french fries
>   1 small soft drink

1. What foods provide calcium?

2. What foods provide phosphorus?

3. Change the menu to eliminate the phosphorus/calcium imbalance.

REFERENCES

Cross, M. Z. *Syllabus for an Introductory Nutrition Course.* 4th ed. Dubuque, IA: Kendall/Hunt Publishing Company, 1984.

de Vries, H. A. *Physiology of Exercise for Education and Athletics.* 3d ed. Dubuque, IA: William C. Brown Company Publisher, 1980.

Lappe, F. M. *Diet for A Small Planet.* rev. ed. New York: Ballantine, 1975.

Longacre, D. J. *More-with-Less Cookbook.* Scottsdale, PA: Herald Press, 1976.

Vyhmeister, I. B. "Vegetarian Diets—Issues and Concerns." *Nutrition and the M.D.,* May 1984.

Unit 16
NUTRIENTS THAT REGULATE BODY FUNCTIONS

Terms to Know

toxicity
acuity
hormones
catalyst
catalyze
milligram
microgram
adenosine
  triphosphate (ATP)

microcytic anemia
macrocytic anemia
RNA
DNA
synthesis
neuromuscular
megadose

Objectives

After studying this unit, you will be able to:
- Name general types of body functions regulated by nutrients.
- Identify nutrients which perform regulatory functions in the body.
- List at least one specific function performed by each of the four nutrient classes identified as regulators.

Energy cannot be produced or released from carbohydrates, proteins, and fats without specific nutrients catalyzing sequential steps. New tissues such as bone, blood, or muscles cannot be formed unless specific vitamins, minerals, and proteins are available for their specific functions in each of these processes. Nerve impulses will not travel from one nerve cell to another, nor muscles contract unless the required nutrients are available in adequate amounts at the appropriate times. Some body functions may be regulated by one or two nutrients in one or two reactions. Many other functions involve intricate sequences of reactions which require many nutrients. All body functions are subject to regulation by nutrients.

Regulation of body functions is an extremely complex process. While much has been learned about the role of nutrients in regulation, there is still much that is unknown. It is important to remember that nutrients and functions are intricately interrelated. No single nutrient can function alone; thus regulation of body functions depends on many nutrients. This unit briefly discusses four nutrient classes involved in regulating body functions:

- vitamins
- minerals
- proteins
- water

Protein has been discussed earlier in terms of both energy and growth. Minerals and water were introduced as tissue-building nutrients and will now be considered as regulatory nutrients. Vitamins are able to perform only regulatory functions. They do not yield energy directly, nor do they become part of body structure. However, no energy can be released or any tissue built without benefit of the specific regulatory activities performed by vitamins.

The regulatory functions discussed in this unit are crucial to the normal growth and development of young children. Generally these functions are:

- energy metabolism
- cellular reproduction and growth
- bone growth
- *neuromuscular* function

Other functions are also crucial to normal development. However, these functions were chosen because of their critical relationship to normal growth, learning, and general good health of infants, toddlers, and young children.

VITAMINS AS REGULATORS

Vitamins are needed in extremely small amounts but they are essential for normal body function. Each vitamin plays a specific role in a variety of body activities, Table 16–1. Vitamins frequently depend upon one another to perform their functions. For example, the vitamins, thiamin and niacin, are both needed as crucial coenzymes for the release of energy, but thiamin cannot function in the place of niacin, nor can niacin function in the absence of thiamin's action in a prior step.

Vitamins are needed and used in specific amounts. Large excesses do not serve any useful function and in some instances are known to be harmful. Toxic effects have long been known for excesses of vitamin A and vitamin D. Recent research has described neurological damage resulting from large amounts of vitamin B_6 and kidney stone formation and destruction of vitamin B_{12} stores as a result of *megadoses* of vitamin C (ascorbic acid). Megadoses are usually defined

TABLE 16-1   Vitamin Summary

VITAMIN	FUNCTIONS	RDA	SOURCES	DEFICIENCY SYMPTOMS	TOXICITY SYMPTOMS
Fat-soluble Vitamins Vitamin A	Maintenance of: • remodeling of bones • all cell membranes • epithelial cells; skin • mucous membranes, glands Regulation of vision in dim light.	1–3 yrs—400 R.E. 4–6 yrs—500 R.E.	Liver, whole milk, butter, fortified margarine, orange and dark green vegetables, orange fruits (apricots, nectarines, peaches).	Depressed bone and tooth formation, lack of visual acuity, dry epithelial tissue, increased frequency of infections related to epithelial cell vulnerability.	Headaches, nausea, vomiting, fragile bones, loss of hair, dry skin. Infant: hydrocephalus, hyperirritability.
Vitamin D	Regulates calcium/phosphorus absorption Mineralization of bone.	1–3 yrs—10 mcg 4–6 yrs—10 mcg	Vitamin D fortified milk, exposure of skin to sunlight.	Rickets (soft, easily bent bones), bone deformities.	Elevated blood calcium; deposition of calcium in soft tissues resulting in cerebral, renal and cardiovascular damage (Dubick and Rucker 1983).
Vitamin E	Antioxidant	1–3 yrs—5 T.E. 4–6 yrs—6 T.E.	Vegetable oils, wheat germ, egg yolk, leafy vegetables, legumes, margarine.	Red blood cell destruction; creatinuria.	Fatigue, skin rash, abdominal discomfort.
Vitamin K	Normal blood coagulation.	Estimated safe range: 1–3 yrs—15–30 mcg 4–6 yrs—20–40 mcg	Leafy vegetables, vegetable oils, liver, pork; synthesis by intestinal bacteria.	Hemorrhage	None reported for naturally-occurring vitamin K.

	Function	Amount	Food Sources	Deficiency	Excess
Water-soluble Vitamins Vitamin C (Ascorbic Acid)	Formation of collagen for: • bones/teeth • intercellular cement • wound healing Aid to calcium/iron absorption Conversion of folacin to active form Neurotransmitter synthesis.	1–3 yrs—45 mg 4–6 yrs—45 mg	Citrus fruits, strawberries, melons, cabbage, peppers, greens, tomatoes.	Poor wound healing, bleeding gums, pinpoint hemorrhages, sore joints, scurvy.	Nausea, abdominal cramps, diarrhea. Precipitation of kidney stones in susceptible persons; "conditioned scurvy" (Dubick and Rucker 1983).
Thiamin	Carbohydrate metabolism Energy metabolism Neurotransmitter synthesis.	1–3 yrs—0.7 mg 4–6 yrs—0.9 mg	Whole or enriched grain products, organ meats, pork.	Loss of appetite, depression, poor neuromuscular control, Beri-Beri.	None reported.
Riboflavin	Hydrogen transport in metabolism of carbohydrates, fats, and proteins. Energy metabolism.	1–3 yrs—0.8 mg 4–6 yrs—1.0 mg	Dairy foods, meat products, enriched or whole grains, green vegetables.	Sore tongue, cracks at corners of the mouth (cheilosis).	None reported.
Niacin	Carbohydrate, protein, and fat metabolism; energy metabolism; conversion of folacin to its active form.	1–3 yrs— 9 mg 4–6 yrs—11 mg	Meat products, whole or enriched grain products, legumes.	Dermatitis, diarrhea, depression, and paranoia.	Flushing, itching, nausea, vomiting, diarrhea, low blood pressure, rapid heart beat, low blood sugar, liver damage (Dubick and Rucker 1983).
Pantothenic Acid	Energy metabolism; fatty acid metabolism; neurotransmitter synthesis.	Estimated safe range: 3–4 mg	Nearly all foods.	Uncommon in humans.	None reported.
Vitamin B₆ (Pyridoxine)	Protein and fatty acid synthesis; neurotransmitter synthesis; hemoglobin synthesis.	1–3 yrs—0.9 mg 4–6 yrs—1.3 mg	Meats, organ meats, whole grains, legumes, bananas.	Nervous system: • irritability • tremors • convulsions } infants Anemia.	Unstable gait, numbness, lack of coordination (Schaumberg, 1983).

TABLE 16–1 Vitamin Summary (Continued)

VITAMIN	FUNCTIONS	RDA	SOURCES	DEFICIENCY SYMPTOMS	TOXICITY SYMPTOMS
Folacin	Synthesis of DNA and RNA; cell replication protein synthesis	1–3 yrs—100 mcg 4–6 yrs—200 mcg	Liver, other meats, green vegetables.	*Macrocytic* anemia characterized by unusually large red blood cells; sore tongue, diarrhea.	None reported. (Large amount may hide a B_{12} deficiency).
Vitamin B_{12} (Cobalamin)	Synthesis of DNA and RNA; conversion of folacin to active form; synthesis of myelin (fatty covering of nerve cells); carbohydrate metabolism.	1–3 yrs—2.0 mcg 4–6 yrs—2.5 mcg	Animal foods, liver, other meats, dairy products, eggs.	Macrocytic anemia, nervous system damage, sore mouth and tongue, loss of appetite, nausea, vomiting. (Pernicious anemia results from faulty absorption of B_{12}.)	None reported.
Biotin	Carbohydrate and fat metabolism; amino acid metabolism.	Estimated safe range: 1–3 yrs—65 mcg 4–6 yrs—85 mcg	Organ meats, milk, egg yolk, yeast; synthesis by intestinal bacteria.	Nervous disorders, skin disorders, anorexia, muscle pain.	None reported.

as ten times the recommended daily amount for an adult. There is not enough information to define toxic doses of all vitamins for young children; it is certainly smaller than the amount required to produce *toxicity* symptoms in an adult. Therefore, extreme caution should be used if giving children vitamin supplements without the advice of a physician. "If a little bit is good, a lot is better" is a dangerous practice relative to vitamins.

Vitamins have been the subject of much attention in the press, having been promoted as "cures" for numerous conditions including cancer, common colds, and mental illness (Consumer Reports 1980). Many people take vitamins and give them to their children as an "insurance policy." Vitamins can supplement a "hit-or-miss" diet, but should not be given as a replacement for an adequate diet. There are a number of reasons why supplements cannot add up to an adequate diet by themselves. Vitamin and/or mineral supplements do not provide all of the nutrients known to be needed by humans nor do they provide any calories, a primary need. Poor diets may lack fiber or essential amino acids or the essential fatty acid which will not be corrected by vitamin/mineral supplements. Also, there may be substances as yet unknown but essential which are derived from foods that are not included in vitamin/mineral preparations. The best means of obtaining nutrients is by "judicious selection of foods" (Williams and Calienda 1984).

Vitamins are classified as fat-soluble (dissolved in or carried in fats) or water-soluble (dissolved in water). Fat-soluble vitamins behave differently chemically than water-soluble vitamins. Table 16–2 provides a summary of the characteristics of vitamins.

TABLE 16–2 Characteristics of Vitamins

	FAT-SOLUBLE VITAMINS	WATER-SOLUBLE VITAMINS
Examples	A, D, E, K	C, Thiamin, Niacin, Riboflavin, Pantothenic Acid, B_6 (Pyridoxine), Biotin, Folacin, B_{12} (Cobalamin)
Stored in body	Yes	No (B_{12} is an exception)
Excreted in urine	No	Yes
Needed daily	No	Yes
Deficiency	Develop slowly	Develop rapidly
Toxicity from increased amounts	A, D, E (research is continuing)	C, B_6 (research is continuing)

Vitamins in Energy Metabolism

A slow steady release of energy is important to body needs. If energy is released in a haphazard fashion, much of it is lost as heat. Since young children require greater amounts of energy per pound, they cannot afford to lose energy in such a fashion. The primary vitamins involved in the regulation of metabolism for release of energy are:

- thiamin
- niacin
- riboflavin
- pantothenic acid

These four vitamins are not the only nutrients involved in this process; all the other nutrients required must also be available in adequate amounts at the time needed. The absence of enough of any of the required nutrients causes the process of energy release to operate inefficiently, abnormally, or not at all.

Vitamins in Cellular Reproduction and Growth

Two vitamins which are absolutely essential for cell growth are folacin and cobalamin (B_{12}). Both vitamins participate in the *synthesis* of DNA and RNA, which are the chemicals that provide the pattern for cell division and growth. So crucial are these vitamins for cell division and growth that deficiencies of them are quickly noticeable in tissues which are frequently replaced, such as red blood cells or the cells lining the intestine.

Young children may be considered at risk for both folacin and B_{12} deficiency. Requirements for these nutrients are always increased during periods of rapid growth such as that typical of early childhood. Another factor which must be considered is the fact that B_{12} is found only in food from animal sources. Parents who are vegetarians will find that very careful planning is required in order to meet their child's needs for vitamin B_{12}, Table 16–3.

In addition to needs for folacin and B_{12}, cellular reproduction and increase in cell size are also dependent on proteins. One vitamin which is essential to the metabolism of proteins is pyridoxine (B_6). Pyridoxine *catalyzes* the chemical changes which permit the building of proteins from amino acids, or the breakdown of proteins to provide needed amino acids.

Vitamins Which Regulate Bone Growth

The minerals calcium and phosphorus are the major structural components of bones and teeth. However, bone growth also depends on a number of other nutrients as regulators including vitamins A, C, and D, Figure 16–1.

Vitamin A regulates the destruction of old bone cells and their replacement by new ones. This process is known as "remodeling."

TABLE 16–3 Facts about Vegetarianism

1. The choice of vegetarianism as a life-style is based on many very personal reasons—philosophical, religious, or economic.
2. *Ovo-lactovegetarians* use no meat, fish, or poultry but do use dairy products and eggs.
3. *Lactovegetarians* limit use of animal foods to milk and dairy products but use no eggs. Lactovegetarian diets can be adequate at all stages of life and can provide the necessary nutrients with careful planning.
4. *Vegans* are vegetarians who use no animal products; all foods come from plant sources such as fruits, vegetables, legumes, grains, nuts, and seeds.
5. The vegan diet is not recommended for infants and young children. These diets may not supply enough calories per volume of food in relation to the young child's small stomach capacity.
6. Important nutrients such as cobalamin (B_{12}), calcium, iron, and riboflavin may occur in reduced amounts in the vegan diet.

Adapted from "Getting Enough to Grow On" by Patricia K. Johnston, Assistant Professor of Nutrition, School of Public Health, Loma Linda University. In the *American Journal of Nursing.*

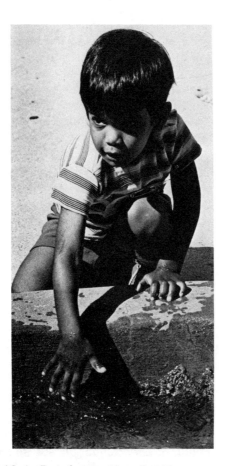

FIGURE 16–1 Body function is regulated by many nutrients.

Vitamin C functions in two ways in the formation of bone tissue:

- maintains the solubility of calcium, making it more available for absorption
- aids in the formation of collagen, the flexible protein foundation upon which phosphorus and calcium are deposited

Vitamin D is necessary for the absorption of calcium and phosphorus, the major constituents of bones and teeth. It is also needed to assure blood levels of calcium and phosphorus that allow for deposition of these minerals in bones and teeth.

Vitamins Which Regulate Neuromuscular Function

Vitamins play a role in neuromuscular function either through the synthesis of neurotransmitters (chemical messengers) or through growth or maintenance of nerve cells.

Vitamin B_6 and vitamin C catalyze the synthesis of neurotransmitters such as serotonin, dopamine, and norepinephrine.

Thiamin and niacin are also involved in neurological function. Thiamin is required for synthesis of the neurotransmitter, acetylcholine. The exact role played by niacin is not clear. Deficiencies of these vitamins result in neurological abnormalities.

B_6 and B_{12} are necessary for the formation and maintenance of the myelin sheath, the insulative layer surrounding nerve cells. Faulty myelin sheath formation and maintenance results in abnormal passage of nerve impulses, which may result in numbness, tremors, or loss of coordination.

MINERALS AS REGULATORS

Many body functions require the presence of specific minerals, Table 16–4. The amounts of minerals required for regulatory purposes are smaller than those required directly to build or repair body tissue. Minerals used by the body for regulatory purposes are usually parts of enzymes or coenzymes or catalyze their action.

Minerals in Energy Metabolism

Minerals also play an important role in the steady, efficient release of energy. This process of energy metabolism (production, storage, and release) depends on adequate amounts of:

- phosphorus
- magnesium
- iodine
- iron

Phosphorus is necessary for the formation of *adenosine triphosphate (ATP)*, the chemical substance in which potential energy is stored in body cells. Another

TABLE 16-4   Mineral Summary

MINERAL	FUNCTIONS	RDA	SOURCES	DEFICIENCY SYMPTOMS	TOXICITY SYMPTOMS
Calcium	Major component of bones and teeth; collagen formation; muscle contraction; secretion/release of neurotransmitters; blood clotting.	1–3 yrs—800 mg 4–6 yrs—800 mg	Dairy products, turnip or collard greens, canned salmon or sardines, soybeans or soybean curd (tofu).	Poor growth, small adult size, fragile and deformed bones, some forms of rickets.	Unlikely. Absorption is controlled; symptoms usually result from excess vitamin D or hormonal imbalance.
Phosphorus	Major component of bones and teeth; energy metabolism; component of DNA and RNA.	1–3 yrs—800 mg 4–6 yrs—800 mg	Dairy products, meats, legumes, grains, additive in soft drinks.	Rare with normal diet.	Large amounts may depress calcium absorption.
Magnesium	Major component of bones and teeth; activator of enzymes for ATP use; required for synthesis of DNA and RNA and for synthesis of proteins by RNA.	1–3 yrs—150 mg 4–6 yrs—200 mg	Nuts, seeds, green vegetables, legumes, whole grains.	Poor neuromuscular coordination, tremors, convulsions.	Unlikely.
Sodium	Nerve impulse transmission; fluid balance; acid-base balance.	Estimated safe range: 1–3 yrs—325–925 mg 4–6 yrs—450–1350 mg	Meats, fish, poultry, eggs, milk, (naturally-occurring sodium); many processed and cured foods (added sodium), salt, MSG.	Rare. (Losses from sweat may cause dizziness, nausea, muscle cramps.)	Linked to high blood pressure in some persons; confusion; coma.
Potassium	Nerve impulse transmission; fluid balance; acid-base balance.	1–3 yrs—550–1650 mg 4–6 yrs—775–2335 mg	Fruits (bananas, orange juice), vegetables, whole grains, fresh meats, fish.	Weakness, irregular heart beat.	Unlikely from food sources.

TABLE 16-4 Mineral Summary (Continued)

MINERAL	FUNCTIONS	RDA	SOURCES	DEFICIENCY SYMPTOMS	TOXICITY SYMPTOMS
Iron	Component of hemoglobin; enzymes involved in oxygen utilization.	1-3 yrs—15 mg 4-6 yrs—10 mg	Liver and other meats, enriched and whole grains, leafy green vegetables.	*Microcytic anemia* (characterized by small, pale red blood cells), fatigue, pallor, shortness of breath.	Unlikely. (May be due to genetic defect.)
Zinc	Component of many enzymes involved in: protein metabolism DNA/RNA syntheses collagen formation wound healing.	1-3 yrs—10 mg 4-6 yrs—10 mg	Liver, oysters, meats, eggs, whole grains, legumes.	Retarded growth, loss of senses of taste and smell, delayed wound healing.	Excess supplementation may interfere with iron/copper metabolism. Nausea, vomiting, diarrhea, gastric ulcers.
Iodine	Component of thyroxin, which regulates basal metabolic rate.	1-3 yrs—70 mcg 4-6 yrs—90 mcg	Iodized salt, seafoods, many processed foods.	Goiter, physical dwarfing, cretinism if deficiency occurs during fetal life.	Iodism; rashes; bronchitis.

mineral, magnesium, is necessary for both the storage and the release of the energy trapped in ATP. Iron functions as part of one of the key enzyme systems in the final stages of energy metabolism. Iodine is a component of the hormone, thyroxin. As such, iodine aids in the control of the rate at which the body uses energy (the basal metabolic rate).

Minerals in Cellular Reproduction and Growth

Minerals required for cellular reproduction and growth include:

- phosphorus
- magnesium
- zinc

Phosphorus is a structural component of both DNA and RNA. Magnesium is required both for the synthesis of DNA and for synthesis of proteins from the pattern provided by DNA. Zinc functions as part of an enzyme system which must be active during DNA and RNA synthesis.

The effect of an inadequate zinc supply is reflected by signs and symptoms such as stunted growth, decreased *acuity* of taste and smell which may further decrease food intake, and delayed sexual maturity. Zinc is chemically similar to iron; its absorption is affected by many of the same factors.

Minerals Which Regulate Neuromuscular Function

Passage of nerve impulses from nerve cell to nerve cell or from nerve cell to muscle is dependent on the presence of:

- sodium
- potassium
- calcium

Sodium and potassium act to change the electrical charge on the surface of the nerve cell, allowing the passage of the nerve impulse. Calcium is required for the release of many neurotransmitters from nerve cells. The passage of a nerve impulse to a muscle cell causes the contraction of muscles. Calcium is required for the actual contraction of a muscle, while ATP which contains phosphorus as a structural component provides the energy for the contraction to take place.

Sodium is an essential mineral in neuromuscular function, fluid, and mineral balance. It is one essential nutrient for which there is little problem in obtaining enough. In fact, many people receive too much sodium in their diets, especially in the form of salt (sodium chloride). Excess sodium intake has been tentatively related to the incidence of high blood pressure and fluid retention. Salt has been omitted from most commercial baby foods and should be omitted from home-prepared baby foods. Foods served to young children should be prepared without salt or only lightly salted, since the taste for salt seems to be acquired. No seasoning, or mild seasoning with lemon juice, lime juice, herbs, or spices teaches the young child to appreciate the actual flavor of food, rather than that of salt.

PROTEINS AS REGULATORS

Proteins are the only class of nutrients that can perform all three general functions of nutrients. They build and repair body tissue, regulate body functions, and provide energy.

Proteins in Energy Metabolism

Proteins (amino acids) are important components of enzymes and some hormones and thus play a major role in regulation of energy metabolism. The body must have an adequate supply of protein in order to produce these important enzymes and hormones.

All body functions are dependent on the presence and activity of enzymes. Enzymes are defined as protein catalysts. A catalyst is a substance which regulates a chemical reaction without becoming part of that reaction. The sequential metabolism for release of energy requires many steps; each step requires at least one enzyme specific for that particular reaction.

Hormones are substances which are secreted by glands for action on tissue elsewhere in the body. As such, they regulate many body functions. While not all hormones are composed of amino acids, two amino-acid dependent hormones are required in energy metabolism. These hormones are thyroxin and insulin.

Thyroxin regulates the rate at which energy is used for involuntary activities. It is secreted by the thyroid gland. Insulin is secreted by the pancreas. Its presence is necessary for glucose to be absorbed by many of the body cells. Before energy can be derived from glucose, it must be inside the cell.

Other hormones derived from amino acids which are important in body function are calcitonin and parathormone which regulate blood calcium and phosphorus levels and ultimately the growth and hardness of bones. Human growth hormone is also made up of amino acids.

WATER AS A REGULATOR

The initial step of processing food for use by the body is digestion. Digestion is the process by which food is broken down mechanically and chemically into nutrients that can be used by the body. Food composition is changed during chemical digestion through the breaking down of food molecules and the addition of water. Water is essential for this process as it is the medium in which chemical reactions take place, Figure 16–2.

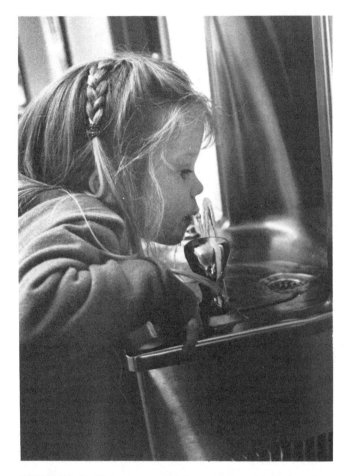

FIGURE 16-2 Water is essential for regulation of body functions.

After food is digested and the nutrients absorbed, the nutrients are carried in solution by the blood and lymph to the cells of the body. Water again is necessary as it is the main transporting agent of the body comprising all body fluids including blood, lymph and tissue fluid. Water also is the major component of body secretions such as salivary juice, gastric juice, bile, perspiration, and expirations from the lungs. Urine is comprised of approximately 95 percent water.

SUMMARY

Nutrient classes which regulate body functions are vitamins, minerals, proteins, and water. Vitamins can perform only regulatory functions. Some functions regulated by vitamins are energy metabolism, cellular reproduction and growth, bone growth, and neuromuscular activities.

Minerals are also required for the regulation of energy metabolism, cellular reproduction and growth, and normal nerve and muscle function.

Proteins (amino acids) function as regulatory substances in the form of enzymes and some hormones. Most body reactions depend on the activity of specific enzymes at specific steps of the process. Hormones, in turn, may regulate the rate of many of these reactions. Thyroxin and insulin are examples of hormones which are synthesized from amino acids.

Water is required as a medium in which most body functions take place. It also performs some specific regulatory activities.

LEARNING ACTIVITIES

1. Using the summary tables for vitamins and minerals, list two specific foods or types of foods which are rich sources of each of the following nutrients:

   | magnesium | thiamin |
   | calcium | riboflavin |

   a. What foods are good sources of more than one of these nutrients?
   b. Which nutrients occur in the same types of foods?
   c. Which nutrients do not occur in the same types of foods?

2. Calculate the INQ for thiamin for an adult female requiring 2000 calories and for a young child requiring 1600 calories per day for each of the following foods. (Refer to Unit 13 for instructions for INQ calculations.)

   • A two-slice serving of whole grain bread containing 15 percent of the USRDA for thiamin, and 150 calories.

   • A two-slice serving of enriched white bread containing 15 percent of USRDA for thiamin, and 150 calories.

   • A one-cup serving of 2% milk containing 8 percent of USRDA for thiamin, and 120 calories.

   • A two-tablespoon serving of peanut butter containing less than 2 percent of USRDA for thiamin, and 200 calories.

   a. Which foods are nutrient-dense?
   b. Which foods are calorie-dense?
   c. Rank the foods from best source to least good source of thiamin.

UNIT REVIEW

A. Multiple Choice. Select the best answer.

   1. Vitamins which regulate energy metabolism are
      a. magnesium, iron, and iodine
      b. thiamin, niacin, and riboflavin
      c. folacin, cobalamin, and pyridoxine
      d. calcium, phosphorus, and iron

2. Vitamins which regulate cell division and growth and metabolize protein are
   a. cobalamin, folacin, and pyridoxine
   b. magnesium, phosphorus, and zinc
   c. vitamin A, vitamin C, and vitamin D
   d. thiamin, niacin, and riboflavin

3. Vitamins which regulate normal bone growth are
   a. calcium, phosphorus, and fluoride
   b. vitamin A, vitamin C, and vitamin D
   c. pyridoxine, iron, and thiamin
   d. magnesium, niacin, and riboflavin

4. Which of the following foods are considered the best contributors of vitamin A?
   a. sweet potatoes, liver, broccoli
   b. peas, bananas, apples
   c. cherries, turnips, potatoes
   d. rice, beans, corn

5. Which of the following foods are considered the best contributors of vitamin C?
   a. milk, liver, whole wheat bread
   b. oranges, strawberries, tomatoes
   c. peas, bananas, apples
   d. cabbage, peanuts, grapes

6. Muscle contraction is regulated by the mineral
   a. calcium
   b. vitamin C
   c. vitamin A
   d. zinc

7. Milk and dairy foods are good sources of
   a. calcium, riboflavin, protein
   b. vitamin C, zinc, copper
   c. niacin, iron, magnesium
   d. pyridoxine, folacin, thiamin

8. Grains and cereals are good sources of
   a. thiamin, phosphorus
   b. calcium, vitamin C
   c. vitamin A, calcium
   d. cobalamin

9. Nutrients which regulate energy metabolism and are furnished by green leafy vegetables include
   a. niacin and phosphorus
   b. magnesium and riboflavin
   c. vitamin D and vitamin B$_{12}$
   d. zinc and cobalamin

10. Vitamins which are essential for cellular division and growth and are provided by liver and other meats are
    a. folacin and cobalamin
    b. iron and copper
    c. vitamin C and vitamin D
    d. pantothenic acid and iodine

B. Briefly answer the following questions.

1. What two minerals are required for energy metabolism?

2. What two minerals are required for cellular division and growth?

3. What is the medium in which chemical reactions take place?

4. Name an important component of enzymes and some hormones.

C. Case Study

   Tony, age 4½, is allergic to citrus fruits. Even a few drops of juice cause him to break out in hives.

1. For what nutrient should Tony's diet be closely monitored?

2. a. If Tony's diet is actually deficient in this nutrient, would symptoms appear rapidly or slowly?
   b. Why?

3. Suggest foods other than citrus fruits which could also provide this nutrient.

4. List two symptoms which Tony might display.

5. a. Should Tony be given large doses of this nutrient to offset possible deficiencies?
   b. Why or why not?

REFERENCES

Dubnick, M. A., and Rucker, R. B. "Dietary Supplements and Health Aids—A Critical Evaluation. Part I Vitamins and Minerals." *Journal of Nutrition Education* 15:47–51, February 1983.

Johnston, P. K. "Getting Enough To Grow On." *American Journal of Nursing* 1:336–39, March 1984.

Nutrition as Therapy. *Consumer Reports* 45:21–24, January 1980.

Schaumberg, H. A., et al. "Sensory Neuropathy from Pyridoxine Abuse." *New England Journal of Medicine* 309:445–48, August 25, 1983.

Williams, E. R., and Calienda, M. A. *Nutrition: Principles, Issues, and Applications.* New York: McGraw-Hill Book Company, 1984.

Additional Readings

Endres, J. E., and Rockwell, R. E. *Food, Nutrition and the Young Child.* St. Louis: The C.V. Mosby Company, 1980.

Kreutler, P. A. *Nutrition in Perspective.* Englewood Cliffs, NJ: Prentice-Hall, Inc., 1980.

Hamilton, E. M. N., and Whitney, E. N. *Nutrition: Concepts and Controversies.* 2d ed. St. Paul: West Publishing Company, 1981.

Labuza, T. P., and Sloan, A. E. *Contemporary Nutrition Controversies.* St. Paul: West Publishing Co., 1979.

Pipes, P. *Nutrition in Infancy and Childhood.* St. Louis: The C.V. Mosby Company, 1981.

Reed, P. B. *Nutrition: An Applied Science.* St. Paul: West Publishing Company, 1980.

Satter, E. *Child of Mine.* Palo Alto, CA: Bull Publishing Company, 1983.

Whitney, E. N., and Hamilton, E. M. N. *Understanding Nutrition.* 3d ed. St. Louis: West Publishing Company, 1984.

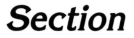

Section

SEVEN

NUTRITION AND THE YOUNG CHILD

Unit 17
NUTRITIONAL
ASSESSMENT

Terms to Know

pallor	clinical
lethargy	biochemical
assessment	24-hour recall
mottling	skin fold
anthropometric	deficiency

Objectives

After studying this unit, you will be able to:
- List four methods of assessing nutritional status.
- Identify the physical signs of common nutritional deficiencies.
- State physical characteristics of a healthy, well-nourished child.
- Describe anthropometric assessment.
- Define biochemical assessment.
- Explain dietary assessment.

Knowledge of the functions that various nutrients perform in the body can be used to assess the dietary intakes of individual children or groups of children. The care provider is in a position to observe young children on a daily basis, both as part of checking children upon arrival each day and through interaction with the child throughout the day. Observations provide unique opportunities to note behaviors that are unusual for individual children or are unusual in comparison to other children. Through observation techniques, care providers may be the first to note unusual behavior or physical problems which might stem from nutritional inadequacies. The care provider can also reassure parents that short-term deficiencies probably are not harmful; malnutrition results from long-term deficiencies of nutrients. The care provider is in a position to observe facial *pallor* and *lethargy* in a young child. This observation and the child's food habits while at the care center should be brought to the attention of the child's parents. Discussion should center on mutual committment to the child's good health and normal growth and development. The care provider must be careful to avoid implied criticism of the parents' care. ("We have noticed that Susie seems very tired lately and has not seemed hungry for her meals and snacks while with us. She does usually drink her milk and often asks for seconds. Have you noticed anything unusual in her eating habits or her behavior at home recently?")

NUTRITIONAL ASSESSMENT AS PART OF PHYSICAL ASSESSMENT

Nutritional *assessment* is useful in evaluating the total physical health status of a child. The healthy, well-nourished child displays the following visible physical signs which are directly related to nutrition:

- height appropriate for age
- weight appropriate for height
- bright, clear eyes—no puffiness or crusting
- clear skin—good color; no pallor, no scaliness
- teeth—appropriate number for age; no evidence of decay or *mottling*
- gums—pink and firm; not puffy, dark red, or bleeding
- lips—soft, moist; no cracking at corners of mouth
- tongue—pink; no cracking, smooth spots, or deep red color

Many of these signs should be noted as part of the daily check-in routine when the child arrives at the care center. Height and weight should be recorded periodically in order to evaluate growth rate (Alford and Bogle 1982). The child's height and weight should be compared to that of the child's previous measurements and not to that of other children. Comparisons with other children do not allow for consideration of the child's individual growth rate.

Height and weight measurements may be incorporated into classroom activities, such as playing "doctor's office," Figure 17–1. Making silhouettes on paper and then talking about individual differences is another effective classroom activity. Such class activities should stress that differences in children are desirable and are what makes each child unique.

ASSESSMENT METHODS

Choice of the method for assessment depends upon the age of the children, the reason for evaluation, and the resources available. Assessment methods used to determine nutritional status, include:

- dietary assessment
- *anthropometric* assessment
- *clinical* assessment
- *biochemical* assessment

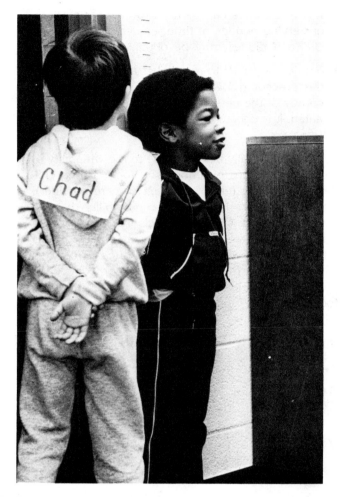

FIGURE 17-1   Height measurements can be incorporated into classroom activities.

Dietary Assessment

Dietary assessment is essential to determine adequacy of nutrient intake. Careful dietary assessment determines the possible causes of nutritional health problems. If nutrient intake appears to be adequate, the possibilities of increased requirements, faulty absorption, faulty transport, or increased destruction or excretion of nutrients should be seriously considered as a cause.

Gathering dietary information may be done in a variety of ways, depending on the number of children being evaluated and the reasons for evaluation. Looking for dietary deficiencies in a single child requires a different means of assessment than one used to determine the adequacy of menus served in a child care center.

Obtaining Dietary Information. Food diaries can be used to obtain dietary information. They may be kept for varying periods of time, as determined necessary for the information needed. Food diaries may be obtained in two ways.

- *24-hour recall* in which the subject is asked to remember all foods and beverages consumed during the preceding 24 hours. The accuracy of this method depends on the accuracy of the person's memory.
- Foods may be recorded as eaten. It is debatable that this means of recording results in typical eating patterns.

Neither method of keeping food diaries is totally accurate due to the variability of the human memory and individual perceptions of amounts of food. Young children's diaries must be recorded by an adult (either a parent or care provider). Even this does not ensure accuracy as there is always the possibility that the child has eaten something of which the adult is unaware. This inaccuracy could result in the recording of lower levels of nutrients than are actually obtained. This becomes crucial in cases in which intake of a dietary element such as calories must be limited.

To be really meaningful, food diary entries must be accompanied by information pertaining to family food practices, Figure 17–2. Pertinent information

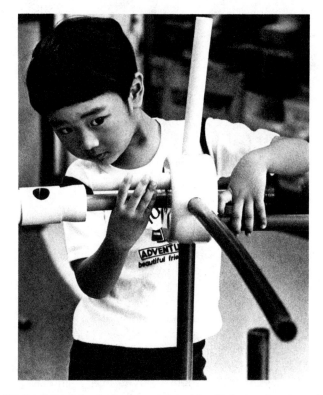

FIGURE 17–2 Cultural food practices must be identified when keeping a food diary.

NUTRITIONAL ASSESSMENT

Dear Parent:

Nutrition is a very important part of our program. In order for us to plan appropriate nutrition-education activities and menus to meet your child's needs, we need to know your child's eating patterns. Please take the time to fill out this questionnaire providing us with the needed information. This information will also help us obtain an overview of the eating habits of preschool children as a group.

NAME_____ DATE_____

1. How many days a week does your child eat the following meals or snacks?
   - a morning meal _____   a midafternoon snack _____
   - a lunch or midday meal _____   an evening snack _____
   - an evening meal _____   snack during the night _____
   - a midmorning snack _____

2. When is your child most hungry?
   - morning _____
   - noon _____
   - evening _____

3. What foods does your child dislike?
   _____

4. Is your child on a diet?   Yes_____   No_____
   - If yes, why?_____
   - Describe diet_____
   - Diet prescribed by whom?_____

5. Does your child eat things not usually considered food e.g., paste, dirt, paper?_____
   - If yes, how often?_____
   - What is eaten?_____

6. Is your child taking a vitamin or mineral supplement?
   Yes_____   No_____   If yes, what kind?_____

7. Does your child have any dental problems that might create a problem when eating certain foods?_____

8. Has your child ever been treated by a dentist?_____

9. Does your child have any diet-related health problems?
   - Diabetes_____   Allergies_____
   - Other_____

10. Is your child taking any medication for a diet-related health problem?_____

11. How much water does your child normally drink throughout the day?_____

12. Please list as accurately as possible what your child eats and drinks on a typical day. If yesterday was a typical day, you may use foods and drinks consumed yesterday.

TIME	PLACE	FOOD	AMOUNT

FIGURE 17–3 Sample questionnaire for obtaining information about a child's eating habits.

includes identifying who does the cooking for the family, times when meals are served, number of meals or snacks each day, ethnic or religious food practices, and family interactions at meal times. An example of family interactions might be whether the child is required to eat all food served before leaving the table, or whether desserts are used as rewards for other behaviors. Figure 17–3 shows a questionnaire which might be used for obtaining information about the child's eating habits.

Analyzing Dietary Information. Once dietary information is obtained, the task remains to analyze the information. Recording foods and eating habits is not enough; the nutritional content of the foods eaten must be calculated. Again, the method chosen depends on the reason for doing the assessment.

The Basic Four Food Groups are an adequate means of assessing food intake for most purposes, Table 17–1. (The Basic Four Food Groups were discussed in Unit 13.) The Food Groups are useful in analyzing the adequacy of menus fed to a group or for general screening purposes when evaluating the overall adequacy of an individual child's diet. This method is not accurate for short periods of time. However, it becomes more accurate as the number of days for which intake is recorded increases.

Careful attention must be paid to serving sizes. Serving sizes must be the same as those that constitute a serving from a specific food group; otherwise, appropriate adjustments must be made in the analysis. Appropriate serving sizes for small children are approximately one-half those recommended for adults.

When using the Basic Four Food Groups as a means of assessment, it is important to remember the nutrient strengths and weaknesses of each group of

TABLE 17–1 Use of the Basic Four Food Groups to Analyze Dietary Intake

	DAIRY GROUP	HIGH PROTEIN GROUP	FRUIT AND VEGETABLE GROUP	GRAIN GROUP	OTHER FOODS
Toast, 1 slice				✓✓	
Margarine, 1 tsp					✓
Egg, 1		✓			
Bacon, 2 slices					✓✓
Orange Juice, ½ c			✓		
Milk, 1 c	✓✓				

TABLE 17-2 Nutrient Strengths and Weaknesses of the Basic Four Food Groups

If fewer than:	Of this group:	These nutrients may be deficient:
2 cups (adults) 3 cups (children)	Dairy	calcium, riboflavin, good quality protein
2 servings 2-3 oz servings (adult) 1-1½ oz serving (children)	High Protein	iron, thiamin, niacin, protein

4 servings
    1 citrus
    1 dark green leafy or
        yellow
    2 others
	Fruit and Vegetable	vitamin A, ascorbic acid

4 servings	Grain	thiamin, niacin, riboflavin, iron

foods, Table 17-2. For example, a child who selects too few servings of fruits and vegetables may receive too little vitamin A and ascorbic acid. Another who does not drink milk or eat dairy products has little chance of getting enough calcium.

Nutrient analysis consists of determining the nutrient content of all foods and beverages consumed during the recording period. Food consumption tables must be used and amounts of food carefully noted. Some suggested publications which are useful for this task are:

- *Nutritive Value of Foods,* House and Garden Bulletin, No. 72, Washington, DC, 1978 (See Appendix A).
- *Food Values of Portions Commonly Used,* Church and Church, J.B. Lippincott and Company, 1975.
- *Composition of Foods,* Agriculture Handbook No. 8, Agriculture Research, USDA

These publications do not contain information for such nutrients as vitamins B_{12}, B_6, or folacin.

Information on nutrient content of packaged foods may be obtained from their labels. This process consists of three simple steps:

1. Determine the percentage of U.S. RDA of nutrients from the label.

2. Compare this percentage to the U.S. RDA tables.

3. Calculate the nutrient content (percent of U.S. RDA times U.S. RDA).

Nutrient content of some "fast" foods is shown in Table 17-3.

TABLE 17–3 Nutrition Analysis of Fast Foods

	Weight (g)	Energy (kcal)	Protein (g)	Fat (g)	Carbo-hydrate (g)	Calcium (mg)	Iron (mg)	Vitamin A value (IU)	Thiamin (mg)	Ribo-flavin (mg)	Niacin (mg)	Vitamin C (mg)
BURGER CHEF												
Big Shef	186	542	23	34	35	189	3.4	282	0.34	0.35	5.4	2
Cheeseburger	104	304	14	17	24	156	2.0	266	0.22	0.23	3.2	1
Double Cheeseburger	145	434	24	26	24	246	3.1	430	0.25	0.34	4.8	1
French Fries	68	187	3	9	25	10	0.9	tr	0.09	0.05	2.1	14
Hamburger, Regular	91	258	11	13	24	69	1.9	114	0.22	0.18	3.2	1
Mariner Platter	373	680	32	24	85	137	4.7	448	0.37	0.40	7.3	24
Rancher Platter	316	640	30	38	44	57	5.1	367	0.30	0.37	8.7	24
Shake	305	326	11	11	47	411	0.2	10	0.11	0.57	0.3	2
Skipper's Treat	179	604	21	37	47	201	2.5	303	0.29	0.30	3.7	1
Super Shef	252	600	29	37	39	240	4.2	763	0.37	0.43	6.7	9

Source: Burger Chef Systems, Inc, Indianapolis, Ind, 1978 (Analyses obtained from USDA Handbook No. 8).

	Weight (g)	Energy (kcal)	Protein (g)	Fat (g)	Carbo-hydrate (g)	Calcium (mg)	Iron (mg)	Vitamin A value (IU)	Thiamin (mg)	Ribo-flavin (mg)	Niacin (mg)	Vitamin C (mg)
BURGER KING												
Cheeseburger	—	305	17	13	29	141	2.0	195	0.01	0.02	2.20	0.5
Hamburger	—	252	14	9	29	45	2.0	21	0.01	0.01	2.20	0.5
Whopper	—	606	29	32	51	37	6.0	641	0.02	0.03	5.20	13.0
French Fries	—	214	3	10	28	12	1.0	0	0.01	0.01	2.42	16.0
Vanilla Shake	—	332	11	11	50	390	0.2	9	0.01	0.05	0.27	tr
Whaler	—	486	18	46	64	70	1.0	141	0.01	0.01	1.04	1.3
Hot dog	—	291	11	17	23	40	2.0	0	0.04	0.02	2.00	0

Source: Chart House, Inc, Oak Brook, Ill, 1978.

	Weight (g)	Energy (kcal)	Protein (g)	Fat (g)	Carbo-hydrate (g)	Calcium (mg)	Iron (mg)	Vitamin A value (IU)	Thiamin (mg)	Ribo-flavin (mg)	Niacin (mg)	Vitamin C (mg)
LONG JOHN SILVER'S												
Breaded Oysters, 6 pc	—	460	14	19	58	—	—	—	—	—	—	—
Breaded Clams, 5 oz	—	465	13	25	46	—	—	—	—	—	—	—
Chicken Planks, 4 pc	—	458	27	23	35	—	—	—	—	—	—	—
Cole Slaw, 4 oz	—	138	1	8	16	—	—	—	—	—	—	—
Corn on the Cob, 1 pc	—	174	5	4	29	—	—	—	—	—	—	—
Fish W/Batter, 2 pc	—	318	19	19	19	—	—	—	—	—	—	—
Fish W/Batter, 3 pc	—	477	28	28	28	—	—	—	—	—	—	—
Fryes, 3 oz	—	275	4	15	32	—	—	—	—	—	—	—

Hush Puppies, 3 pc	—	153	1	7	20	—	—	—	—	—	—	—
Ocean Scallops, 6 pc	—	257	10	12	27	—	—	—	—	—	—	—
Peg Leg W/Batter, 5 pc	—	514	25	33	30	—	—	—	—	—	—	—
Shrimp W/Batter, 6 pc	—	269	9	13	31	—	—	—	—	—	—	—
Treasure Chest, 2 pc fish, 2 Peg Legs	—	467	25	29	27	—	—	—	—	—	—	—

Source: Long John Silver's Seafood Shoppes, Jan 8, 1978 (nutritional analysis information furnished in study conducted by the Department of Nutrition and Food Science, University of Kentucky).

DAIRY QUEEN

Big Brazier Deluxe	213	470	28	24	36	111	5.2	—	0.34	0.37	9.6	<2.5
Big Brazier Regular	184	457	27	23	37	113	5.2	—	0.37	0.39	9.6	<2.0
Big Brazier W/Cheese	213	553	32	30	38	268	5.2	495	0.34	0.53	9.5	<2.3
Brazier W/Cheese	121	318	18	14	30	163	3.5	—	0.29	0.29	5.7	<1.2
Brazier Cheese Dog	113	330	15	19	24	168	1.6	—	—	0.18	3.3	11.0
Brazier Chili Dog	128	330	13	20	25	86	2.0	—	0.15	0.23	3.9	11.0
Brazier Dog	99	273	11	15	23	75	1.5	—	0.12	0.15	2.6	11.0
Brazier French Fries, 2.5 oz	71	200	2	10	25	tr	0.4	tr	0.06	tr	0.8	3.6
Brazier French Fries, 4.0 oz	113	320	3	16	40	tr	0.4	tr	0.09	0.03	1.2	4.8
Brazier Onion Rings	85	300	6	17	33	20	0.4	tr	0.09	tr	0.4	2.4
Brazier Regular	106	260	13	9	28	70	3.5	—	0.28	0.26	5.0	<1.0
Fish Sandwich	170	400	20	17	41	60	1.1	tr	0.15	0.26	3.0	tr
Fish Sandwich W/Cheese	177	440	24	21	39	150	0.4	100	0.15	0.26	3.0	tr
Super Brazier	298	783	53	48	35	282	7.3	—	0.39	0.69	15.6	<3.2
Super Brazier Dog	182	518	20	30	41	158	4.3	tr	0.42	0.44	7.0	14.0
Super Brazier Dog W/Cheese	203	593	26	36	43	297	4.4	—	0.43	0.48	8.1	14.0
Super Brazier Chili Dog	210	555	23	33	42	158	4.0	—	0.42	0.48	8.8	18.0
Banana Split	383	540	10	15	91	350	1.8	750	0.60	0.60	0.8	18.0
Buster Bar	149	390	10	22	37	200	0.7	300	0.09	0.34	1.6	tr
DQ Chocolate Dipped Cone, sm	78	150	3	7	20	100	tr	100	0.03	0.17	tr	tr
DQ Chocolate Dipped Cone, med	156	300	7	13	40	200	0.4	300	0.09	0.34	tr	tr
DQ Chocolate Dipped Cone, lg	234	450	10	20	58	300	0.4	400	0.12	0.51	tr	tr
DQ Chocolate Malt, sm	241	340	10	11	51	300	1.8	400	0.06	0.34	0.4	2.4
DQ Chocolate Malt, med	418	600	15	20	89	500	3.6	750	0.12	0.60	0.8	3.6
DQ Chocolate Malt, lg	588	840	22	28	125	600	5.4	750	0.15	0.85	1.2	6.0
DQ Chocolate Sundae, sm	106	170	4	4	30	100	0.7	100	0.03	0.17	tr	tr
DQ Chocolate Sundae, med	184	300	6	7	53	200	1.1	300	0.06	0.26	tr	tr
DQ Chocolate Sundae, lg	248	400	9	9	71	300	1.8	400	0.09	0.43	0.4	tr
DQ Cone, sm	71	110	3	3	18	100	tr	100	0.03	0.14	tr	tr
DQ Cone, med	142	230	6	7	35	200	tr	300	0.09	0.26	tr	tr
DQ Cone, lg	213	340	52	10	10	300	tr	400	0.15	0.43	tr	tr

TABLE 17–3 Nutrition Analysis of Fast Foods (Continued)

	Weight (g)	Energy (kcal)	Protein (g)	Fat (g)	Carbo-hydrate (g)	Calcium (mg)	Iron (mg)	Vitamin A value (IU)	Thiamin (mg)	Ribo-flavin (mg)	Niacin (mg)	Vitamin C (mg)
Dairy Queen Parfait	284	460	10	11	81	300	1.8	400	0.12	0.43	0.4	tr
Dilly Bar	85	240	4	15	22	100	0.4	100	0.06	0.17	tr	tr
DQ Float	397	330	6	8	59	200	tr	100	0.12	0.17	tr	tr
DQ Freeze	397	520	11	13	89	300	tr	200	0.15	0.34	tr	tr
DQ Sandwich	60	140	3	4	24	60	0.4	100	0.03	0.14	0.4	tr
Fiesta Sundae	269	570	9	22	84	200	tr	200	0.23	0.26	tr	tr
Hot Fudge Brownie Delight	266	570	11	22	83	300	1.1	500	0.45	0.43	0.8	tr
Mr. Misty Float	404	440	6	8	85	200	tr	120	0.12	0.17	tr	tr
Mr. Misty Freeze	411	500	10	12	87	300	tr	200	0.15	0.34	tr	tr

Source: International Dairy Queen, Inc, Minneapolis, Minn, 1978. Dairy Queen stores in the State of Texas do not conform to Dairy Queen-approved products. Any nutritional information shown does not necessarily pertain to their products.

McDONALD'S

	Weight (g)	Energy (kcal)	Protein (g)	Fat (g)	Carbo-hydrate (g)	Calcium (mg)	Iron (mg)	Vitamin A value (IU)	Thiamin (mg)	Ribo-flavin (mg)	Niacin (mg)	Vitamin C (mg)
Egg McMuffin	132	352	18	20	26	187	3.2	361	0.36	0.60	4.3	1.6
English Muffin, Buttered	62	186	6	6	28	87	1.6	106	0.22	0.14	6.4	<0.7
Hot Cakes, W/Butter & Syrup	206	472	8	9	89	54	2.4	255	0.31	0.43	4.0	<2.1
Sausage (Pork)	48	184	9	17	tr	13	0.9	36	0.22	0.13	5.9	<0.5
Scrambled Eggs	77	162	12	12	2	49	2.2	514	0.07	0.60	0.4	<0.8
Big Mac	187	541	26	31	39	175	4.3	327	0.35	0.37	8.2	2.4
Cheeseburger	114	306	16	13	31	158	2.9	372	0.24	0.30	5.5	1.6
Filet O Fish	131	402	15	23	34	105	1.8	152	0.28	0.28	3.9	4.2
French Fries	69	211	3	11	26	10	0.5	<52	0.15	0.03	2.9	11.0
Hamburger	99	257	13	9	30	63	3.0	231	0.23	0.23	5.1	1.8
Quarter Pounder	164	418	26	21	33	79	5.1	164	0.31	0.41	9.8	2.3
Quarter Pounder W/Cheese	193	518	31	29	34	251	4.6	683	0.35	0.59	15.1	2.9
Apple Pie	91	300	2	19	31	12	0.6	<69	0.02	0.03	1.3	2.7
Cherry Pie	92	298	2	18	33	12	0.4	213	0.02	0.03	0.4	1.3
McDonaldland Cookies	63	294	4	11	45	10	1.4	<48	0.28	0.23	0.8	1.4
Chocolate Shake	289	364	11	9	60	338	1.0	318	0.12	0.89	0.8	<2.9
Strawberry Shake	293	345	10	9	57	339	0.2	322	0.12	0.66	0.5	<2.9
Vanilla Shake	289	323	10	8	52	346	0.2	346	0.12	0.66	0.6	<2.9

Source: "Nutritional analysis of food served at McDonald's restaurants." WARF Institute, Inc, Madison, Wisc, June 1977.

TACO BELL

Bean Burrito	166	343	11	12	48	98	2.8	1657	0.37	0.22	2.2	15.2
Beef Burrito	184	466	30	21	37	83	4.6	1675	0.30	0.39	7.0	15.2
Beefy Tostada	184	291	19	15	21	208	3.4	3450	0.16	0.27	3.3	12.7
Bellbeefer	123	221	15	7	23	40	2.6	2961	0.15	0.20	3.7	10.0
Bellbeefer W/Cheese	137	278	19	12	23	147	2.7	3146	0.16	0.27	3.7	10.0
Burrito Supreme	225	457	21	22	43	121	3.8	3462	0.33	0.35	4.7	16.0
Combination Burrito	175	404	21	16	43	91	3.7	1666	0.34	0.31	4.6	15.2
Enchirito	207	454	25	21	42	259	3.8	1178	0.31	0.37	4.7	9.5
Pintos' N Cheese	158	168	11	5	21	150	2.3	3123	0.26	0.16	0.9	9.3
Taco	83	186	15	8	14	120	2.5	120	0.09	0.16	2.9	0.2
Tostada	138	179	9	6	25	191	2.3	3152	0.18	0.15	0.8	9.7

Sources: Menu Item Portions, July 1976. Taco Bell Co, San Antonio, Tex.
Adams CF: *Nutritive Value of American Foods in Common Units.* USDA Agricultural Research Service, Agricultural Handbook No. 456, November 1975.
Church CF, Church HN: *Food Values of Portions Commonly Used,* ed 12. Philadelphia, JB Lippincott Co, 1975.
Valley Baptist Medical Center, Food Service Department: Descriptions of Mexican-American Foods, NASCO, Fort Atkinson, Wisc.

KENTUCKY FRIED CHICKEN

Original Recipe Dinner*	425	830	52	46	56	150‡	4.5‡	750‡	0.38‡	0.56‡	15.0‡	27.0‡
Extra Crispy Dinner*	437	950	52	54	63	150‡	3.6‡	750‡	0.38‡	0.56‡	14.0‡	27.0‡
Individual Pieces†												
(Original Recipe)												
Drumstick	54	136	14	8	2	20	0.9	30	0.04	0.12	2.7	0.6
Keel	96	283	25	13	6	—	0.9	50	0.07	0.13	—	1.2
Rib	82	241	19	15	8	55	1.0	58	0.06	0.14	5.8	<1.0
Thigh	97	276	20	19	12	39	1.4	74	0.08	0.24	4.9	<1.0
Wing	45	151	11	10	4	—	0.6	—	0.03	0.07	—	<1.0
9 Pieces	652	1892	152	116	59	—	8.8	—	0.49	1.27	—	—

Source: Nutritional Content of Average Serving, Heublein Food Service and Franchising Group, June 1976.
*Dinner comprises mashed potatoes and gravy, cole slaw, roll, and three pieces of chicken, either 1) wing, rib, and thigh; 2) wing, drumstick, and thigh; or 3) wing, drumstick, and keel.
†Edible portion of chicken.
‡Calculated from percentage of US RDA.

From Young, E. A., Brennan, E. H., and Irving, G. L.: "Perspective on Fast Foods," *Dietetic Currents* 5:24-29, 1978 (Ross Laboratories, Columbus, Ohio). Reprinted by permission.
Nutritional Analysis of Fast Foods
(Dashes indicate information not provided by sources)

The second step of nutrient analysis is of comparing the nutrient totals to the Recommended Daily Dietary Allowances for the appropriate age group. Seventy-five percent or more of the recommended allowance for at least seven of the ten leader nutrients is one possible criteria for judging overall adequacy.

Family or Group Food Accounts describe the kinds and amounts of food purchased. This information is useful in determining whether enough total food and the right types of foods are being purchased. Food accounts indicate if adequate amounts of food are being provided for the group.

Food records indicate the amount of food on hand at the beginning of the assessment period, plate waste, and the amount of food on hand at the end of the assessment period. This type of system determines the average amounts per person of food actually used. It is useful for determining food intake of groups and whether or not the amounts eaten were adequate. Food records are frequently used in child care settings; they are the means of reporting used by federally-funded school food services and child care food programs.

Anthropometric Assessment

Anthropometric assessment is accomplished through the following physical measurements which give an indication of the child's growth:

- height
- weight
- head circumference
- skin fold thickness

In many instances, height and weight are sufficient measurements of growth. These measurements require a minimum of training to do and the necessary equipment is readily available. Height and weight measurements should be taken periodically in order to detect growth spurts, slowing of growth, and rapid weight gains or losses. The heights and weights of individual children may be compared to norms for age and sex.

Skin fold, and head circumference measurements are frequently used assessment tools, although their use in the actual child care setting is minimal. Skin fold measurements are one method of determining the fat content of the body, Figure 17–4. It may be used as a determinant of obesity. Head circumference measurements are a method of monitoring the rate of cranial growth (Pipes 1981). Both procedures require special equipment and some training in their use. Interpretation depends on the availability of tables showing ranges of normal values. These procedures are mentioned so that the care provider will be aware of their use as assessment tools.

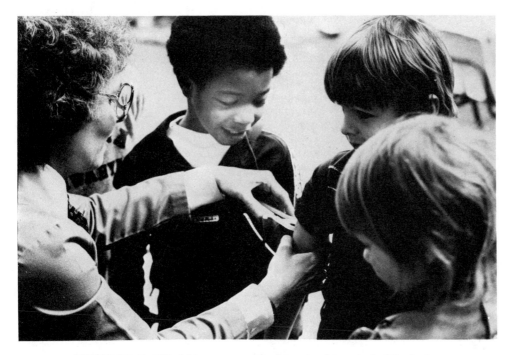

FIGURE 17-4 Skin fold measurements determine fat content of the body.

Clinical Assessment

Physical signs of nutrient deficiency vary according to the nutrient which is deficient. Since nutrients perform specific functions, deficiency symptoms arise from the reduction or absence of those functions. Tissues which are experiencing rapid growth or which are frequently replaced are often good indicators of nutritional status. Examples of such tissues are lips, tongue, nose and eye linings and skin. Table 17-4 lists some physical signs of malnutrition and their possible causes.

Biochemical Assessment

Biochemical assessment may be done by measuring nutrients or their derivatives in body tissues or fluids. An example is measurement of hemoglobin as an indicator of iron status. Biochemical techniques are performed by professionals, usually under orders from a physician. The need for biochemical assessment may be indicated by the discovery of health problems which are thought to be related to malnutrition. Discovery of these health problems may be the result of any or all of the previously discussed means of nutritional assessment.

TABLE 17-4 Physical Signs of Malnutrition

TISSUE	SIGN	CAUSE
Face	Pallor.	Niacin, iron deficiency
	Scaling of skin around nostrils	Riboflavin, B_6 deficiency
Eyes	Hardening of cornea and lining; pale lining.	Iron deficiency
	Foamy spots in cornea	Vitamin A deficiency
Lips	Redness; swelling of mouth and lips; cracking at corners of mouth	Riboflavin deficiency
Teeth	Decayed or missing.	Excess sugar (or poor dental hygiene)
	Mottled enamel.	Excess fluoride
Tongue	Red, raw, cracked, swollen.	Niacin deficiency
	Magenta color.	Riboflavin deficiency
	Pale.	Iron deficiency
Gums	Spongy, red, bleeding	Ascorbic acid deficiency
Skin	Dry, flaking.	Vitamin A deficiency
	Small underskin hemorrhages.	Ascorbic acid deficiency
Nails	Brittle, ridged.	Iron deficiency

SUMMARY

Nutritional adequacy may be assessed by several means. Nutritional assessment is a means of determining the adequacy of dietary intakes. Assessment may be made of group intakes or of individual intakes. Recorded dietary intakes may be analyzed in terms of nutrients or food groups. Analysis on the basis of nutrients is more accurate, but is time-consuming and requires the use of food composition tables. Tabulation of some nutrients requires resources beyond the standard food composition tables. Analysis on the basis of Food Groups becomes more accurate with increasing numbers of days recorded. It is important to remember that a nutritional deficiency can exist even with adequate intake if absorption, transport, or utilization are abnormal.

Anthropometric assessment may be accomplished merely by accurately recording height and weight, although additional measurements such as head circumference and skin fold thickness may also be valuable. Growth charts and tables of ranges of normal values for age and sex are helpful in interpreting anthropometric assessments.

Clinical assessment of nutritional status involves observation of physical signs. This assessment can be included as part of the daily health check done by the care provider. Parts of the body which are visibly indicative of nutritional health include eyes, mouth, teeth, tongue, nails, and skin.

Biochemical assessment involves the measurement of nutrients or their derivatives in body tissues or fluids. These assessments and their interpretation are done by professional health personnel.

LEARNING ACTIVITIES

1. Place a check mark in the appropriate food group column for each of the listed foods.

Food	Dairy Group	Protein Group	Fruit and Vegetable Group	Grain Group	Other Foods
Toast					
Margarine					
Jelly					
Dry Cereal					
Sugar					
Milk					
Peanut Butter and Honey Sandwich					
Carrot Sticks					
Milk					
Pizza					
Cola Drink					

   a. Assume that a full child-size serving of each listed food is consumed. Is this diet adequate in terms of the Basic Four Food Groups?

   b. Based on nutrient strengths and weaknesses, what nutrients may not be provided in adequate amounts?

   c. How many servings of other foods are there?

2. Devise a monitoring system whereby daily food intakes are recorded for each child. This information is primarily intended to provide information about daily food consumption to parents. Factors to consider are:

    a. What nutritional information is needed? In what form?
    b. Who is responsible for obtaining this data?
    c. How can this information be obtained efficiently?
    d. How can food intake records increase opportunities for communication with parents?
    e. What other uses are food intake records to the care provider?

UNIT REVIEW

A. Match the physical sign in column I with the probable deficient (or excess) nutrient in column II.

Column I	Column II
1. skin pallor, pale eye linings, ridged nails	a. ascorbic acid
2. spongy, bleeding gums	b. iron
3. mottled teeth	c. excess fluoride
4. cracks at corners of mouth	d. excess sugar
5. decayed teeth	e. riboflavin

B. Multiple Choice. Select the best answer.

1. Diets which contain inadequate servings of dairy products are low in
   a. iron
   b. vitamin A
   c. vitamin C
   d. calcium

2. Diets which contain inadequate servings from the Fruit and Vegetable Food Group are low in
   a. vitamin A and vitamin C
   b. calcium and iron
   c. iron and thiamin
   d. riboflavin and calcium

3. A physical sign resulting from a deficiency of niacin in the diet is
   a. cracks at corner of the mouth
   b. cracked, swollen tongue
   c. dry, flaking skin
   d. brittle nails

4. In comparison to the Basic Four Food Groups, nutrient analysis
   a. is more accurate
   b. requires the use of food composition tables
   c. is more time consuming
   d. all of these

C. Briefly answer the following questions.

1. List four methods of assessing nutritional status.

2. Name four physical signs of a healthy, well-nourished child.

3. How is anthropometric assessment accomplished?

4. List four means of analyzing dietary information.

5. What is biochemical assessment?

6. Name two possible causes for nutritional deficiencies.

REFERENCES

Alford, B. B., and Bogle, M. L. *Nutrition During the Life Cycle.* Englewood Cliffs, NJ: Prentice-Hall, Inc., 1982.

Pipes, P. L. *Nutrition in Infancy and Childhood.* St. Louis: C.V. Mosby Company, 1981.

Guidelines for Anthropometric Measurement. Columbus, OH: Ross Laboratories, 1978.

Additional Reading

Brody, J. *Jane Brody's Nutrition Book.* New York: Bantam Books, 1982.

Christakin, G. "Community Assessment of Nutritional Status." In *Community Nutrition: People, Policies and Programs.* Edited by H.S. Wright and L.S. Sims. Monterey, CA: Wadsworth Health Sciences Division, 1981.

Unit 18
PLANNING AND SERVING MEALS

Terms to Know

cycle menus	full-strength
weekly menus	fruit drinks
whole grains	sensory qualities
enriched	odd-day cycle menus
ethnic	bottle-mouth syndrome

Objectives

After studying this unit, you will be able to:
- Identify the criteria for adequate menus for young children.
- List the eight steps in preparing menus.
- State three methods of writing menus.
- Name four sensory qualities that help to make food appealing.
- State where information regarding licensing requirements for food and nutrition services can be obtained.
- Plan meals and snacks which meet nutritional requirements for young children.
- Describe the proper way to bottle feed an infant.
- Explain how to make mealtimes pleasant experiences for young children.

One of the basic human needs is nourishing the body. This is an activity that most people, including infants and young children, enjoy. Eating is a sensory, emotional, social, and learning experience. It is associated with the young child's feeling of well-being. As many infants and young children spend much of their early years in the care of care providers other than parents, it is important that care providers help the children establish proper attitudes towards meals. This can be accomplished by planning nourishing meals that are acceptable to the children and serving these meals in a pleasant atmosphere that builds the children both socially and emotionally.

FEEDING THE INFANT

Infant feeding is a highly individual relationship between infant, parent, pediatrician, and care provider. Many mothers choose breast feeding for the first two or three months; breast milk contains all the nutrients known to be needed by an infant until about three months of age. However, care providers are more likely to be concerned with bottle feeding and added solid foods. The suggested feeding guide given in Table 18–1, shows approximate amounts of formula and added solid foods for baby's first year. Decisions as to amounts of foods and when to add them are made by the pediatrician and the parent. An infant should never be forced to eat or drink more than it desires.

Bottle Feeding

The pediatrician usually advises the parents on the formula to use for their infant. Formulas may be prepared by either the aseptic method or the terminal method, Table 18–2. The baby may also be prescribed one of the commercially-prepared formulas. The parents should bring a supply of formula to the center each day to meet the needs of the infant while the infant is at the center.

The care provider's hands must be washed prior to feeding an infant. The infant should be cuddled and talked to with close eye-to-eye contact while feeding. This makes feeding time a pleasant, social time for the infant. It also gives the infant needed close human contact. The nipple of the bottle should be kept full of formula so the infant does not swallow air. **Caution:** The bottle should never be propped and the baby left unattended. The infant does not have the motor control to remove the bottle and may aspirate formula if it falls asleep. Also, propping the bottle can foster tooth decay by allowing the liquid to lie in the mouth thus coating the teeth with sugar. This is often referred to as "bottle-mouth syndrome." Propping the bottle may also lead to ear infections due to bacteria growth in the pooled liquid which travel up the eustachian tubes.

The infant should not be hurried when feeding. The baby should be allowed at least 20 minutes to feed. The amount and frequency of the feedings vary with each infant.

After feeding, the infant should be placed on its stomach or right side to aid the passage of the feeding into the stomach; this also prevents distention and regurgitation of the feeding. A pillow may be propped behind the infant's back to maintain the side-lying position. Any remaining contents of the bottle should be discarded and the bottle rinsed in cold water.

Introducing Solid Foods

The care provider, parent, and health care professional must cooperate closely in introducing solid foods to the infant. Solid foods are usually introduced at approximately four to six months of age. The need for formula decreases as the amount of solid foods increases. New foods should be introduced slowly with a few baby spoonfuls offered one or two times daily. Iron-fortified baby cereal is

TABLE 18–1   Infant Feeding Guide

FOODS	0–4 MONTHS OF AGE	5–6 MONTHS OF AGE	7–9 MONTHS OF AGE	10–12 MONTHS OF AGE
FORMULA (if not breast-fed)	22–29 oz (660–870 mL)	If no other food, 29–32 oz (about 1 quart); decrease amount as other foods are introduced.	2–2½ cups (480–600 mL) per day	2–3 cups (480–720 mL) per day
ADDITIONS Iron-fortified baby cereals		1–2 baby spoons, 1–2 times/day	2–3 tablespoons, 2 times per day	2–4 tablespoons, 2 times per day
Vegetables (include dark green)		1–2 baby spoons, 1–2 times/day	2–3 tablespoons, 2 times per day	3–4 tablespoons, 2 times per day
Fruits		1–2 baby spoons, 1–2 times/day	2–3 tablespoons, 2 times per day	3–4 tablespoons, 2 times per day
Fruit juices (include 1 citrus fruit such as orange or grapefruit juice)			3–4 oz (90–120 mL) per day	3–4 oz (90–120 mL) per day
Meats Examples: meat, poultry, fish, egg (use yolk only until 12 months of age)			1–2 tablespoons, 2 times per day	2–3 tablespoons, 2 times per day
Breads whole grain or enriched Examples: toast, crackers, hard biscuits			½–1 serving, as desired	½–1 serving, as desired
Additional Vitamins and Minerals		Check with your health care provider		

FLUIDS—The baby needs more fluids for good health than is in the formula and juice suggested above. Water is the best drink to use.

Source: "A Guide for Feeding Your Baby," Kansas State University Extension Service C–594, 1978.

TABLE 18-2 Formula Preparation Methods

Terminal Method
- Wash the bottles, nipples, caps and all utensils used for preparing the formula.
- Prepare the formula and place it into clean bottles.
- Place inverted nipples and caps loosely on bottles (this allows the steam to escape while sterilizing).
- Place bottles on rack in a kettle containing four inches of water; cover with a tight-fitting lid.
- Bring the water to a boil; boil for 25 minutes.
- Let bottles cool then tighten caps and refrigerate.

Aseptic Method
- Boil clean bottles, nipples, caps, and all utensils used for preparing the formula for 20 minutes.
- Boil the water used to make the formula for 5 minutes.
- Prepare formula using sterilized utensils.
- Pour formula into sterilized bottles.
- Place inverted nipples and caps on bottles being careful to touch only the outer rim of the nipples and caps.
- Refrigerate until ready to use.

---

usually the first addition. It is wiser to introduce single foods rather than mixtures; in case of allergy or sensitivity, the offending food can be more readily identified. Neither sugar nor salt should be added to foods given to infants.

MEAL PLANNING

A menu is a list of foods which are to be served; it is the basis of any food service. Menu planning requires thought and careful evaluation of the physical, developmental, and social needs of those for whom it is planned. Thought and planning are as necessary for a menu designed to feed a family of three as they are for an institution serving thousands of meals a day. The difference between the two situations is largely one of scale. The same careful planning must be applied to the development of menus suitable for young children. To be adequate, a menu planned for children must:

- meet the nutritional needs of children
- meet any existing funding or licensing requirements
- be appealing (have taste, texture, and eye appeal)
- make children comfortable by serving familiar foods
- encourage healthy food habits by introducing new foods
- provide safe food cooked and served in clean surroundings
- stay within budgetary limits

A Good Menu Meets Nutritional Needs

The primary criterion for a good menu is nutritional adequacy. A menu must meet the nutritional needs of those for whom it is intended. When planning menus for young children in a care center, it is important to first determine what share of the day's total intake must be included in the menu. To determine the

TABLE 18-3   Sources of Iron and Suggested Preparation

Liver
    Strips, baked
    Loaf
    Braised, with tomato sauce
    Braised, with apple slices and onion

Beef
    Ground beef and macaroni casserole
    Ground beef patty
    Meat loaf
    Roast beef
    Hot beef sandwich with gravy
    Beef stew
    Meat balls and spaghetti
    Meat sauce and spaghetti
    Roast beef sandwich

Ham
    Creamed ham and peas
    Ham salad
    Ham and sweet potato casserole
    Scalloped ham and potatoes
    Sliced baked ham
    Ham sandwich

Prunes
    Stewed
    Whip
    Fruit soup

Chicken
    Chicken and rice
    Chicken and dumplings
    Chicken and noodles
    Creamed chicken
    Baked chicken
    Chicken salad

Pastas (whole grain or enriched)
    Buttered
    In bouillon
    With cheese
    With tomato sauce
    With meat sauce
    With tuna
    With chicken

Raisins
    In bread or rice pudding
    Plain
    Stewed

Spinach
    Raw
        Salad with onions and bacon
    Cooked and Buttered
        With hard cooked eggs
        With cheese sauce
        With onions and bacon

nutritional needs of young children, the Basic Four Food Groups and/or the Recommended Daily Dietary Allowances for that age group should be reviewed. Menus should be planned around servings from the Basic Four Food Groups.

Iron, calcium, and vitamin C are nutrients for which young children are most at risk; these nutrients should be provided daily. Tables 18–3 through 18–5 give

TABLE 18-4   Sources of Calcium and Suggested Preparation

Milk
    Plain
    In custards
    In puddings

Cheese
    In sandwiches
    In cream sauce
    Cubes
    In salads

Yogurt
    Plain
    With fruit
    As dip for fruits or vegetables

Salmon
    Patties
    Loaf

TABLE 18–5 Sources of Vitamin C and Suggested Preparation

Rich Sources

Oranges
  Juice
  Sections
  Slices
  Wedges
  Juice in gelatin

Strawberries
  Plain
  With milk
  In fruit cup

Cauliflower
  Raw
    Florets
    With yogurt dip
  Cooked
    Buttered
    With cheese sauce
    With cream sauce

Green Pepper
  Strips
  Rings
  Seasoning in sauces, casseroles

Broccoli
  Raw
    Strips
    Chunks
    Florets with yogurt dip
  Cooked
    Buttered
    With cheese sauce
    With lemon sauce

Tomatoes
  Raw
    Slices
    Wedges
    Cherry
    Juice
    In tossed salad
  Cooked
    Baked
    Broiled
    Sauce
    Scalloped
    Stewed

Good Sources

Cabbage
  Raw
    Coleslaw
    Wedges
    In tossed salad
  Cooked
    Buttered
    In stew

Spinach
  Raw
    Salad with onions and bacon

Tangerine
  Sections
  Slices
  In fruit cup

sources for these nutrients and suggestions for preparation. Every other day is often enough to provide sources of vitamin A since it is stored in the body, Table 18–6.

Federally-funded food programs for children are required to provide one-third of the recommended daily nutrient requirements for children (Egan 1981). However, it is recommended that nearly one-half the day's nutrients be included in the event that meals at home do not provide the other two-thirds of the needed nutrients. Federal guidelines for child care centers receiving federal reimbursement require the following menu pattern in order to ensure minimum nutritional adequacy:

1. Minimum Breakfast Requirement
   - whole grain or enriched bread or substitute
   - full-strength fruit or vegetable juice, or fruit or vegetable
   - milk, fluid
2. Minimum Snack Requirement (Choose two)
   - whole grain or enriched bread or substitute
   - milk, fluid
   - full-strength fruit or vegetable juice, fruit or vegetable
   - meat or alternate

TABLE 18-6 Sources of Vitamin A and Suggested Preparation

Rich Sources
Liver
  Strips, baked
  Loaf
  Braised, with tomato sauce

Carrots
  Raw
  Sticks, curls, coins
  Salad, with raisins
  Cooked
    With celery
    With peas
    Creamed

Pumpkin
  Mashed
  Bread
  Custard

Sweet Potatoes
  Baked
  Mashed
  Bread

Spinach
  Raw
    Salad with onions and bacon
  Cooked
    Buttered
      With hard cooked eggs
      With cheese sauce
      With onions and bacon

Good sources
Apricots
  Raw
  Canned
    Plain
    In fruit cup
    Whip
    Nectar

Watermelon
  Balls
  Cubes
  In fruit cup

Broccoli
  Raw
    Strips
    Chunks
    Florets with yogurt dip
  Cooked
    Buttered
    With cheese sauce
    With lemon sauce
    Stir-fried with celery, onions

3. Minimum Lunch or Supper Requirement

- meat or substitute

- fruits and/or vegetables, two or more

- whole grain or enriched bread or substitute

- milk, fluid

Minimum serving sizes are determined by the child's age in categories of 1 to 3 years and 3 to 6 years (USDA, FNS-64 1981).

TABLE 18-7 Child Care Food Program Meal Pattern

	Children 1 up to 3 years	Children 3 up to 6 years
Breakfast		
Milk, fluid	1/2 cup	3/4 cup
Juice or **fruit** or **vegetable**	1/4 cup	1/2 cup
Bread and/or **cereal,** enriched or whole grain		
Bread or	1/2 slice	1/2 slice
Cereal: Cold dry or	1/4 cup[1]	1/3 cup[2]
Hot cooked	1/4 cup	1/4 cup
Midmorning or midafternoon snack (supplement)		
(Select 2 of these 4 components)		
Milk, fluid	1/2 cup	1/2 cup
Meat or **meat alternate**	1/2 ounce	1/2 ounce
Juice or **fruit** or **vegetable**	1/2 cup	1/2 cup
Bread and/or **cereal,** enriched or whole grain		
Bread or	1/2 slice	1/2 slice
Cereal: Cold dry or	1/4 cup[1]	1/3 cup[2]
Hot cooked	1/4 cup	1/4 cup
Lunch or supper		
Milk, fluid	1/2 cup	3/4 cup
Meat or **meat alternate**		
Meat, poultry, or fish, cooked		
(lean meat without bone)	1 ounce	1 1/2 ounces
Cheese	1 ounce	1 1/2 ounces
Egg	1	1
Cooked dry beans and peas	1/4 cup	3/8 cup
Peanut butter	2 tablespoons	3 tablespoons
Vegetable and/or **fruit** (two or more)	1/4 cup	1/2 cup
Bread or **bread alternate,** enriched or whole grain	1/2 slice	1/2 slice

[1] 1/4 cup (volume) or 1/3 ounce (weight), whichever is less.
[2] 1/3 cup (volume) or 1/2 ounce (weight), whichever is less.
Source: *A Planning Guide for Food Service in Child Care Centers.* USDA, FNS-64, January 1981.

A Good Menu Meets Funding or Licensing Requirements

Many child care organizations depend on some form of government monies for their funding. Perhaps the best known of these government programs is the Child Care Food Program. This is a program which provides reimbursement for meals served to children in child care centers and home child care programs. This program provides support to child care centers for meal service. Meal service includes cost of food, labor, and administration. Funds are provided by the Food and Nutrition Service of the U. S. Department of Agriculture; the program is administered at the state level by the Department of Education. The meal plan cited in Table 18-7 is the minimum which must be served in order to qualify for reimbursement under this program. The guidelines are quite specific as to the minimum amounts of food required to fulfill a serving. Guidelines are also available listing specific foods which are permitted as alternatives within each food group, Table 18-8. The menu planner working within these guidelines must take great care to keep up with the current information as this program undergoes frequent and sometimes sweeping changes.

Licensing of child care facilities is administered by state agencies, usually the Department of Health. Each state has its own licensing requirements with regard to nutrition and food service. Care providers who provide food for children should check the licensing requirements for their particular state. Figure 18-1 gives the food service licensing requirements for the State of Kansas. Aspects pertaining to nutrition often covered by licensing regulations include:

1. Administration and record keeping

   • sample menus

   • number of meals served daily

TABLE 18-8   Acceptable Bread and Bread Alternates

Important Notes:

■ All products must be made of whole grain or enriched flour or meal.

■ Serving sizes listed below are specified for children under 6 years of age.

■ A "full" serving (defined below) is required for children 6 years of age and older.

■ USDA recommends that cookies be served in a snack no more than twice a week. They may be used for a snack only when:

   ■ whole grain or enriched meal or flour is the predominant ingredient as specified on the label or according to the recipe; and

   ■ the total weight of a serving for children under 6 years of age is a minimum of 18 grams (0.6 oz.) and for children over 6 years, a minimum of 35 grams (1.2 oz.).

■ To determine serving sizes for products in Group I that are made at child care centers, refer to "Cereal products" in FNS-86, "Quantity Recipes for Child Care Centers."

■ Doughnuts and sweet rolls are allowed as a bread item in breakfasts and snacks only.

■ French, Vienna, Italian, and Syrian breads are commercially prepared products that often are made with unenriched flour. Check the label or manufacturer to be sure the product is made with *enriched* flour.

■ The amount of bread in a serving of stuffing should weigh at least 13 grams (0.5 ounces).

TABLE 18-8   Acceptable Bread and Bread Alternates (Continued)

Group I
When you obtain these items commercially, a *full* serving should have a minimum weight of 25 grams (0.9 ounces). The serving sizes specified below should have a minimum weight of 13 grams (0.5 ounces).

Item	Serving Size
Bagels	1/2 bagel
Biscuits	1 biscuit
Boston brown bread	1/2 serving
Buns (all types)	1/2 bun
Cornbread	1 serving
Doughnuts (all types)	1/2 doughnut
English muffins	1/2 muffin
French or Vienna bread	1/2 serving
"Fry" bread	1/2 piece
Italian bread	1/2 serving
Muffins	1/2 muffin
Pretzels, Dutch (soft) twisted	1 pretzel
Pumpernickel	1/2 slice
Raisin bread	1/2 slice
Rolls (all types)	1 roll
Rye bread	1/2 slice
Salt sticks	1/2 stick
Stuffing (bread)	1/2 serving
Sweet rolls	1/2 roll
Syrian bread (flat)	1/2 section
White bread	1/2 slice
Whole wheat bread	1/2 slice

Group II
When you obtain these items commercially, a *full* serving should have a minimum weight of 20 grams (0.7 ounces). The serving sizes specified below should have a minimum weight of 10 grams (0.4 ounces).

Item	Serving Size
Bread sticks (dry)	2 sticks
Graham crackers	2 crackers
Melba toast	3 pieces
"Pilot" bread	1 piece
Rye wafers (whole-grain)	2 wafers
Saltine crackers	4 crackers
Soda crackers	2 crackers
Taco shells	1 shell
Zwieback	2 pieces

Group III
When you obtain these items commercially, a *full* serving should have a minimum weight of 30 grams (1.1 ounces). The serving sizes specified below should have a minimum weight of 15 grams (0.6 ounces).

Item	Serving Size
Dumplings	1/2 dumpling
Hush puppies	1/2 serving
Meat or meat alternate pie crust	1/2 serving
Meat or meat alternate turnover crust	1/2 serving
Pancakes	1/2 pancake
Pizza crust	1/2 serving
Popovers	1/2 popover
Sopapillas	1/2 serving
Spoonbread	1/2 serving
Tortillas	1 tortilla
Waffles	1/2 serving

Group IV
When you serve these items, a *full* serving should have a minimum of 1/2 cup cooked product. The serving sizes specified below are the minimum *half* servings of cooked product.

Item	Serving Size
Bulgur	1/4 cup
Corn grits	1/4 cup
Macaroni or spaghetti	1/4 cup
Noodles	1/4 cup
Rice (white or brown)	1/4 cup

Source: *A Planning Guide for Food Service in Child Care Centers.* USDA, FNS–64, January 1981.

2. Food service

   • specifications for kitchens and equipment

   • sanitation of dishes, utensils and equipment

   • requirements for transport of food when kitchen facilities are not available

   • feeding equipment required for specific age groups

3. Staffing

   • requirements of person in charge of food service

28-4-439. Child care centers: food service.

(a) Single or multi-unit centers serving a meal prepared at the center to 13 or more children shall employ a staff person who:
   (1) Has knowledge of nutritional needs of children;
   (2) understands quantity food preparation and service;
   (3) practices sanitary methods of food handling and storage;
   (4) is sensitive to individual and cultural food tastes of children; and
   (5) is willing to work with the program director in planning learning experiences for children relative to nutrition.

(b) Centers shall serve meals and snacks as follows:

Length of Time at Center	Food Served
2½ to 4 hours	1 snack
4 to 8 hours	1 snack & 1 meal
8 to 10 hours	2 snacks & 1 meal or
	1 snack & 2 meals
10 hours or more	2 meals & 2 or 3 snacks

(c) Meals and snacks.
   (1) Breakfasts shall include:
       (A) A fruit, vegetable, or full strength fruit or vegetable juice;
       (B) bread, bread product or cereal; and
       (C) milk.
   (2) Noon or evening meals shall include one item from each of the following:
       (A) Meat, poultry, fish, egg, cheese, cooked dried peas or beans, or peanut butter;
       (B) two vegetables, 2 fruits, or one vegetable and one fruit;
       (C) bread, bread product or cereal; and
       (D) milk.
   (3) Mid-morning and mid-afternoon snacks shall include at least two of the following:
       (A) Milk, milk product or food made with milk;
       (B) fruit, vegetable, or full-strength fruit or vegetable juice;
       (C) meat or a meat alternate; or
       (D) bread, bread product or cereal.

(d) A sufficient quantity of food shall be prepared for each meal to allow the children second portions of vegetables or fruit, bread, and milk.

(e) Food allergies of specific children shall be known to cooks, staff members, child care workers, and substitutes.

FIGURE 18-1 Sample licensing requirements for food service for young children.

(f) Menus shall be posted where parents can see them. Copies of menus served the previous month shall be kept on file.

(g) Staff shall sit at the table with the children, and socialization shall be encouraged. Children shall be encouraged to serve themselves. Spoons and forks shall be provided for each child's use. Appropriate service shall be used for meals and snacks.

(h) Children's food shall not be placed on the bare table.

(i) Toothbrushes shall be provided for each child's use. They shall be used daily after meals, and shall be stored in a sanitary manner out of children's reach.

(j) When meals are prepared on the premises, the kitchen shall be separate from the eating, play, and bathroom areas, and shall not be used as a passageway while food is being prepared.

(k) Food shall be stored as follows:

(1) Poisonous or toxic materials shall not be stored with food. Medications requiring refrigeration shall be labeled and kept in locked storage in the refrigerator.

(2) All perishables and potentially hazardous foods shall be continuously maintained at 45°F or lower in the refrigerator, or 10°F or lower in the freezer, with 0°F recommended. Each cold storage facility shall be provided with a clearly visible, accurate thermometer.

(3) All foods stored in the refrigerator shall be covered.

(4) Foods not requiring refrigeration shall be stored at least six inches above the floor in clean, dry, well-ventilated storerooms or other areas.

(5) Dry bulk foods which are not in their original unopened containers shall be stored in metal, glass or food-grade plastic containers with tight-fitting covers, and shall be labeled.

(l) Table service shall be maintained in sanitary condition using one of the following methods:

(1) Disposable plates and cups, and plastic utensils of food grade, medium weight; or

(2) a three-compartment sink supplied with hot and cold running water and a drainboard for washing, rinsing, sanitizing, and airdrying; or

(3) a mechanical dishwasher.

(m) Dishes shall have smooth, hard-glazed surfaces, and shall be entirely free from cracks or chips.

(n) Tables shall be washed before and after meals, and floors shall be swept after meals.

(o) If meals are catered:

(1) Food shall be obtained from sources licensed by the Kansas department of health and environment; and

(2) food shall be transported in covered and temperature-controlled containers, and not allowed to stand. Hot foods shall be maintained at not less than 140°F, and cold foods shall be maintained at 45°F or less.

(p) Fluid dairy products shall be Grade A pasteurized. Solid dairy products shall be pasteurized. Dry milk shall be used only for cooking.

(q) Meat shall be from government-inspected sources.

(r) Home-canned food, food from dented, rusted, bulging, or leaking cans, or food from cans without labels shall not be used.

(s) Garbage shall be placed in covered containers inaccessible to children, and removed from the kitchen daily. (Authorized by and implementing K.S.A. 65–508; effective May 1, 1983; amended May 1, 1984.)

FIGURE 18–1   Continued

4. Nutrition Policies

  • number of meals to be served within given time spans

  • posting of menus and their availability to parents

  • seating of adults at the table with children

A Good Menu is Appealing

The French have an old saying, "We eat with our eyes." Menu planners who take into consideration how the food will look on the plate are likely to develop meals that are appealing and accepted by the children to whom they are served. Figure 18–2 shows an interesting way to serve orange slices that will make them more appealing to children. Appeal can be increased by contrasting the following *sensory qualities:*

  • color
  • flavor (strong or mild; sweet or sour)
  • texture (crisp or soft)
  • shape (round, cubed, strings)

These sensory qualities of foods play an important part in a young child's choice of foods. Toddlers and young children think of foods in terms of color, flavor, texture, and shape rather than the nutrient content. Color plays a major role in children's knowledge of food (Rush 1984; Contento 1981). Using sensory qualities of food to appeal to young children takes advantage of their developmental level of interpreting their environment through the physical senses.

A comparison of the following two menus illustrates how menus can be made more appealing:

Menu # 1
Grilled Cheese Sandwiches
Deviled Eggs
French Fried Potatoes
Banana Chunks
Milk

Menu #2
Grilled Cheese Sandwiches
Deviled Eggs
Buttered Broccoli
Red Apple Wedges
Milk

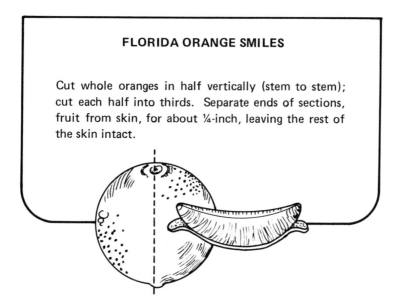

FLORIDA ORANGE SMILES

Cut whole oranges in half vertically (stem to stem); cut each half into thirds. Separate ends of sections, fruit from skin, for about ¼-inch, leaving the rest of the skin intact.

FIGURE 18-2 Orange "smiles" are a novel way to serve a familiar food in order to make it more appealing to children (Courtesy of State of Florida, Department of Citrus).

Menu #1 is essentially tones of yellow and light brown. Substituting broccoli for french fried potatoes adds color and increases the amount of vitamin A and C. Substituting red apples for bananas improves color contrast and adds a crunchier texture.

The sensory contrasts which contribute to the attractiveness of a meal also provide many opportunities for the care provider or parent to expand the young child's language development. The child can be encouraged to identify foods and describe their qualities such as round, rectangular, red, yellow, hot, or cold.

A Good Menu Includes Familiar Foods and New Foods

While it is important to introduce nutritious new foods to children, it is also important to use many foods with which the children in the group are familiar. Familiarity plays a large part in young children's food choices.

Acceptance of a meal may depend on the number of familiar foods included. When introducing new foods, it is a good idea to include them along with familiar ones. It is a good idea to back up one unfamiliar new food with familiar foods; if the new food is not well-accepted, the children will not leave the table hungry.

The menu planner might also consider introducing unfamiliar foods at snack time. Introducing unfamiliar foods at snack time prevents the new food from being labeled ''breakfast food'' or ''lunch food.''

When feeding young children, it is wise to include numerous finger foods, Table 18–9. Some children may not be skilled in the use of tableware and find finger foods to be reassuring. New foods should be introduced with little fanfare. Child involvement in preparation of an unfamiliar food may enhance its acceptance.

STEPS IN MENU PLANNING

Menu planning should be organized so that it may be done efficiently and effectively. Some of the materials which are helpful· in menu planning are:

- menu forms
- a list of foods on hand which need to be used
- recipe file
- old menus with notes and suggestions
- calendar
- grocery ads for short-term planning

TABLE 18–9   Suggested Finger Foods

Apple wedges
Banana slices
Berries
Cabbage wedges
Carrot sticks
Cauliflowerets
Celery sticks*
Cheese cubes
Dried peaches
Dried pears
Fresh peach wedges
Fresh pear wedges
Fresh pineapple sticks
Grapefruit sections (seeded)
Green pepper sticks
Meat cubes
Melon cubes
Orange sections
Pitted plums
Pitted prunes
Raisins
Tangerine sections
Tomato wedges
Turnip sticks
Zucchini sticks

*May be stuffed with cheese or peanut butter

Source: *A Planning Guide for Food Service in Child Care Centers.* USDA, FNS–64, 1981.

The menu form shown in Figure 18–3 could be used for a child care center or home. The form may be adapted to provide only the meals which are served in the individual center. Components of each meal or snack are included in the form to serve as reminders of kinds of foods which should be included to provide a nutritious menu.

Step 1. List the main dishes to be served for lunch during the week. These should include protein foods or appropriate substitutes.

Tuna noodle casserole with cheese	BBQ beef	Scrambled eggs	Chili	Macaroni and cheese	Protein

Step 2. List vegetables and fruits, including salads, for the main meal. Be sure to use fruits and vegetables in season. Fresh produce in season is less expensive and more nutritious than canned and some frozen foods. Fresh fruits and vegetables also offer excellent materials for learning activities. If planning seasonal menus months in advance, local County Extension Offices can provide information concerning produce in season and predicted supplies.

Peas Orange wedges	Broccoli Peach slices	Tomato juice ½ banana	Carrots and celery Canned pear slices	Green beans Apple wedges	Fruits and Vegetables

Step 3. Add enriched or whole grain breads and cereal products.

Enriched noodles (in casserole)	Enriched bun	Whole wheat toast	Corn muffin	Enriched macaroni (in casserole)	Bread

Step 4. Add beverage. Be sure to include the required amount of milk.

Milk	Milk	Milk	Milk	Milk	Milk

	Monday	Tuesday	Wednesday	Thursday	Friday
Breakfast Fruit/Vegetable Bread Milk					
Snack Bread Fruit/Vegetable or Milk					
Lunch Protein Fruit/Vegetable Fruit/Vegetable Bread Milk					
Snack Bread Fruit/Vegetable or Milk					
# Served					
Notes					

FIGURE 18-3   A sample menu form

Step 5. Plan snacks to balance the main meal. Especially check for vitamin C, vitamin A, iron, and calcium.

A.M. Snack Prepared oat cereal Milk	Bran muffin Apple juice	Pumpkin bread Milk	Raisin toast Orange juice	Rye cracker Milk
P.M. Snack Carrot curls Wheat crackers	Cheese crackers Peanut butter Milk	Pizza biscuits Pineapple juice	Oatmeal cookies Milk	Brown-white sandwich Apricot-orange juice

Step 6. Review your menu. Be sure it includes the required amounts from the Basic Four Food Groups.

- Does it meet funding or licensing requirements?
- Does it include a variety of contrasting foods?
- Does it contain familiar foods?
- Does it contain new foods?

Step 7. Post the menu where it can be seen by staff and parents, Figure 18–4. Be sure to note any changes made and the likes and dislikes of the children.

Step 8. Evaluate the menu. Did the children appear to like the foods that were served? Was there much plate waste? Keep a copy of the notes with menu planning materials.

WRITING MENUS

There are several methods of writing menus which the planner may wish to consider: weekly menus, cycle menus, and odd-day cycle menus. Among the factors that influence the method chosen are the child care center's schedule and hours, and the personnel who will be preparing the foods on the menu. The means of buying food and sources of food supply also influence the chosen method of menu planning.

Weekly menus list the foods that are to be prepared and eaten for one week at a time. This is a very time-consuming method and should be extended to include a minimum of two or three weeks at a time. Planning more than one week allows utilization of larger, more economical amounts of food. It also permits an outline of all the foods to be served over a period of time, so that too frequent repetitions of foods may be avoided.

Cycle menus incorporate a series of weekly menus which are re-used or cycled over a period of two or three months. Frequently, cycle menus are written to parallel the seasons, with heavier, more filling foods being selected in winter and the plentiful raw fruits and vegetables being included in spring and summer.

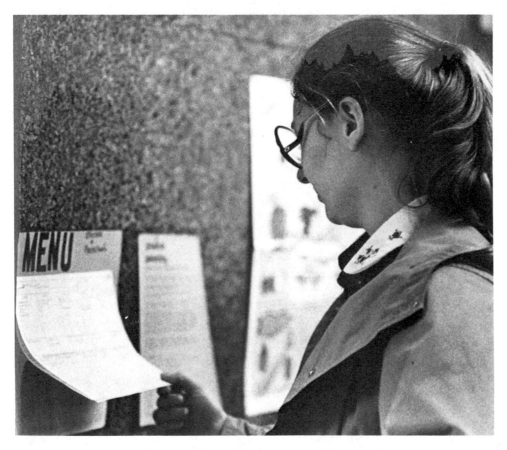

FIGURE 18-4 Menus should be available to the parents.

A well-planned cycle menu is quite efficient since, after the initial expenditure of time in planning the cycle, little additional time is required for menu planning. Food ordering also becomes less time consuming and the use of food is more efficient. However, the planner should not hesitate to change parts of the cycle that prove difficult to produce or that are not well accepted by the children. Seasonal cycle menus may be used for a period of years with timely revisions.

Odd-day cycle menus involve planning menus for periods of days other than a week. Cycles of any number of days may be used. This type of cycling avoids the association of specific foods with certain days of the week. This type of menu requires very careful planning to avoid dishes or foods that require advance preparation in Monday to Friday child care centers.

Menus That Include Ethnic Foods

Most centers care for children from a variety of cultural and *ethnic* backgrounds. A good menu planner draws on this wealth of backgrounds and includes foods that are familiar to a number of cultures. The inclusion of ethnic foods serves several purposes:

- The children from that culture feel familiar with these foods and are likely to accept them at meal or snack times.
- They add variety to the meals offered children from other cultures and may serve as bases for related educational activities.
- Preparation of ethnic foods may foster increased parental participation.

NUTRITIOUS SNACKS

Snacks should contribute to the child's daily food needs and educational experiences. Snacks should contribute vitamins, minerals and other nutrients important in health, growth and development, Figure 18-5. Snack foods should include nutrients which were not adequately provided by lunch and/or breakfast.

New or unusual foods can often be better introduced at snack time. This may often be accomplished in a party atmosphere such as a taste-testing party.

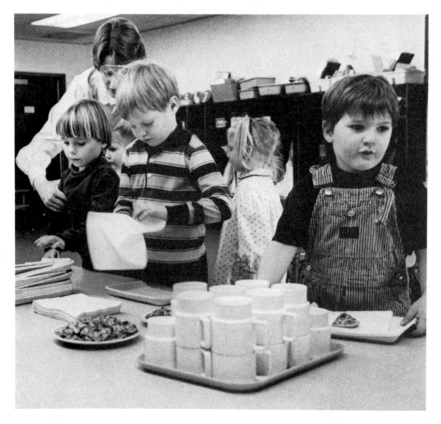

FIGURE 18-5 Snacks should provide nutrients to balance the meals.

Snacks are a means of providing nutrients and energy between meals, since children have small stomach capacities and may not be able to eat enough at one meal to sustain them until the next meal. One and one-half or two hours between meals seems to be the best spacing for most children in order to prevent them from becoming too hungry or spoiling their appetite.

Suitable Snack Foods

A variety of raw fruits and vegetables are ideal for snack foods. Raw fruits and vegetables are excellent sources of vitamin C and vitamin A, and should be included often. The care provider must be sure the fruits and vegetables are sectioned or sliced so the children can chew them. The crispness of fruits and vegetables helps to remove food clinging to the teeth. The crispness and texture also stimulate the gums so they stay healthy. Fresh fruits and vegetables provide cellulose which aids elimination. Another important factor not to be forgotten is exposure to the subtle flavors of fruits and vegetables.

Whole grains and cereal products or enriched breads and grain products are also good snack foods. The flavor of *whole grains* adds variety to the diet. Whole grain products also add fiber, which aids elimination. *Enriched* breads and cereals are refined products to which iron, thiamin, niacin and riboflavin are added in amounts equal to the whole grain product.

Unsweetened beverages such as full-strength fruit and vegetable juices are good choices for snacks. Juices made from oranges, grapefruits, tangerines, and tomatoes are rich in vitamin C. Vitamin C may also be added to apple, grape and pineapple juices. Check the labels of these juices to determine if they are fortified with vitamin C. Carbonated beverages, *fruit drinks,* and some fruit ades are unacceptable for snacks. These beverages contain large amounts of sugar and no other nutrients, except perhaps some added vitamin C. Water is also essential for good health; children should drink 6 to 8 small glasses of water a day, Figure 18–6.

SERVING MEALS

A nutritious meal is of no value to the child if the child does not eat the meal. The atmosphere in which meals are served can forestall or enhance eating problems. All meals should be served in a relaxed, social atmosphere. The classroom should be cleaned up prior to mealtimes; this eliminates the distraction of toys or unfinished games lying around. It also makes for an uncluttered environment which is more restful.

The table should be made as attractive as possible. Placemats made by the children add interest and neatness to the meal. Centerpieces also add to the attractiveness of the meal setting. Simple centerpieces can be made by the children thereby adding interest. Plates, cups, utensils and napkins should be laid out neatly and appropriately. The proper way to set a table can also be a learning

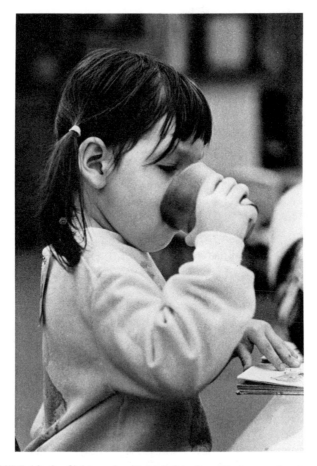

FIGURE 18-6   Children should drink 6 to 8 small glasses of water daily.

experience for the children. The food served should be made attractive and appealing to the children.

It is important that teachers and care providers eat meals with the children as this offers the children role models for appropriate behavior and attitudes. Mealtime should be a time when teachers and care providers sit and engage in pleasant conversation with the children about things that interest the children. Children should also be encouraged to talk with one another. Dwelling on table manners and behavior during meals should be avoided as much as possible. Only positive reinforcement of good behavior should be mentioned. Problem eaters need special positive reinforcement of good eating behavior; all negative behavior should be ignored during mealtime.

Children may find it fun to have a chart on which a star or sticker can be placed beside the child's name each time the child finishes a meal. Table 18-10 gives some additional ideas on making mealtimes happy times.

TABLE 18–10   Make Mealtime a Happy Time

Feeding young children can be fun if you know:
- What foods children should have.
- How to bring children and foods together happily. Pleasant eating experiences are as important as nutritious foods. They provide pleasant associations with food and eating. Food habits and attitudes that form during the preschool years remain with most people throughout life.
- Try to understand each child's personality and reaction to foods.
- Children need to do as much for themselves as they are able to do. First efforts may be awkward, but encourage them. These efforts are a step toward growth.
- Children may be in no hurry to eat once the first edge is taken off their hunger. They do not have adults' sense of time. Urging them to hurry may spoil their pleasure in eating.
- Most 1-year-old children can handle bite-sized pieces of food with their fingers. Later they can handle a spoon by themselves. Since they are growing slower than infants, they may be less hungry. They may be choosy and refuse certain foods. Don't worry or force them to eat. Keep on offering different foods.
- Sometimes children 3 to 6 years old go on food "jags." They may want two or three servings of one food at one meal. Given time they will settle down and eat a normal meal. The overall pattern from week to week and month to month is more important.

Source: *A Planning Guide for Food Service in Child Care Centers*. USDA, FNS–64, January 1981.

SUMMARY

The atmosphere in which meals are served is very important. Mealtimes should be happy, social times free from reprimands about table manners and behavior. Infants should be cuddled and talked to when being fed to provide socialization and needed close human contact; they should not be hurried when feeding. Solid foods should be introduced into the infant's diet one at a time in small quantities as indicated by the pediatrician.

The menu is the basic tool of any food service. It is the plan for what is served when. The primary requirement for a good menu is that it meet the nutritional needs of those for whom it is intended. Other considerations when planning menus are: the satisfaction of funding and licensing requirements, providing for nutritious familiar foods, introduction of nutritious new foods, planning appealing foods, providing safe food cooked and served in clean surroundings, and staying within budgetary limits. Menus which contrast sensory qualities of foods such as color, texture, flavor and shape are more appealing than those which do not.

Menu planning should be made as efficient as possible through the use of a routine method and sequence of operations. The finished menu should be checked for nutritional adequacy, fulfillment of existing funding and/or licensing requirements, sensory contrasts, and inclusion of new foods, familiar foods, and foods rich in vitamin A, vitamin C, calcium and iron.

Types of menus may vary from center to center. Some types which might be used are weekly menus, cycle menus, and odd-day cycle menus. Foods from different cultures contribute further variety to the menu and also provide opportunities for extended learning experiences. Preparation of ethnic foods can promote increased parental participation.

Snacks should be planned as a nutritional contribution to the overall menu. Fresh fruits and vegetables, full-strength juices, and whole grain or enriched bread or cereal products are good snack foods.

LEARNING ACTIVITIES

1. Plan a five-day menu appropriate for 4-year-old children that includes morning snack, lunch, and afternoon snack. The menu should provide one-half of the foods needed according to the Basic Four Food Groups. Provide one good source each of vitamin C, calcium, and iron daily. Provide at least three good sources of vitamin A during the five-day period.

2. Four-year-old Jamie often comes to the child care center without having had breakfast at home (both his parents work and must leave early every day). His mother often buys him a doughnut on the way to the center, explaining that she felt "he should have something to eat." During circle times, he's often inattentive and seems to be "in his own world" and somewhat lethargic. He rarely engages in large-motor activities voluntarily. At snack times and mealtimes, he tends to select only milk or juices and is resistant to eating vegetables and meats.
   a. What may be the cause of Jamie's behavior during circle times?
   b. How would you characterize Jamie's nutritional status?
   c. What eating patterns need to be corrected?
   d. What steps should be taken to improve Jamie's participation in activities, as well as his nutritional patterns and status?

3. Review the criteria given for menus. Rank the criteria as you perceive their degree of importance. Are there other factors which you feel should also be considered in planning adequate menus? Consider the needs of individual child care centers, child care homes, or family homes. Are the important factors the same or different for each situation?

UNIT REVIEW

A. Multiple Choice. Select the best answer.

1. The *primary* criterion for a good menu is
   a. sensory contrasts
   b. nutritional adequacy
   c. meeting funding requirements
   d. meeting licensing requirements

2. Nutrients for which young children's menus must be carefully monitored
   are
   a. vitamin A, vitamin C, thiamin, iron
   b. vitamin A, vitamin D, calcium, iron
   c. vitamin A, vitamin C, calcium, iron
   d. vitamin C, niacin, vitamin D, iron

3. The recommended daily allowance of nutrients that federally-funded food
   programs for children are required to provide is a minimum of
   a. one-half
   b. one-third
   c. three-fourths
   d. one-fourth

4. Menu planning requires careful evaluation of
   a. physical needs
   b. developmental needs
   c. social needs
   d. all of these

5. Items appropriate for snacks include
   a. carbonated beverages
   b. fresh fruit slices
   c. fruit drinks
   d. potato chips

6. Foods rich in vitamin A include
   a. tomatoes and cabbage
   b. apricots and carrots
   c. salmon and yogurt
   d. ham and raisins

B. Briefly answer the following questions.

1. State the serving size for a child 3 to 6 years old for each of the following
   foods:
   a. milk
   b. dry cereal
   c. fruit
   d. vegetable
   e. bread

2. Where can information relative to licensing requirements for nutrition and
   food services for young children be obtained?

3. Name four sensory qualities that can be contrasted to make food appealing.

4. What are two reasons for using fresh fruits and vegetables in season?

5. Name three methods of writing menus.

6. List the eight steps in preparing a menu.

7. List three reasons for not propping an infant's bottle when the infant is feeding.

8. Name three ways that mealtimes can be made pleasant for the children.

REFERENCES

Contento, I. "Children's Thinking About Food and Eating—A Piagetian-based Study." *Proceedings of the Workshop on Nutrition Education Research,* 1981.

Egan, M. C. "Federal Nutrition Support Programs for Children." In *Community Nutrition: People, Policies, and Programs.* Edited by H. S. Wright and L. S. Sims. Belmont, CA: Wadsworth, Inc., 1981.

Pamphlets

Conserving the Nutritive Value in Foods, USDA Home and Garden Bulletin No. 90. Superintendent of Documents, U. S. Government Printing Office, Washington, DC 20402.

Food is More than Just Something to Eat, Nutrition, Pueblo, CO 81009.

Growing Up with Breakfast, Kellogg Company, Department of Home Economics Services, 235 Porter Street, Battle Creek, MI 49016.

Buying Food, Superintendent of Documents, U. S. Government Printing Office, Washington, DC 20402.

Fun With Good Foods, USDA, PA–1204. Superintendent of Documents, U. S. Government Printing Office, Washington, DC 20402.

A Planning Guide for Food Service in Child Care Centers, USDA, FNS–64. Food Nutrition Service, Washington, DC.

Unit 19
FOOD SAFETY
AND ECONOMY

Terms to Know

pasteurized
sanitized
food-borne illness
food infection
food intoxication

bacteria
parasites
cost control
viruses

Objectives

After studying this unit, you will be able to:
- State aspects of personal hygiene that relate to food safety.
- Describe proper ways to store food.
- Describe methods of sanitizing food preparation areas and equipment.
- Identify proper dish washing practices.
- Explain how to prevent contamination of food.
- Cite examples of food-borne illnesses.
- Describe five ways to keep food costs within the budget.

This unit introduces factors other than the menu which contribute to effective food service in the child care setting. The success of a carefully planned menu depends upon the food being safe to eat. The menu must also stay within the allotted food budget.

FOOD SAFETY DEPENDS ON SANITATION

The safety of meals prepared for young children should be of great concern. Food-borne illnesses are unpleasant and may be very dangerous or even fatal to young children. Common illnesses such as colds and influenza can be better controlled by careful sanitary practices. Personal hygiene, proper handling of food, and sanitation of food preparation and serving areas and equipment are essential for food safety.

Personal Hygiene and Food Safety

Those who are involved in food preparation and service must take great care to maintain a high level of personal hygiene. Food-borne illnesses can be transmitted by failure to wash one's hands carefully.

The food handler must meet health standards. Those working in licensed child care facilities are required to supply to the school or child care center written proof that they are currently free of tuberculosis. Sufficient evidence of their tuberculosis-free status is afforded by a negative skin test or a negative chest X ray. Food handlers should also undergo periodic physical examinations to document their state of general good health. Health standards for food service workers vary according to the regulations of individual states.

Everyone who is involved in food preparation and service should be free of communicable diseases. Those suffering from colds, respiratory or intestinal types of influenza, gastrointestinal upsets, or severe throat infections should not be involved in food handling. Even though persons suffering from mild forms of these diseases frequently feel that they are well enough to work, to do so may transmit their illness to others. Those suffering from any communicable disease should refrain from handling food (Hospital Research and Educational Trust 1976). An emergency store of simply prepared foods can solve the problem of what to feed the children when the cook is ill. Foods which could be available for emergency use are:

- canned soups
- peanut butter
- pre-prepared macaroni and cheese
- instant puddings
- canned fruits
- tuna

An adequate supply of these foods can provide meals which require a minimum of time or cooking skill to prepare.

Food handlers should wear clean, washable clothing and should change aprons frequently if they become soiled. Clothing should be comfortable and allow ease of movement. Hair should be covered by a net, cap, or scarf while the worker is handling food. Head coverings should be put on and shoulders checked carefully for loose hair prior to entering the kitchen.

Food handlers should refrain from chewing gum or smoking while working with food. Both practices can introduce saliva to the food handling area.

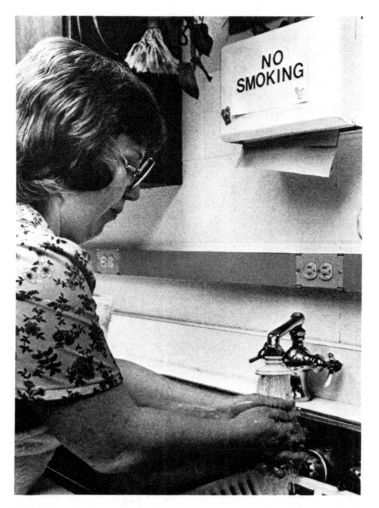

FIGURE 19-1 Hands should be washed thoroughly before handling food.

Handwashing is of utmost importance to personal hygiene, Figure 19-1. Hands should be washed thoroughly:

- before work
- before touching food
- after handling nonfood items, such as cleaning or laundry supplies
- between handling different food items
- after using the bathroom
- after coughing, sneezing, or blowing the nose

Safe Food Handling

Food. All raw produce should be inspected for spoilage upon delivery and should be thoroughly washed before use. Careful washing removes sprays and other contaminants. All dairy products should be *pasteurized.* Tops of cans should be washed before opening; contaminants on cans can be passed to other cans or work surfaces by a dirty can opener. The can opener should also be washed daily.

Food storage.   Careful storage and handling of food at appropriate temperatures are essential factors of food safety. Refrigerators should be maintained at 38°F to 40°F. A thermometer hung from a shelf in the warmest area of the refrigerator can be used to check whether appropriate temperatures are being maintained. Freezers should be maintained at 0°F or below. Frozen foods should be thawed:

- in the refrigerator
- under cold running water
- while cooking

Caution: Frozen food should never be thawed at room temperature!

Transport. Food should be covered or wrapped during transport. Covering provides additional temperature control and avoids the possibility of contamination during transport. When serving foods, each serving bowl, dish, or pan should have a spoon; spoons should not be used to serve more than one food.

Food Service. Food which has been on the tables should not be saved. An exception to this rule is fresh fruits and vegetables which may be washed after removal from the table and served later. Food which has been held in the kitchen at safe temperatures (160°F for hot food or 40°F or below for cold foods) may be saved. Foods which are to be saved should be placed in shallow pans and refrigerated or frozen immediately. Spreading food in a thin layer in shallow pans allows it to cool more rapidly.

Foods such as creamed dishes, meat, poultry, or egg salads which are especially prone to spoilage should be prepared from chilled ingredients as quickly as possible and served or refrigerated in shallow containers immediately. All such foods should be maintained at temperatures below 40°F until cooked or served.

Sanitation of Food Preparation Areas and Equipment

The cleanliness of the kitchen and kitchen equipment is a vital factor of safe food service. These areas should be cleaned on a regular schedule. Minimizing traffic through the kitchen reduces the amount of dirt brought in. Schedules, such as that shown in Figure 19–2, should be maintained for the cleaning of floors, walls, ranges, ovens, and refrigerators. The equipment used in the direct handling of food must receive extra care. Surfaces on which food is prepared should be *sanitized* with chlorine bleach solution each time a different food is prepared on it. Cutting boards should be nonporous and should be sanitized with bleach solution or boiling water after cutting any meat. A separate cutting board should be used exclusively for poultry products. Sanitizing may be done with either a liquid chlorine bleach solution (1/4 cup bleach to each gallon of water, made up daily) or with boiling water.

CLEANING SCHEDULE

Daily
- Cutting boards sanitized after each use
- Counter tops washed and sanitized between preparation of different foods
- Tables washed with sanitizing solution
- Can openers washed and sanitized
- Range tops cleaned
- Floors damp mopped

Weekly
- Ovens cleaned
- Refrigerator cleaned and rinsed with vinegar water

As Needed
- Refrigerator/freezer defrosted
- Walls washed
- Floors scrubbed

FIGURE 19-2   Kitchen sanitation depends on frequent, systematic cleaning.

Dish washing. Dishes may be washed by hand or with a mechanical dish-washer. If washing by hand:

- wash dishes with hot water and detergent
- rinse dishes in hot, clear water
- sanitize dishes with chlorine bleach solution or scald with boiling water

All dishes, utensils, and surfaces must be air dried (not dried with a towel), Figure 19-3.

If dishes are washed by a mechanical dishwasher, the machine must meet local health department standards. Some state licensing regulations provide guidelines as to the method of dishwashing to be used based on the number of persons served.

Sanitation of Food Service Areas

The eating area requires special attention. Cleanliness of the tables can be a problem, especially if they are also used as classroom tables. In order to maintain adequate sanitation, the tables should be washed with chlorine bleach solution:

- before each meal
- after each meal
- before each snack
- after each snack

The children should be taught to wash their hands carefully before eating. They should also be taught that serving spoons should be used to serve food and

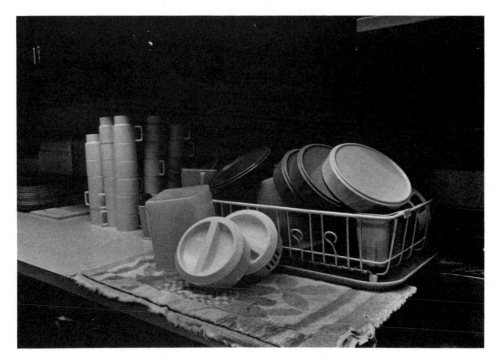

FIGURE 19-3 Hand-washed dishes should be air dried.

then replaced in the serving dishes. Children should never be allowed to eat from serving spoons.

The guidelines for sanitation evaluation shown in Figure 19–4 are a useful tool in assessing food service sanitation on a regular basis.

FOOD-BORNE ILLNESSES

Food poisoning refers to a variety of *food-borne illnesses* which may be caused by the presence of *bacteria, viruses, parasites,* or some kinds of molds growing on foods. Foods which are visibly molded, soured, or beginning to liquify should not be used; nor should food from bulging cans or cans in which the liquid is foamy or smells strangely. Foods containing most food poisoning organisms may carry few signs of spoilage. The food usually appears and smells safe, but still can cause severe illness. Proper sanitation procedures, preparation, and food handling should prevent most food-borne illnesses (Labuza and Erdman 1984).

Bacterial Food-borne Illness

Bacteria thrive especially well on protein foods such as meats, poultry, eggs, custards, and salads containing eggs (Harvard Medical School Health Letter June

SANITATION EVALUATION

	EX	GOOD	FAIR	POOR
FOOD				
1. Supplies of food and beverages must meet local, state and federal codes.				
2. Meats and poultry must be inspected and passed for wholesomeness by federal or state inspectors.				
3. Milk and milk products must be pasteurized.				
4. Home canned foods must not be used.				
FOOD STORAGE				
1. Perishable foods are stored at temperatures which will prevent spoilage: a. Refrigerator temperature: 40°F or below				
b. Freezer temperature: 0°F or below				
2. Thermometers are located in the warmest part of each refrigerator and freezer and are checked daily.				
3. Refrigerator has enough shelves to allow space between foods for air circulation to maintain proper temperatures.				
4. Frozen foods are thawed in refrigerator or quick-thawed under cold running water for immediate preparation, or thawed as part of the cooking process. (Never thawed at room temperature.)				
5. Food is examined when brought to center to make sure it is not spoiled, dirty, or infested with insects.				

FIGURE 19–4 Guidelines for sanitation evaluation

	EX	GOOD	FAIR	POOR
6. Foods are stored in rodent-proof and insect proof covered metal, glass or hard plastic containers.				
7. Containers of food are stored above the floor (6 inches) on racks which permit moving for easy cleaning.				
8. Storerooms are dry and free from leaky plumbing or drainage problems. All holes and cracks in storeroom are repaired.				
9. Storerooms are kept cool (60°F to 70°F).				
10. All food items are stored separately from nonfood items.				
11. Inventory system is used to be sure that stored food is rotated.				
FOOD PREPARATION AND HANDLING 1. All raw fruits and vegetables are washed before use. Tops of cans are washed before opening.				
2. Thermometers are used to check internal temperatures of: a. Poultry—minimum 165°F				
b. Pork and pork products— minimum 150°F				
3. Meat salads, poultry salads, potato salads, egg salad, cream-filled pastries and other potentially hazardous prepared food are prepared from chilled products as quickly as possible and refrigerated in shallow containers or served immediately.				
4. All potentially hazardous foods are maintained below 40°F or above 140°F during transportation and holding until service.				

FIGURE 19-4   Continued

	EX	GOOD	FAIR	POOR
5. Foods are covered or completely wrapped during transportation.				
6. Two spoons are used for tasting foods.				
7. Each serving bowl has a serving spoon.				
8. Leftover food from serving bowls on the tables is not saved. An exception would be raw fruits and vegetables that could be washed. Food held in kitchen at safe temperatures is used for refilling bowls as needed.				
9. Food held in the kitchen at safe temperatures is re-used.				
10. Foods stored for re-use are placed in shallow pans and refrigerated or frozen immediately.				
11. Leftovers or prepared casseroles are not held in refrigerator or frozen immediately.				
STORAGE OF NONFOOD SUPPLIES 1. All cleaning supplies (including dish sanitizers) and other poisonous materials are stored in locked compartments or in compartment well above the reach of children and separate from food, dishes and utensils.				
2. Poisonous and toxic materials other than those needed for kitchen sanitation are stored in locked compartments outside the kitchen area.				
3. Insect and rodent poisons are stored in locked compartments in an area apart from other cleaning compounds				

FIGURE 19–4 Continued

	EX	GOOD	FAIR	POOR
to avoid contamination or mistaken usage.				
CLEANING AND CARE OF EQUIPMENT 1. A cleaning schedule is followed: a. Floors are wet mopped daily; scrubbed as needed.				
b. Food preparation surfaces are washed and sanitized between preparation of different food items (as between meat and salad preparation).				
c. Cutting boards are made of hard nontoxic material, and are smooth and free from cracks, crevices and open seams.				
d. After cutting any single meat, fish or poultry item, the cutting board is thoroughly washed and sanitized.				
e. Can openers are washed and sanitized daily.				
f. Utensils are cleaned and sanitized between uses on different food items.				
2. Dishwashing is done by an approved method: a. *Hand washed*—3-step operation including sanitizing rinse.				
b. *Mechanical*—by machine that meets local health department standards.				
3. Range tops are washed daily and as needed to keep them clean during preparation.				
4. Ovens are cleaned weekly or as needed.				
5. Refrigerator is washed once a week with vinegar.				

FIGURE 19-4   Continued

	EX	GOOD	FAIR	POOR
6. Refrigerator is defrosted when there is about 1/4″ thickness of frost.				
7. Tables and other eating surfaces are washed with a mild disinfectant solution before and after each meal.				
8. All food contact surfaces are air-dried after cleaning and sanitizing.				
9. Cracked or chipped utensils or dishes are not used; they are disposed of.				
10. Garbage cans are leakproof and have tight-fitting lids.				
11. Garbage cans are lined with plastic liners and emptied and cleaned frequently.				
12. There is a sufficient number of garbage containers available.				
INSECT AND RODENT CONTROL 1. Only an approved pyrithren base insecticide or fly swatter is used in the food preparation area.				
2. The insecticides do not come in contact with raw or cooked food, utensils or equipment used in food preparation and serving, or with any other food contact surface.				
3. Doors and windows have screens in proper repair and are closed at all times. All openings to the outside are closed or properly screened to prevent entrance of rodents or insects.				

FIGURE 19–4   Continued

	EX	GOOD	FAIR	POOR
PERSONAL SANITATION 1. Health of food service personnel meets standards: a. TB test is current				
b. Physical examination is up to date				
2. Everyone who works with or near food is free from communicable disease.				
3. Clean washable clothing is worn.				
4. Hairnets or hair caps are worn in the kitchen.				
5. There is no use of tobacco or chewing gum in the kitchen.				
6. Hands are washed thoroughly before touching food, before work, after handling nonfood items, between handling of different food items, after using bathroom, after coughing, sneezing, blowing nose.				

FIGURE 19–4 Continued

1984). In order for bacteria to grow they must have food, moisture, darkness, and temperatures between 40°F and 140°F. Bacterial food-borne illnesses are of two general types:

- food infections
- food intoxications

Food Infections. *Food infections* result from ingestion of large amounts of viable bacteria in foods which cause infectious disease. Symptoms usually develop relatively slowly (12–24 hours) since incubation of the bacteria takes time.

Salmonellosis is a food infection that is transmitted through foods contaminated by unwashed hands or the presence of rodents or insects in the food service area. Salmonella infection is marked by severe gastrointestinal distress including abdominal cramps, vomiting, and nausea which begins within 12–24 hours after eating. It lasts for two to three days.

Food Intoxications. *Food intoxications* result from eating food containing toxins which are produced in the food by bacterial growth. Symptoms develop more rapidly (within 1–6 hours) than those associated with infections (Williams 1981).

Staphylococcal food intoxication occurs in foods which have been contami-nated from sores or boils on the food handler's skin. As the Staphylococcus bacteria grow, they produce a toxin which is the actual cause of the illness. Severe symptoms, including nausea, diarrhea, headache, and fever, begin from one to six hours after eating the affected food. It lasts for one to three days.

Clostridium botulinum causes a rare but serious form of food poisoning called botulism. Botulism can result from eating improperly canned, low-acid foods. In recent years, several cases of botulism have been linked to the ingestion of raw honey. Onset of symptoms takes three to six days and is marked by respiratory paralysis. The current fatality rate from botulism is approximately 20 percent of those contracting it (Labuza and Erdman 1984).

Viral Food-borne Illness

Upper respiratory diseases such as colds or influenza can be transmitted through foods. Prevention includes careful, frequent handwashing, covering coughs and sneezes, and disposal of used tissues.

Another viral disease which may be transmitted through foods is infectious hepatitis. Contaminated foods, milk, or water may be the source of the disease. Stringent personal hygiene and sanitary practices by food handlers are essential to the prevention of infectious hepatitis by food (Williams 1981).

Parasitic Food-borne Illness

Another food-borne illness which should be considered is trichinosis. The parasitic food infection is caused by the presence of Trichinella spiralis parasites in muscle meats such as pork or game. Cooking these meats to the well-done stage destroys the Trichinella organism. Chronic symptoms of infection are chills, muscular aches, and weakness.

Molds

Food-borne illnesses caused by molds are uncommon in the United States. However, there are some species of molds which produce toxins that can cause severe diarrhea and even death (Labuza and Erdman 1984).

Aflatoxins, first found in peanut meal, are examples of food contamination caused by Aspergillus molds. The toxins are apparently produced immediately after harvesting of the peanuts and early in the storage period. Rapid drying, improved storage conditions, and possible use of fungicides are important control measures (Williams 1981).

THE MENU MUST STAY WITHIN THE BUDGET

While the menu lists what foods are to be served, the budget defines the resources allotted for preparation of the menu. Items which must be included in the budget are food, personnel, and equipment. The food budget can be controlled through careful attention to:

- menu planning
- food purchasing
- food preparation
- food service
- record keeping

Cost control is essential if a food service is to stay within the budget. The goal is to feed the children appetizing, nutritious meals at a reasonably low cost. Cost control should never be attempted at the expense of good nutrition.

Menu Planning

Cost control begins at the menu-planning stage. To plan menus that stay within a budget, it is important to begin by including inexpensive foods. To do so, the planner must be aware of current prices and seasonal supplies.

In order to lower food costs, the menu planner should make careful use of leftovers and supplies on hand. To ensure that quality foods are selected from supplies on hand, a storage system should be devised which places newly purchased foods at the back of storage and older foods at the front so they can be used first. This method of rotating stocks of food can be facilitated by dating all supplies as they come into the storage area.

Food Purchasing

Food purchasing is a crucial step in cost control. Purchase of too much food or of inappropriate foods can transform a menu that is planned around inexpensive foods to an expensive menu at service. The key step is to determine as accurately as possible the amount of food which is needed to feed everyone an adequate amount. The use of standardized recipes can be a great help in determining how much and what kinds of food is needed. One such set of recipes is that developed by the United States Department of Agriculture for use in school lunches or Child Care Food Programs. These recipes provide the ingredients needed as well as the amounts required to produce the recipe for groups of various sizes.

Before purchasing food, a written food order should be prepared listing the following:

- market units—ounces, pounds, can size, cases, etc.
- quantity (number) of units needed
- style of food desired—pieces, slices, halves, chunks, etc.

For those who purchase food at local retail stores, a simple form which follows the floor plan of the store(s) where food is purchased may be helpful. When completing the market order, list the foods needed for the entire period of time for which food must be purchased in the following order:

- main dishes
- fruits and vegetables
- breads, cereals, pastas
- dairy products

Frozen foods should be selected last in order to minimize thawing between store freezer and food service freezer.

Food Preparation

Careful preparation methods that are appropriate for the specific food contribute both to the nutritional quality of the food and to cost control. Fruits and vegetables should be peeled only if necessary, as more nutrients are retained if the skin is left intact. If peeling is necessary, as it may be for very young children, only a thin layer of skin should be removed.

Correct heat and cooking time are important factors in cost control as well as nutrient retention. Foods cooked too long or at excessively high heat may undergo shrinkage or be burned. In either case, food costs increase because burned food is not usable and shrinkage results in fewer portions than originally planned. Nutrients, such as thiamin and vitamin C, are readily destroyed when exposed to heat.

Tested standardized recipes, such as those available from the U.S. Department of Agriculture, help to ensure correct amounts of ingredients and to reduce leftovers. Leftover foods which have not been placed on the table may be promptly frozen and used when serving the same dish again. Leftovers should be reheated in a separate pan and not mixed with freshly-prepared portions. Leftovers should be reheated only once.

Food Service

If the recipe specifies a serving size, that amount should be served, for example, "one-half cup or 1 1/2" X 1 1/2" square." In child care centers using family style service, the staff may serve standard portions to the children as a means of portion control. In centers where children are encouraged to serve themselves, each child should be asked to take only as much as can be eaten.

Serving utensils which are made to serve specific portions are an aid to portion and cost control. Examples of such utensils are soup ladles and ice cream scoops, which are available in a number of standardized sizes. These tools are available at restaurant supply companies.

Record Keeping

Complete, accurate records should be kept of the amount of money spent for food, and the number of children and staff served daily. These records provide an idea of how much money is being spent for food and whether this amount is within the projected budget. Figure 19–5 shows an example of a form used to report the number of meals served.

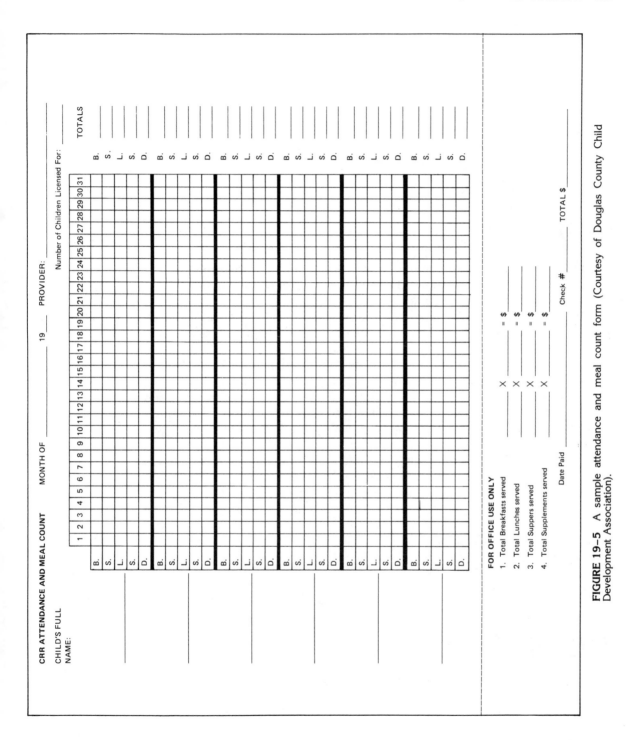

FIGURE 19-5 A sample attendance and meal count form (Courtesy of Douglas County Child Development Association).

A record of expenses for each month should be kept. For further accuracy, an inventory of foods on hand should be done and the cost of the inventory determined and deducted from the raw food cost for that month. (If inventories tend not to differ much from month to month, this last step may be omitted.) At the end of each month:

- calculate the total number of individuals served
- calculate the total food bills
- divide the total dollars spent by the total number served to determine monthly food costs per person

SUMMARY

Factors other than menu planning contribute to effective food service in the child care setting. Sanitation and cost control are integral factors in the success or failure of the total food service operation.

An important aspect of sanitation is the personal health and hygiene of personnel preparing and serving the food. A state of acceptable good health is confirmed by negative tuberculosis tests and periodic physical examinations. Cleanliness of work clothing, use of head coverings, and frequent handwashing are essential to the maintenance of good personal sanitation in food service.

Cleanliness of the food preparation and service areas requires frequent and systematic attention. Cleaning schedules are helpful in achieving a desirable degree of cleanliness. Counter tops, table tops, walls, floors, equipment, and utensils must all be kept clean.

Food safety refers to the handling of foods. Foods must be kept hot enough to kill bacteria (above 140°F) or cold enough to prevent bacterial growth (below 40°F). Bacteria which lead to food-borne illnesses include Salmonella, Staphylococcus, and Clostridium botulinum. Trichinella infection is a parasitic infection transmitted by improperly cooked pork and game meats. Viruses and molds can also cause food-borne illnesses.

Food costs can be controlled by careful attention to: menu planning, food purchasing and storage, food preparation and storage, serving standard portions and accurate recordkeeping.

LEARNING ACTIVITIES

1. The following menu is planned for a child care center for one week in January.

   Meat Loaf   Bread with margarine
   Creamed new peas and potatoes   Fresh strawberry-banana fruit cup
   Peach half in cherry gelatin   Milk

a. Evaluate this menu and suggest changes which could make it less expensive but equally or more nutritious.
b. How would the cost of this menu served in January compare to the cost of the same menu served in June?

2. Which of the following foods would probably be safe to eat? Why are the remaining foods unsafe?
a. Corn from a can with a slight bulge
b. Cake dropped on a just-cleaned table
c. Hard cooked eggs with a grayish green circle around the yolk
d. Unheated pork and beans from a can with a small leak
e. Stuffed turkey partially roasted one day and finished the next day to save time

3. Invite a laboratory technician to class to make culture plates of a
a. hand before washing
b. hand after washing with water only
c. hand after washing with soap and water
d. strand of hair
The technician should then return to the class with the cultures after the cultures have incubated for 2 to 3 days.
e. Is there bacterial growth on any of the culture plates?
f. Which cultures have the most bacterial growth?
g. Discuss how these results could be best utilized in terms of
   (1) food preparation and service
   (2) child care center meal and snack times

4. Suggest market order descriptions for the following foods. Example: canned pineapple for fruit cup, # 10 can.
a. canned peaches for fruit cup
b. canned tomatoes for spaghetti sauce
c. carrots for vegetable soup
d. chicken for chicken casserole

UNIT REVIEW

A. Multiple Choice. Select the best answer.

1. Sanitation relative to food service refers to
   a. safe food handling
   b. personal hygiene
   c. cleanliness of the service area
   d. all of these

2. Food-borne bacterial infections include
   a. salmonellosis
   b. trichinosis
   c. infectious hepatitis
   d. all of these

3. Refrigerator temperatures should be maintained at
   a. 28°F to 30°F
   b. 38°F to 40°F
   c. 45°F to 50°F
   d. 0°F

4. Bacterial growth requires the following condition(s)
   a. temperatures between 40°F and 140°F
   b. moisture
   c. darkness
   d. all of these

5. Milk served in child care centers should be
   a. homogenized
   b. skim
   c. pasteurized
   d. two percent

6. Hands should be carefully washed
   a. after using the bathroom
   b. before touching food
   c. between handling different foods
   d. all of these

7. Easily spoiled foods such as custards and creamed dishes should be
   a. placed in a shallow pan and cooled slowly to prevent curdling
   b. cooled on the counter to avoid warming the refrigerator
   c. placed in a shallow pan and refrigerated immediately
   d. both a and b

8. Frozen foods may be thawed safely
   a. in the refrigerator
   b. under hot running water
   c. at room temperature
   d. both a and b

9. Dishes or pots and pans that are washed by hand may be sanitized with
   a. hot tap water
   b. a chlorine bleach solution
   c. sudsy water
   d. all of these

10. Dishes and utensils that have been washed by hand must be
    a. air dried
    b. dried with a clean towel
    c. rinsed in cold water
    d. put in cupboards immediately

B. Briefly answer the following questions.

1. Name two ways the menu planner can control food costs.

2. What is the key step in cost control when purchasing food?

3. Name three ways to control food costs when preparing food.

4. How can food costs be controlled when serving food.

5. Of what value is keeping accurate food records?

6. List three means of keeping the food preparation area clean and germfree.

REFERENCES

"Food poisoning: Worse Than Ants At A Picnic." *The Harvard Medical School Health Letter* 9:5, June 1984.

Hospital Research and Education Trust. *Being a Food Service Worker.* Washington, DC: Robert J. Brady Company, 1976.

Labuza, T. P., and Erdman, J. W. *Food Science and Nutritional Health.* St. Paul: West Publishing Company, 1984.

Williams, S. R. *Nutrition and Diet Therapy.* 4th ed. St. Louis: The C. V. Mosby Company, 1981.

Additional Reading

Rucker, M. H., Tom, P. Y., and York, G. K. "Food Safety—What Do The Experts Say?" *Journal of Nutrition Education* 9:158, October–December 1977.

Day, H. G. "Food Safety—Then and Now." *Journal of the American Dietetic Association* 69:229, September 1976.

Unit 20

FEDERAL FOOD PROGRAMS

Terms to Know

child nutrition
  programs
reduced price meals
poverty guidelines

tax-exempt
lactation
allowed foods

Objectives

After studying this unit, you will be able to:
- List two reasons why nutritional adequacy is important in child development.
- State the purpose of federally-funded food programs.
- Describe five nutrition programs which provide food assistance directly to children.
- Describe two family nutrition programs.
- State eligibility requirements for the Child Care Food Program.

Nutritional adequacy is recognized as a crucial aspect of normal child development. Well-fed children grow more rapidly than poorly-fed children; nutritional adequacy also enhances effective learning (Winick 1980). Many children receive most of their meals in schools or child care centers, Figure 20–1. This trend will continue and increase in magnitude as more women join the labor force. Economic stress makes it even more difficult for many families to purchase adequate amounts of nutritious food. A number of governmental programs have been developed to provide adequate food for children and to families who lack the money to purchase sufficient nutritious food to feed their children.

CHILD NUTRITION PROGRAMS

Child nutrition programs provide cash and/or food assistance for children in public schools, nonprofit private schools, child care centers, home care day cen-

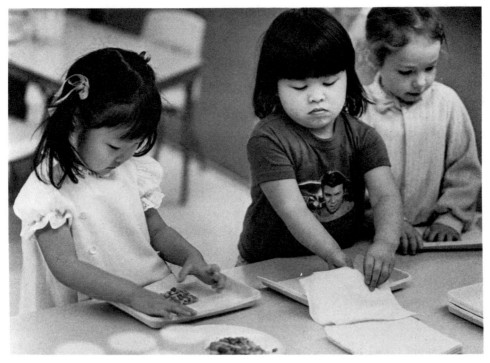

FIGURE 20-1   Many children receive most of their meals in child care centers.

ters, and summer day camps (Egan 1981). When dealing with federal programs, it is important to remember that there is always the prospect of changed funding requirements and/or criteria for benefits. Changes in guidelines and qualifications affect both the funding for food received by many child care centers and care homes, and the families whose children are served by those centers and homes.

National School Lunch Program (NSLP)

The National School Lunch Program is the oldest and largest federal child feeding program in existence, both in terms of number of children reached and dollars spent. The National School Lunch Program is administered at the national level by the United States Department of Agriculture and at the state level by the Department of Education. The U.S. Department of Agriculture reimburses the states for nutritionally adequate lunches served according to federal regulations. The amount of money received per meal depends upon whether the student must receive free meals or is able to pay either full or reduced price. The families of those students receiving free or *reduced price meals* must submit statements of income and meet family size and income guidelines to be eligible. These guidelines are adjusted periodically according to national *poverty guidelines.* Statements of family income must be submitted to the local school district at the beginning of each school year (Dairy Council Digest 1981).

The meal provided daily includes five food components:

- meat or meat alternate, such as peanut butter, eggs or beans
- two or more fruits and/or vegetables
- bread
- milk

The meals must provide at least one-third of the Recommended Daily Dietary Allowances for the age group served. Meal patterns available from the Department of Education and lists of allowed foods within each food group help to ensure that nutritional adequacy is met.

In an effort to reduce the amount of plate waste often found in school lunch programs, many schools are introducing "offer versus serve" in which the child may select as few as three of the five components of the meal. The effect of this practice on nutritional adequacy remains to be determined.

School Breakfast Program (SBP)

The School Breakfast Program was authorized by the Child Nutrition Act of 1966. This program also makes provision for free or reduced price meals along with full price meals. The same income guidelines are used for the School Breakfast Program as for the School Lunch Program. The School Breakfast Program includes schools and public or licensed nonprofit residential child care facilities.

Special Milk Program (SMP)

The Special Milk Program began in 1954. Its original purpose was to encourage the consumption of milk. It has been found to contribute to the nutritional well-being of children since milk provides calcium and good quality protein. The Special Milk Program is limited to schools and institutions which do not participate in other federally-funded meal programs. Schools which charge a yearly tuition of more than $1500 per child are excluded.

Child Care Food Program (CCFP)

The Child Care Food Program provides money for food and commodities for meals served to children in licensed child care centers and group child care homes (Federal Register August 20, 1982). The program is restricted to children 12 years old and under. Exceptions to the age limit are handicapped persons in an institution serving a majority of persons 18 years old and under, and migrant children 15 years old and younger. Infant meal patterns are different, and include infant formula, milk, and other foods.

Reimbursement is for two meals and one snack or one meal and two snacks. Reimbursements are the same as those paid for lunches and breakfasts in the National School Lunch Program and School Breakfast Program respectively. The meal pattern is the same as that required in the National School Lunch Program, adjusted by age in categories of 1–3 years, 3–6 years and 6–12 years of age.

Eligibility Requirements. In order to be eligible for Child Care Food Program assistance, the following requirements must be met.

Program Eligibility

- Centers must provide organized, nonresidential child care.
- Centers must show they are nonprofit (family day care homes may have a *tax-exempt* sponsor in lieu of establishing their own tax-exempt status).
- Centers must have local or state licensing, or official approval as a child care center if required by the state. If unlicensed, they must have met federal interagency day care requirements.

Sponsoring Organization

- assumes responsibility for administration of a center or a number of centers or homes
- responsible for paperwork and all administrative requirements
- assumes financial responsibility
- must have tax-exempt status
- must assure that all programs under its sponsorship meet the licensing or day care standards requirements
- must submit a management plan for review and approval

The following information must be submitted annually by independent centers, or by the sponsoring organization for each center under its sponsorship:

- family size and income data
- application; a separate application must be submitted from each child care center or family day care program sponsored by an organization

Children's Eligibility

- All children in a center approved for the program are eligible.
- Eligibility for free, reduced price, or paid lunches is based on the same family size guidelines used for the National School Lunch Program and the School Breakfast Program.
- Hardship deductions can be taken for extremely high medical, housing and education expenses.
- Family income data must be supplied unless the data is already available through school enrollment. A short family size and income statement is sufficient.

Reimbursement

- Centers must fill out monthly reimbursement claim forms.
- Centers must be reimbursed for meals served no later than 30 days after state receives claim form.
- Centers must receive reimbursement for every meal served, as many days as they are served, for all children served.

- The U.S. Department of Agriculture will reimburse centers for the cost of meal service up to a maximum rate. Included in meal service costs are food, labor and administrative costs.

Summer Food Service Program for Children

The Summer Food Service Program for Children provides free meals and snacks to children in economically depressed areas during the summer months. Eligible sponsors include school food authorities, and state, city or private summer camps. The program is restricted to areas where at least 50 percent of the children meet criteria for free or reduced price meals. Summer camps receive payment only for children who are eligible for free and reduced price meals.

FAMILY NUTRITION PROGRAMS

Two governmental programs that help to provide the family with adequate food are the Special Supplemental Program for Women, Infants and Children, better known as WIC, and the Food Stamp Program.

Special Supplemental Program for Women, Infants and Children (WIC)

The WIC program may be operated by either public or nonprofit health agencies. It provides nutrition counseling and supplemental foods rich in protein, iron and vitamin C to pregnant or *lactating* women, infants, and children up to 5 years of age who are determined to be at risk by professional health assessment. Participants receive specified amounts of the following foods:

- iron-fortified infant formula
- iron-fortified cereal
- fruit/vegetable juices high in vitamin C
- fortified milk
- cheese
- eggs

The Food Stamp Program

The Food Stamp Program may be administered by either state or local welfare agencies. It is the major form of food assistance in the United States. Its purpose is to increase the food purchasing power of low income persons. Those who meet eligibility standards may buy stamps that are worth more than the purchase price. The very poor receive stamps free. Stamps may be used to buy *allowed foods* or seeds from which to grow foods. Items not allowed include soap, cigarettes, paper goods, alcoholic beverages, pet foods or deli foods which may be eaten on the premises (Dairy Council Digest 1981).

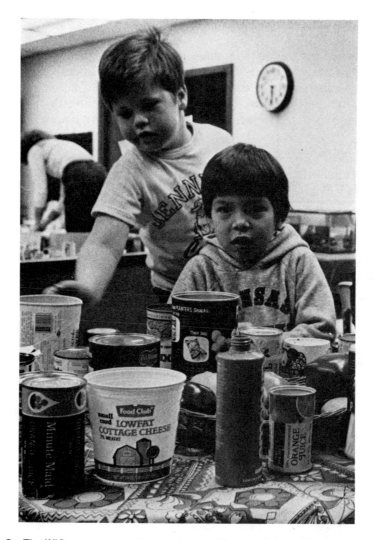

FIGURE 20-2   The WIC program provides supplemental foods rich in protein, iron, and vitamin C.

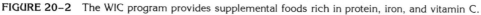

SUMMARY

Nutritional adequacy is recognized as a crucial aspect of child development. During times of economic stress it becomes more difficult to provide enough nutritious food for children. There are several federally-funded programs which provide food assistance for children or their families.

Programs which provide child nutrition assistance are the National School Lunch Program, the School Breakfast Program, Special Milk Program, Summer Food Service Program for Children and the Child Care Food Program. These programs provide funds or food to children through schools, care centers, and camps.

Two programs which provide assistance to families are WIC (Special Supplemental Program for Women, Infants and Children) and the Food Stamp Program. WIC provides specific foods to pregnant or nursing women, infants, and children up to 5 years old. Food Stamps are the major form of food assistance in the United States. Food Stamps are intended to increase the food purchasing power of low income families.

LEARNING ACTIVITIES

1. Contact the food service of the local school district and find out the current family size and income guidelines for eligibility in the school lunch program. Would the two children of a family of four earning $8200 per year be eligible for free, reduced, or full price meals? What is the current rate of reimbursement for each meal served to these children?

2. Consult the *Federal Register* to review the most recent rule changes pertaining to the Child Care Food Program. What changes were made? Did they pertain to funding, eligible foods, or eligibility guidelines? What impact could these changes have on child care centers or care homes?

3. For the following programs, name the agency to contact at the local level:
   a. National School Lunch Program
   b. Child Care Food Program
   c. Special Supplemental Program for Women, Infants and Children (WIC)
   d. Food Stamps

UNIT REVIEW

A. Multiple Choice. Select the best answer.

1. The purpose of federally-funded food programs is to
   a. supplement poverty-level incomes
   b. reduce agricultural surpluses
   c. provide adequate nutrition for children and families
   d. provide nutrition counseling to school-age children

2. Meals supplied through the National School Lunch Program must provide
   a. five food components
   b. at least one-third of the child's daily dietary needs
   c. nutritious foods
   d. all of these

3. Under the Child Care Food Program, child care centers are reimbursed for
   a. two snacks and two meals
   b. two meals and one snack
   c. two snacks and one meal
   d. both b and c

4. Family nutrition programs include
   a. National School Lunch Program
   b. Special Milk Program
   c. Food Stamp Program
   d. all of these

5. To be eligible for Child Care Food Program assistance, the child care center must
   a. be nonprofit
   b. have a local or state license
   c. provide organized, nonresidential child care
   d. all of these

B. Briefly answer the following questions.

   1. Why is nutritional adequacy important in child development?

   2. What limits are placed on the Special Milk Program?

   3. What nutrients does the WIC program focus on providing?

   4. What must a family do to receive free or reduced price meals under the National School Lunch Program?

REFERENCES

"Child Care Food Program. Final Rules." *Federal Register* 47:36524–51, August 20, 1982.
"Child Nutrition Programs." *Dairy Council Digest* 52:1–6, January–February 1981.
Egan, M. C. "Federal Nutrition Support for Children." In *Community Nutrition: People, Policies, and Programs.* Edited by H. S. Wright and L. A. Sims. Monterey, CA: Wadsworth Health Sciences Division, 1981.
Winick, M. "Nutrition and Brain Development." *Natural History,* December 1980.

Additional Reading

Food and Nutrition Service. *Child Care Food Program.* FNS–154. Washington, DC: United States Department of Agriculture, February 1976.
Food and Nutrition Service. *Food Stamp Program.* FNS–118. Washington, DC: United States Department of Agriculture, January 1976.

Food and Nutrition Service. *The National School Lunch Program, Background and Development.* FNS–63. Washington, DC: United States Department of Agriculture, 1971.

"Food and Nutrition." *Newsletter of the Food and Nutrition Service,* March 8, 1976.

Owen, A. L., Owen, G. M., and Lanna, G. "Health and Nutritional Benefits of Federal Food Assistance Programs." In *Community Nutrition: People, Policies, and Programs.* Edited by H. S. Wright and L. A. Sims. Monterey, CA: Wadsworth Health Sciences Division, 1981.

Section

EIGHT

NUTRITION EDUCATION

Unit 21
NUTRITION EDUCATION CONCEPTS AND ACTIVITIES

Terms to Know

nutrition education	objectives
primary goal	evaluation
concepts	harvest
hands-on	pre-plan
attitudes	peer
sensorimotor	serrated

Objectives

After studying this unit, you will be able to:
- Identify the primary goal of nutrition education for preschool children.
- List four basic concepts important to nutrition education.
- List six guidelines for planning nutrition education activities.
- Explain the various roles child care personnel play in nutrition education.
- Name five sources of nutrition information for young children.
- Describe four ways in which nutrition education activities contribute to child development.
- Outline the format used to plan a food experience for young children.
- Describe the general principles of safety that must be observed in planning nutrition education activities for children.
- State the criteria for choosing appropriate nutrition education concepts for young children.

In the simplest of terms, *nutrition education* is any activity which tells a person something about food. These activities may be highly structured, planned activities or very brief, informal happenings. The *primary goal* of nutrition education at the preschool level is to introduce children to some simple basic principles of nutrition and to encourage them to eat and enjoy a variety of nutritious foods.

BASIC CONCEPTS OF NUTRITION EDUCATION

The conceptual framework of any nutrition education program has been outlined by the Interagency Committee on Nutrition Education. It consists of four major *concepts.*

1. Nutrition is the way the body uses food.
   - Food is necessary to live, to grow, to keep healthy and well, and to get energy for work and play.

2. Food is made up of chemical substances called nutrients which are required for health and growth.
   - All nutrients needed by the body are available from food.
   - Nutrients have specific functions.
   - Many kinds and combinations of food can lead to a well-balanced diet.
   - No food by itself has all the nutrients needed for health.
   - Most nutrients work best in combination with other nutrients.

3. All persons throughout life need the same nutrients but in varying amounts.
   - The amounts of nutrients needed are influenced by age, sex, activity and state of health.
   - Suggestions (guidelines) for the kinds and amounts of food (or nutrients) needed are made by trained scientists.

4. The way food is handled influences the amount of nutrients in food, and its safety, appearance, cost and taste.
   - Handling means everything that happens to food while it is being grown, processed, stored and prepared for eating. (Alford and Bogle 1982; Williams 1981).

These conceptual points require that the persons responsible for nutrition education have a basic knowledge of nutrition, in relation to both foods and nutrients.

Many magazine articles and books are available which deal with nutrition. Some are very good, some are very bad, and many fall somewhere in between. The person planning nutrition education must be able to evaluate these resources. A good resource should receive a "yes" to the following questions:

1. Is it from a reliable source?

2. Is it accurate?

3. Is the material at the appropriate level or adaptable?

4. Are the suggested projects nutritious?

5. Are the projects safe?

Beware of some of the so-called "children's" cookbooks which rely on cleverness at the expense of good nutrition and/or safety.

Nutrition knowledge should be combined with a knowledge of educational techniques appropriate for the age group. Food experiences should be planned with consideration for the developmental level of the age group and individual children in the group who will be participating in the activity.

RESPONSIBILITY FOR NUTRITION EDUCATION

All personnel involved in the nutrition program are responsible for nutrition education. Effectiveness of the nutrition education program depends on cooperation between the director, teacher, and cook or food service personnel, Figure 21–1. While programs vary in their organization, these people generally have the responsibility for nutrition education.

The director's role is mainly supportive. The director should stress to the staff the importance of nutritious meals and snacks. The director should see that financial support is available for nutrition education in the curriculum.

The teacher is usually responsible for planning and executing the nutrition education program and for creating a pleasant atmosphere for meals and snacks. For this reason, the preschool teacher should be familiar with the conceptual framework behind nutrition education. The teacher should be aware of the nutritional value of foods and of educational methods and be able to clearly state objectives and realistically evaluate the results of nutrition activities.

The food service personnel are responsible for planning, preparing and serving nutritious, attractive meals. Food service personnel can be a great asset to a

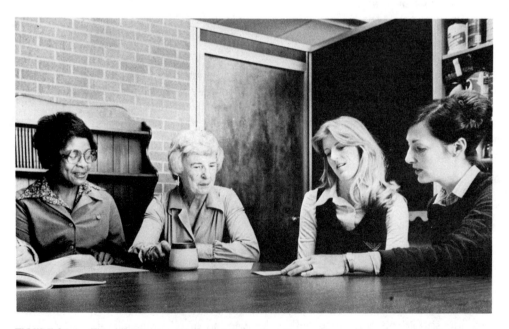

FIGURE 21-1 The effectiveness of the nutrition education program depends on cooperation between the director, teachers and food service personnel.

nutrition education program by including foods in the menu which reinforce what the children have learned from nutrition activities. The cook is a valuable resource person for food preparation methods. Since the cook is also responsible for the kitchen equipment, the cook may determine what is available for use for food preparation experiences.

Parental Involvement in Nutrition Education

Parental involvement is vital to nutrition education. Part of the nutrition program should involve helping parents understand their role in the provision of adequate nutrition for the child and the development of healthful eating habits. Communication between staff and parents is important so that parents may provide additional reinforcement for what has been learned at school.

Parents need to know what steps the staff is taking to meet nutritional responsibility for their children. A simple first step in this direction is posting the menu and serving the menu as it is written. Parents may even be involved in the menu writing process as part of a menu advisory committee. Menu advisory committees serve two purposes:

- the parents have input into the program
- some parents may learn more about good nutritional planning

Copies of the menus with tactful suggestions of general kinds of foods which complete the day nutritionally may be included in newsletters. The newsletter could present nutritional concepts explaining the reasons for the suggested combinations. Family-size recipes for favorite dishes are often appreciated.

Parents are an invaluable resource to the nutrition education program. They can be involved in some nutrition activities by helping to prepare ethnic or traditional foods which are unfamiliar to many of the children in the class.

RATIONALE FOR NUTRITION EDUCATION IN THE EARLY YEARS

There are several reasons for presenting information on nutrition to young children. Simple basic principles of good nutrition and how they relate to health can be effectively taught through nutrition education. Another advantage is that nutrition education activities foster child development in the following areas that relate directly to the preschool curriculum:

- *Promotion of language development*
  Children learn and use food names, food preparation terms, and names of utensils. Children also use language to communicate with their peers and care providers throughout the nutrition activity. A variety of children's literature and music can also be introduced to reinforce both language skills and nutrition concepts, Figure 21–2. (Also see the Appendix.)

Children's Books

Adams, R. *Mr. Picklepaw's Popcorn*. New York: Lothrop, Lee and Shepard Co., 1965.
Aliki. *Green Grass and White Milk*. New York: Thomas Y. Crowell, 1974.
Begley, E. *My Color Game*. Tell-A-Tale Book. Racine, WI: Whitman Publishing Co., 1966.
Benson, H. *Boy the Baker, The Miller and More*. New York: Crown Books, 1975.
Berenstein, J., and Berenstein, S. *The Big Honey Hunt*. Beginner Books. New York: Random House, 1962.
Berenstein, J. *Little Bear's Pancake Party*. New York: Lothrop, Lee and Shepard Co., 1966.
Brown, M. *Stone Soup*. New York: Charles Scribner, 1947.
Buckley, H. *Some Cheese for Charles*. New York: Lothrop, Lee and Shepard Co., 1963.
Buckley, H. *Too Many Crackers*. New York: Lothrop, Lee and Shepard Co., 1966.
Hoben, R. *Bread and Jam for Francis*. New York: Harper and Row, 1964.
Johnson, H. *From Seed to Jack O'Lantern*. New York: Lothrop, Lee and Shepard Co., 1978.
Lenski, L. *Let's Play House*. New York: Henry Z. Walck, Inc., 1944.
Lenski, L. *My Friend the Cow*. Chicago: National Dairy Council, 1975.
LeSieg, T. *Ten Apples Up On Top!* New York: Random House, 1961.
Lionni, L. *Swimmy*. New York: Pantheon Books, 1963.
The Little Red Hen. New York: The Golden Press, 1981.
McCloskey, R. *Blueberries for Sal*. New York: Viking Press, 1966.
Moncure, J. *Magic Monsters Learn About Health*. Chicago: Children's Press, 1980.
———— *The Healthkin Food Train*. Chicago: Children's Press, 1982.
———— *Plants Give Us Many Kinds of Food*. Chicago: Children's Press, 1975.
———— *See My Garden Grow*. Chicago: Children's Press, 1976.
———— *A Tasting Party*. Chicago: Children's Press, 1982.
Pollendorf, Illa. *Food Is for Eating*. New York: Children's Publisher's, 1970.
Potter, B. *The Tale of Peter Rabbit*. London: F. Warne and Co., 1903.
Potter, B. *The Tale of Squirrel Nutkin*. New York: Frederick Warne and Co., 1913.
Sawyer, R. *Journey Cake Ho!* New York: The Viking Press, 1953.
Scott, Elisa. *I See Something Red*. Kansas City, MO: Hallmark, 1970.
Sendak, M. *Chicken Soup With Rice*. New York: Harper and Row, 1962.
Strauss, R. *The Carrot Seed*. New York: Scholastic Book Service, 1971.
Dr. Suess. *Green Eggs and Ham*. New York: Random House, 1960.
Dr. Suess. *One Fish, Two Fish, Red Fish, Blue Fish*. New York: Random House, 1960.
Dr. Suess. *Scrambled Eggs, Super!* New York: Random House, 1953.
Tolstoy, A. *The Great Big Enormous Turnip*. New York: Franklin Watts, Inc., 1968.
Wahl, J. *Cabbage Moon*. New York: Holt, Rinehart and Winston, 1965.
Wilson, G. *Squash Pie*. New York: William Morrow and Co., 1966.
Yezback, S. *Pumpkinseeds*. New York: The Bobbs-Merrill Co., 1969.

Children's Nursery Tales and Rhymes

Here We Go Round The Mulberry Bush
Jack and the Beanstalk
Jack Sprat
Little Miss Muffett
Pease Porridge Hot, Pease Porridge Cold
Peter, Peter, Pumpkin Eater
Polly, Put the Kettle On
Three Billy Goats Gruff
The Gingerbread Boy
The Little Red Hen
The Queen of Hearts
The Three Bears

FIGURE 21-2 Children's literature relating to foods

- *Promotion of cognitive development*
  Children learn to follow step-by-step directions in recipes. Math concepts are learned through activities that involve measurement of food (cups, ounces, teaspoons), counting, and time periods. Science concepts, such as changes in form, are reinforced through activities that involve heating, mixing, cooking, or chilling foods.
- *Promotion of sensorimotor development*
  Hand and finger dexterity are developed through measuring, cutting, mixing, spreading, and serving food. Shapes, textures, and colors are learned through a variety of foods.
- *Promotion of social/emotional development*
  Through nutrition activities, children learn to work as part of a team in either large or small groups. Their knowledge and acceptance of cultural differences may also be enhanced through food activities that feature ethnic foods. In addition, children gain a more positive self-concept when they master such skills as pouring juice into a glass for themselves.

Figure 21–3 illustrates the potential contribution of food experiences to the early childhood curriculum.

PLANNING A NUTRITION EDUCATION PROGRAM

The nutrition education program should consist of well-planned activities which lead to specific outcomes. (A list of resources for children's activities involving nutrition education is given in Figure 21–4.) The desired outcome behaviors are the objectives of the program.

The overall program should be planned around some or all of the four basic nutrition education concepts. Concepts should be chosen which are appropriate for the children in the group according to their age and developmental level.

Nutrition education activities for preschool children should be based primarily on concepts #1 and #4. Young children have the ability to comprehend that food is good. They can benefit from an introduction to a variety of nutritious foods. Older children can begin to understand the concept of food groups based on similar nutrient contributions.

The preschool nutrition program is the ideal place to increase familiarity with a variety of new foods. It is also an effective tool for showing children that common foods may be prepared in a number of ways. The 3 year old, for instance, may not yet realize that a head of lettuce, a leaf of lettuce on a sandwich, and torn lettuce in a salad are all the same food. (Tasting parties are easy ways to introduce new foods, or different forms of the same food.)

Nutrition education activities should be part of a coordinated program designed to explore each of the concepts chosen. They should be planned to meet specified goals rather than simply serving as a means of filling time or keeping the children busy.

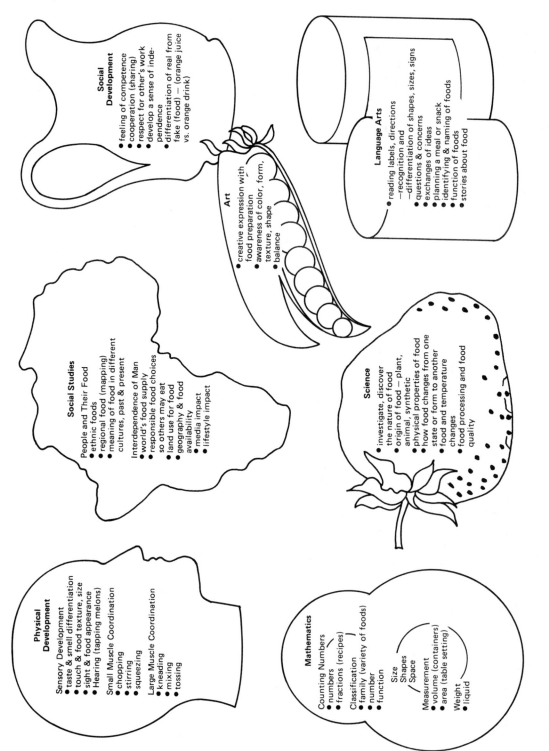

Social Development
- feeling of competence
- cooperation (sharing)
- respect for other's work
- develop a sense of independence
- differentiation of real from fake (food) — (orange juice vs. orange drink)

Art
- creative expression with food preparation
- awareness of color, form, texture, shape
- balance

Language Arts
- reading labels, directions
  —recognition and
  —differentiation of shapes, sizes, signs
- exchanges of ideas
- questions & concerns
- planning a meal or snack
- identifying & naming of foods
- function of foods
- stories about food

Social Studies

People and Their Food
- ethnic foods
- regional food (mapping)
- meaning of food in different cultures, past & present

Interdependence of Man
- world's food supply
- responsible food choices so others may eat
- land use for food
- geography & food availability
- media impact
- lifestyle impact

Science
- investigate, discover the nature of food
- origin of food — plant, animal, synthetic
- physical properties of food
- how food changes from one state or form to another
- food and temperature changes
- food processing and food quality

Physical Development

Sensory Development
- taste & smell differentiation
- touch & food texture, size
- sight & food appearance
- Hearing (tapping melons)

Small Muscle Coordination
- chopping
- stirring
- squeezing

Large Muscle Coordination
- kneading
- mixing
- tossing

Mathematics

Counting Numbers
- numbers
- fractions (recipes)

Classification
- family (variety of foods)
- number
- function

Size
Shapes
Space

Measurement
- volume (containers)
- area (table setting)

Weight
- liquid

FIGURE 21-3 Potential contribution of food experiences to early childhood curriculum. All learning takes place through the senses. Since food appeals to all senses it is a powerful learning tool. (Reprinted from *Creative Food Experiences for Children* which is available from the Center for Science in the Public Interest, 1501 Sixteenth Street, N.W., Washington, DC 20036, for $5.95, copyright 1980.)

Carle, E. *The Very Hungry Caterpillar.* Cleveland, OH: Williams Collins and World Publishing Company, Inc., not dated.

Fraser, J., Farkas, J., and Stimmel, D. *Child Center Nutrition Handbook.* Cleveland, OH: Cleveland State University, 1980.

Food Is Good, Books I–VI. Yakima, WA: The Yakima Home Economics Association, 1973–1981.

Fun With Foods Coloring Book. Denver, CO: American School Food Service Association, 1970.

Naworski, P. *Let's Taste Fruits and Vegetables.* Vallejo, CA: Vallejo Unified School District, 1978.

Palmer, M., and Edmonds, A. *Vegetable Magic: A Preschool and Nutrition Education Source Book.* Storrs, CT: CNETP Publications, Department of Nutritional Sciences, University of Connecticut, 1981.

Spencer, E., and Campbell, J. *Picture Recipes for Beginning Cooks.* Baltimore, MD: Preventive Medicine Administration, Department of Health and Mental Hygiene, not dated.

The Thing the Professor Forgot. Nutrition Department, General Mills, Inc., not dated.

Wanamaker, N., Hearn, K., and Richard, S. *More Than Graham Crackers: Nutrition Education and Food Preparation With Young Children.* Washington, DC: National Association for the Education of Young Children, 1979.

Wilms, B. *Crunchy Bananas—And Other Great Recipes Kids Can Cook.* Salt Lake City, UT: Sagamore Books, 1975.

FIGURE 21-4   Resources for children's activities involving food.

The results of the program should be measurable in order to determine its effectiveness. Results may be evaluated by determining whether any of the desired behaviors outlined in the objectives are observed. Figures 21–5 and 21–6 give examples of how a nutrition concept can be outlined and incorporated into learning experiences for young children.

It should be remembered that setting goals does not imply that the activity should be rigidly imposed, or that the exact activities and discussion topics that are listed in the outline and lesson plans should be followed without deviation. Rather, as in any other curricular activity, the interests of the children and their optimal development, should be the governing factors for planning and extending learning activities.

GUIDELINES FOR NUTRITION EDUCATION ACTIVITIES

1. Nutrition activities should be suitable for the developmental level of the participating children. **Caution:** Special consideration should be given to the chewing ability of the children involved, especially when raw fruits and vegetables are to be used in the food activity.

2. With consideration to food safety, funds, equipment available, and any known food allergies, actual foods should be used in nutrition projects as often as possible. These may be accompanied by pictures, games, and

CONCEPT: NUTRITION IS THE WAY THE BODY USES FOOD
OBJECTIVES: The children should learn that
- all living things need food
- food is important for growth and for good health

SUGGESTED ACTIVITIES:
- Caring for animals in the classroom with special attention to their diets.
- Taking field trips to the zoo or farm to learn what animals eat.
- Caring for plants in the classroom.
- Planting a vegetable garden in containers or a small plot of ground.
- Weighing and measuring the children periodically.
- Tracing outlines of each child on large sheets of paper.

QUESTIONS FOR EXTENDING LEARNING EXPERIENCES:
- What do animals eat?
- Do all animals eat the same foods?
- Do animals eat the same foods as people?
- Do animals grow faster or slower than people?
- What do plants eat?
- Can people see plants eating?
- Do plants eat the same foods as people?
- What does it mean to be healthy?
- Do people need food to be healthy?
- Do children need food to grow?

EVALUATION:
- Children can name what animals and plants eat.
- Children can describe some effects of not feeding plants and animals.

FIGURE 21-5   Sample outline for incorporating nutrition education concept #1 into learning experiences for the young child.

stories to reinforce what is learned in real food activities. **Caution:** The care provider should always check for allergies to any foods (or similar foods) introduced in the nutrition activity.

3. The foods used should be nutritious. Nutrient-density (INQ) is one means of determining if a food is nutritious. Foods from the Basic Four Food Groups are nutritious. Foods from the Other Food Group usually are not nutritious. Cakes, pies, and cookies, although made from grain products, are high in added sugars and fats and should be considered very carefully before inclusion in a nutrition project.

4. The end products of a nutrition activity should be edible and should be eaten by the children. Pasta collages and chocolate pudding finger paintings are not suitable nutrition projects since it is not possible to eat the end product.

5. The children should be involved in the actual food preparation. Hands-on experiences such as cleaning vegetables, rolling dough, spreading butter,

CONCEPT: FOOD HANDLING INFLUENCES NUTRIENTS IN FOODS
OBJECTIVES: Children should understand
  • where foods come from
  • how foods are handled

SUGGESTED ACTIVITIES:
  • Grow, *harvest* and prepare foods from a garden.
  • Sprout alfalfa, radishes, or bean seeds.
  • Discuss and illustrate the different parts of plants used as food (leaves, roots, fruits, seeds).
  • Conduct simple experiments that show change in color or form of food.
  • Play "store" or "farm".
  • Take children on a field trip to a farm, dairy, bakery, or grocery store.

QUESTIONS FOR EXTENDING LEARNING EXPERIENCES:
  • From where does food come?
  • Where do grocery stores get food?
  • Is food always eaten the way it is grown?
  • Who prepares different foods?
  • Does all food come from the store?

EVALUATION:
  • Children can name sources of specific foods.
  • Children can name who handles such foods as bread, milk, etc.

FIGURE 21-6   Sample outline for incorporating nutrition education concept #4 into learning experiences for the young child.

and cutting biscuits increase learning and help to develop a child's positive feelings about food, Figure 21–7. These activities not only enhance food experiences, but aid in the development of other skills such as manual dexterity, counting, or learning to follow directions. Children will often accept new, unfamiliar foods more readily if they have helped in its preparation.

6. Once the nutrition activity is completed, the food should be eaten within a short period of time, Figure 21–8. Delays between the completion of the activity and use of the food lessen the impact of the activity.

SAFETY CONSIDERATIONS

Attention to the following points can contribute to the increased success and safety of all food experiences.

Basic Guidelines

  • Be aware of all food allergies identified in children. Post a list of the names of these children, along with the foods they cannot eat. Some of the more

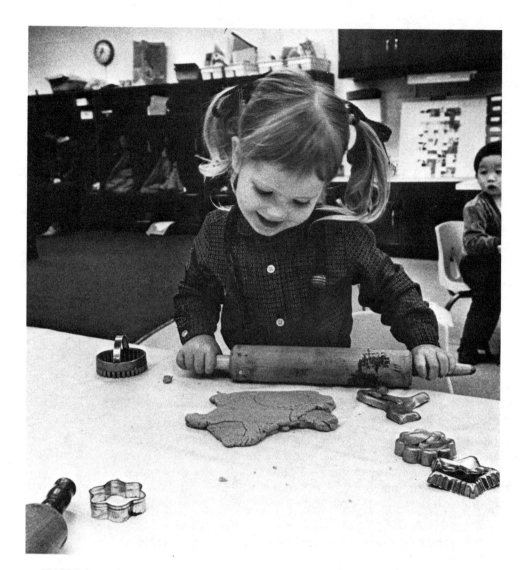

FIGURE 21-7   Hands-on experiences foster the development of positive feelings about food.

common foods to which children may be allergic are: wheat; milk and milk products; juices such as orange or grapefruit juice which have a high acid content; chocolate; eggs; and nuts.

- Avoid serving foods such as nuts, raw vegetables and popcorn which could cause young children to choke.
- Children should always sit down to eat.
- Use low work tables and chairs.
- Use unbreakable equipment whenever possible.
- Supply enough tools and utensils for all of the children in the group.

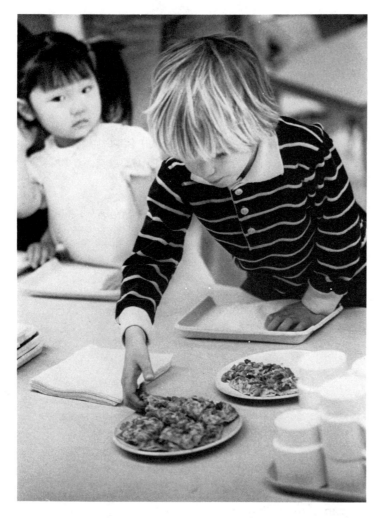

FIGURE 21-8 Foods prepared during nutrition activities should be eaten within a short period of time after the activity is completed.

- Use blunt knives or *serrated* plastic knives for cutting cooked eggs, potatoes, bananas, etc. Vegetable peelers should be used only under supervision and only after demonstrating their proper use to the children.
- Have only the necessary tools, utensils, and ingredients at the work table. All other materials should be removed as soon as they are no longer needed. Plan equipment needs carefully to avoid having to leave the work area during the activity.
- *Preplan* the steps of the cooking project; discuss these steps with the children before beginning. Children should understand what they are expected to do and what the adults will do before the cooking materials are made available to them.

- Long hair should be pulled back and fastened; floppy or cumbersome clothing should not be worn. Aprons are not essential, but may be helpful.
- Wash hands before beginning the activity.
- Begin with simple recipes that require little cooking. Once the children feel comfortable with those cooking projects, move on to slightly more complex ones.
- Allow plenty of time for touching, tasting, looking, and comparing, as well as for discussion. Use every step in the cooking project as an opportunity to expand the learning experience for the children.

Food Safety

- Wash hands before and after cooking project; this applies to care providers as well as children.
- Children and adults with colds should not help with food preparation.
- Keep all cooking utensils clean. Have extra utensils available in case one is dropped or is put into a child's mouth.
- Teach children how to taste foods that are being prepared. Give each child a small plate and spoon to use. Never let the children taste foods directly from the bowl or pan in which the foods are being prepared.
- Avoid using foods that spoil rapidly. Keep sauces, meats, and dairy products refrigerated.

Cooking Safety

- Match the task to the children's developmental levels and attention spans.
- Instruct children carefully regarding the use of utensils.
- Emphasize that all cooking must be supervised by an adult.
- Adults should do the cooking over stove burners. Pot handles should always be turned away from the edge of the stove.
- Use wooden utensils or utensils with wooden handles for cooking. (Metal utensils conduct heat and can cause painful burns.)

DEVELOPING LESSON PLANS FOR NUTRITION ACTIVITIES

Each food activity should be planned as a part of an overall nutrition program; it should also be fun for the children. The success of these activities may be facilitated by the development of a lesson plan for each. The following are some of the points which should be considered (Gahagan, not dated):

- Title (or Subject)
  Nutrition projects should always involve food of high nutrient density.
- Length of Time Required
  This should be both approximate and flexible. If an activity is enthusiastically received, it should be continued for additional time.

- Type of Group

  Is this activity to be done with the entire group, two or three children, or on a one-to-one basis with only one child? To what number of children is this activity most readily applied? Is there enough equipment for all children of a large group to have their own utensils?

- Nutritional Concepts To Be Reinforced

  What concepts have been chosen as the basis for your nutrition program?

- Objectives of Activity

  What concepts or behaviors should children learn from this project? Are they learning to eat a new food? Are they learning different ways of fixing a familiar food? What developmental areas are enhanced by the activity? Sensorimotor skills? Cognitive skills such as the learning of math or science concepts? Language or social skills? Does the activity develop their creativity?

- Motor Skills/Sensory Experiences/Developmental Areas

  What types of activities will be done while preparing the food? What senses do the foods used appeal to? What kinds of math concepts, social learning, language skills, science facts can be introduced with this food activity?

- Materials/Equipment

  What ingredients are needed? What equipment and utensils are needed to complete the activity? Do the children require instruction in the use of the equipment?

- Setting for Activity

  Where will preparation and the actual activity take place? Is the equipment well-suited for this setting? What safety procedures are necessary? (These should be listed in detail.) For instance, if an electric skillet is to be used, is the cord placed so that children will not trip over it? Are knives to be used, and if so, do the children need special instructions or reminders as to how to use them? How much time will be needed to complete the activity? To clean up?

- Pre-lesson Preparation Needed

  Does the activity require any advanced preparation? Is peeling, chopping, soaking, or other preparation necessary? If so, who does it?

- Procedure

  All recipes and directions should be carefully read and each step thought out clearly. A detailed plan should then be developed for giving appropriate instructions to the children.

- Cautions

  Do the children need instruction in the appropriate use of knives? Will heat be used in the preparation of the food? Is the food featured in the activity one that is likely to cause allergic reactions? Is the food in a form which might possibly cause choking?

- Discussion Questions

  What questions could be asked to further extend learning about this food or any of the related concepts?

FOOD ACTIVITY (TITLE):_____

DATE:_____LENGTH OF TIME REQUIRED:_____

TYPE OF GROUP: Individual_____   Small_____   Large_____

NUTRITIONAL CONCEPTS TO BE REINFORCED:

    Nutrition is how the body uses food._____

    Many kinds of food contribute to a balanced diet._____

    Food must be safe to be healthful._____

    Food handling influences the nutrients in food._____

OBJECTIVES OF ACTIVITY (Reasons for choosing activity):

    1.   3.
    2.   4.

Motor Skills Involved:	mixing	dipping	pouring
	beating	peeling	spreading
	grinding	measuring	cutting
	grating	rolling	other_____

Sensory Experiences:	smelling	feeling	tasting
	seeing	hearing	

    Related Concepts/Developmental Areas

MATERIALS/EQUIPMENT:

    1.   5.
    2.   6.
    3.   7.
    4.   8.

SETTING FOR ACTIVITY:

PRE-LESSON PREPARATION NEEDED: _____yes   _____no
    Describe.

PROCEDURE (step-by-step):

    1.   6.
    2.   7.
    3.   8.
    4.   9.
    5.   10.

CAUTIONS:

DISCUSSION QUESTIONS/OPPORTUNITIES FOR EXTENDING LEARNING EXPERIENCE:

EVALUATION AND COMMENTS:

SUGGESTIONS FOR FOLLOW-UP ACTIVITIES:

FIGURE 21-9   Nutrition education lesson planning form

- Evaluation and Comments
  Did the children eat a new food? Do they recognize that foods may be prepared in different ways? Did they become more skilled in peeling, chopping, etc? Did the children learn any new words? Did they use these new terms correctly? In what other ways were their developmental skills enhanced? Were they cooperative and friendly to their peers while working in the group? Did they learn any multicultural concepts through the activity? Is there any carry-over of learned behaviors to other activities?
- Suggestions for Follow-up Activities
  What further activities does this activity suggest?

The lesson plan form depicted in Figure 21–9 serves as a checklist and outline for developing and implementing nutrition education activities. Following are sample lesson plans related to nutrition which may be incorporated into the preschool curriculum. Additional nutrition activities may be found in the Appendix.

Lesson Plan #1 Weighing and Measuring Children

FOOD ACTIVITY (TITLE): Weighing and Measuring Children

DATE:_____ LENGTH OF TIME REQUIRED: 10–15 minutes

TYPE OF GROUP: Individual_____ Small___x___ Large_____

NUTRITIONAL CONCEPTS TO BE REINFORCED:

Nutrition is how the body uses food.___x___

Many kinds of food contribute to a balanced diet._____

Food must be safe to be healthful._____

Food handling influences the nutrients in food._____

OBJECTIVES OF ACTIVITY (Reasons for choosing activity):

1. Children learn that their growth depends on food.
2. Children learn that growth may be measured by (1) height and (2) weight.

Motor Skills Involved:	mixing	dipping	pouring
	beating	peeling	spreading
	grinding	(measuring)	cutting
	grating	rolling	other_____
Sensory Experiences:	smelling	feeling	tasting
	(seeing)	hearing	

Related Concepts/Developmental Areas: Math: numbers on scale, units of measure (pounds, inches). Language: comparisons of size. Social skills: acceptance of individual differences.

MATERIALS/EQUIPMENT:

1. Balance-beam scale or bathroom scale
2. Yardstick
3. Sheets of paper

SETTING FOR ACTIVITY: Classroom or child care center

PRE-LESSON PREPARATION NEEDED: _____yes ___x___no

Describe.

PROCEDURE (step-by-step):

1. Help each child onto scale.
2. Help child read his/her weight.
3. Measure height.
4. Help child read his/her height.
5. Record height.
6. Record weight.

CAUTIONS:

DISCUSSION QUESTIONS/OPPORTUNITIES FOR EXTENDING
LEARNING EXPERIENCE:

Does everybody weigh the same?
Is everyone the same height?
Do children stay the same size? Do adults?
What makes children grow?
Name some foods that help children grow?

EVALUATION AND COMMENTS:

Each child can tell the care provider his/her height and weight.
Children can name foods which contribute to health and growth.

SUGGESTIONS FOR FOLLOW-UP ACTIVITIES:

Trace outline of each child on large sheets of paper.
Repeat this activity periodically to monitor each child's rate of growth.
Discuss individual differences between children, such as concepts of
  tall and short.
(The discussion should be positive—these differences are what make
  each child special.)

Lesson Plan #2 Making Indian Fried Bread

FOOD ACTIVITY (TITLE): Indian Fried Bread

DATE:_____ LENGTH OF TIME
REQUIRED: 20 minutes contact time; 1 hour between kneading and
cooking

TYPE OF GROUP: Individual_____ Small___x___ Large_____

NUTRITIONAL CONCEPTS TO BE REINFORCED:

Nutrition is how the body uses food._____

Many kinds of food contribute to a balanced diet.___x___

Food must be safe to be healthful._____

Food handling influences the nutrients in food._____

OBJECTIVES OF ACTIVITY (Reasons for choosing activity):

1. To introduce foods from another culture.
2. To provide tactile sensations from kneading dough.

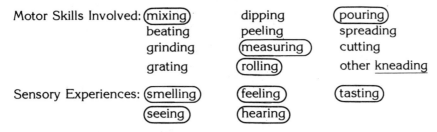

Motor Skills Involved: (mixing)   dipping   (pouring)
   beating   peeling   spreading
   grinding   (measuring)   cutting
   grating   (rolling)   other kneading

Sensory Experiences: (smelling)   (feeling)   (tasting)
   (seeing)   (hearing)

Related Concepts/Developmental Areas: Science: melting butter,
browning bread, addition of water to dough. Language: discussion of
American Indian heritage. Social skills: learning safe cooking procedures.

MATERIALS/EQUIPMENT:

1. Electric skillet
2. Bowl
3. Spoon
4. Measuring cups
5. Measuring spoons

6. Recipe:
   2 c. whole wheat flour
   2 c. unbleached white flour
   1 tsp. salt
   3 Tbsp. corn oil
   Water to make soft dough
   (See picture recipe attached.)

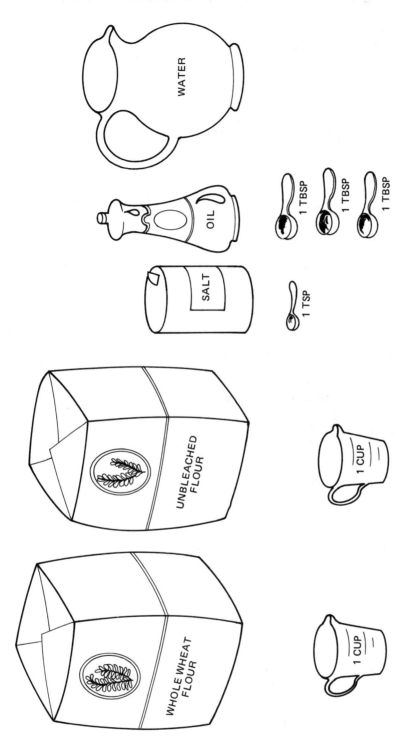

FIGURE 21-10   Picture recipe for Indian fried bread.

SETTING FOR ACTIVITY:

Kitchen (or use electric skillet in the classroom)

PRE-LESSON PREPARATION NEEDED: ___x___yes _____no

Describe. Gather equipment as listed.

PROCEDURE (step-by-step):

1. Wash hands.
2. Mix together and knead dough 5–10 minutes.
3. Put dough in bowl, cover with cloth.
4. Let dough stand for 1 hour.
5. Shape dough into balls the size of a marble and roll and pat them flat.
6. Melt butter in pan.
7. Fry 3–4 pieces of dough at one time.
8. Serve bread warm with butter, jelly, or honey.

CAUTIONS:

Adults must cook the bread.
Table with electric skillet should be against the wall.

DISCUSSION QUESTIONS/OPPORTUNITIES FOR EXTENDING LEARNING EXPERIENCE:

Is this bread like the bread you have at home? Can you describe the bread you usually eat? How did the early Indians make their bread?

EVALUATION AND COMMENTS:

Children's social skills were further developed by working together to make the bread.
The children experienced the feel of dough by kneading it.
Kneading helped to develop motor skills.
Children learned about American Indian food customs.
Children tasted a new food from another culture.

SUGGESTIONS FOR FOLLOW-UP ACTIVITIES:

Have children make another type of bread, e.g., corn pone.

Lesson Plan #3 Tasting Party

FOOD ACTIVITY (TITLE): <u>Tasting Party for Dairy Foods</u>

DATE:_____ LENGTH OF TIME REQUIRED: <u>10–15 minutes</u>

TYPE OF GROUP: Individual_____ Small_____ Large___x___

NUTRITIONAL CONCEPTS TO BE REINFORCED:

Nutrition is how the body uses food._____

Many kinds of food contribute to a balanced diet.____x____

Food must be safe to be healthful.____x____

Food handling influences the nutrients in food.____x____

OBJECTIVES OF ACTIVITY (Reasons for choosing activity):

1. Children learn that common foods may be served in a variety of ways.
2. Children learn to recognize foods that belong to the dairy group.

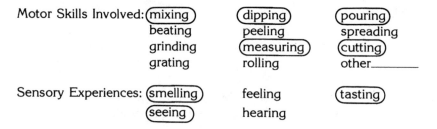

Motor Skills Involved: (mixing)   (dipping)   (pouring)
     beating   peeling   spreading
     grinding   (measuring)   (cutting)
     grating   rolling   other_____

Sensory Experiences: (smelling)   feeling   (tasting)
    (seeing)   hearing

Related Concepts/Developmental Areas: Social skills: task delegation, cooperation. Cognitive skills: classify foods as part of dairy group even though they look different than milk. Science: changes which took place to make cheese, yogurt, etc.

MATERIALS/EQUIPMENT:

1. Pitcher of milk
2. Yogurt, plain
3. Cottage cheese
4. Cheddar cheese
5. Bowl of apple chunks
6. Small bowl of granola
7. Orange juice concentrate
8. Cutting board
9. Bowls
10. Spoons
11. Cups
12. Blender

SETTING FOR ACTIVITY: Classroom or child care center

PRE-LESSON PREPARATION NEEDED: ___x___yes _____no

Describe. Assemble necessary equipment and materials.

PROCEDURE (step-by-step):

1. Wash hands.
2. Blend part of cottage cheese with orange juice, using blender. Leave remainder as is.
3. Spoon yogurt into bowl.
4. Cut cheddar cheese into cubes.
5. Wash tables.
6. Wash hands.
7. Place all foods on table.
8. Taste small servings of each food.

CAUTIONS:

Instruct and demonstrate safe use of knife and blender.
Check for milk or dairy product allergies of any children in group.
Stress that refrigeration and sanitation are very important when working with protein foods, such as milk and milk products.

DISCUSSION QUESTIONS/OPPORTUNITIES FOR EXTENDING LEARNING EXPERIENCE:

Are all these foods made from milk?
Do they look alike?
Do they taste alike?
Is cottage cheese like cheddar cheese? How is it different?
Why were these foods chilled before preparation and why should they be eaten immediately?

EVALUATION AND COMMENTS:

Children can identify foods made from milk.
Children will taste each food served.
Children help with cleaning the tables.

SUGGESTIONS FOR FOLLOW-UP ACTIVITIES

Make yogurt or cheese from milk.
Mix fruit with yogurt and discuss fruit and milk as "healthful" foods.

Lesson Plan #4 Trip to the Grocery Store

FOOD ACTIVITY (TITLE): Trip to the Grocery Store

DATE:_____ LENGTH OF TIME REQUIRED: varies

TYPE OF GROUP: Individual___x___ Small___x___ Large_____

NUTRITIONAL CONCEPTS TO BE REINFORCED:

Nutrition is how the body uses food._____

Many kinds of food contribute to a balanced diet.___x___

Food must be safe to be healthful._____

Food handling influences the nutrients in food.___x___

OBJECTIVES OF ACTIVITY (Reasons for choosing activity):

1. Children are encouraged to make decisions about foods and to taste a variety of foods.
2. Children buy a food with which they are not familiar.

Motor Skills Involved:

mixing	dipping	pouring
beating	peeling	spreading
grinding	measuring	cutting
grating	rolling	other_____

Sensory Experiences: (smelling) (feeling) tasting
(seeing) hearing

Related Concepts/Developmental Areas: Language: names of foods on list, color/shape/size concepts. Cognitive skills: classification (food sections in the store). Math: paying for food, number concepts (pick 2 red fruits). Social skills: working as a team to complete a task, interacting with grocers/clerks.

MATERIALS/EQUIPMENT:

1. Shopping list

SETTING FOR ACTIVITY: Grocery store, child care center

PRE-LESSON PREPARATION NEEDED: ___x___ yes _____no

Describe. Secure parental permission for field trip; make up grocery list.

PROCEDURE (step-by-step):

1. Select 1 to 3 children.
2. Travel to store.
3. Find produce section.
4. Find fruits.
5. Find red fruits.
6. Select 2 varieties of red fruit.
7. Count the number of each fruit needed.

8. Purchase fruit.

9. Return to child care center.

10. Ask cook to prepare fruit for snack or meal.

CAUTIONS:

Permission must be obtained from parents for field trip.
Fasten restraints if driving to store.
If walking to store, review safety rules for walking, crossing streets, etc.

DISCUSSION QUESTIONS/OPPORTUNITIES FOR EXTENDING
LEARNING EXPERIENCE:

What will this fruit taste like?
What is the name of this food?
How does this fruit grow?
Is the skin peeled or eaten?
Will this fruit have seeds?
What ways can this fruit be prepared?

EVALUATION AND COMMENTS:

Children are able to identify two varieties of red fruit.
Children eat and enjoy the prepared fruit.

SUGGESTIONS FOR FOLLOW-UP ACTIVITIES:

Children play "store" with some children acting as grocers, some acting as clerks, and some acting as shoppers. Have children select two
types of green vegetables.

OTHER SOURCES OF INFORMATION ABOUT FOOD

Children learn about food from informal sources as well as from planned
programs of instruction. The family, care providers, other children, and television
are additional sources of information about food and all have an effect on children's eating habits.

The Family

Food preferences and *attitudes* of the family unit are of primary importance
in the formation of the young child's attitudes about and preferences for food.
Family food choices are subject to cultural influences, money available for food,
educational level, and specific preferences of family members. Since familiarity
with a food is often a factor in choices, the child who comes from a family which
eats a wide variety of foods is more willing to try new foods, because that is
acceptable behavior in the home.

Care Providers

Care providers exert considerable influence over children's attitudes about food. For this reason the care provider should display positive attitudes about food and demonstrate both with actions and words enjoyment of food and enthusiasm for trying new foods.

Other Children

Young children's choices of food are frequently made on the basis of approval or disapproval of others within their group. A child with a strong personality who eats a variety of foods can be a positive influence on other children. On the other hand, children who are "picky eaters" can also spread their negative influence. A simple statement from the care provider, such as, "You don't have to eat the broccoli, Jamie, but I can't allow you to spoil it for Tara and Pablo," should be effective in curbing this negative influence. Younger children may base their choices on familiarity of food and its taste. Older children (5–6) are more subject to *peer* influence when deciding whether or not to eat a food.

Television

A major source of many children's information about food is television advertising. Television programs directed toward children are usually sponsored by fast food chains or by companies which make candies, gum, soft drinks, snack items, and sugared cereals. Commercials typically tell the child that these products "taste good" or are "fun." Nutrient-dense foods are less frequently advertised during programs produced for children (Gussow 1972). Both parents and care providers can help counteract the influence of television by monitoring the programs viewed and by discussing with their children the difference between programs and commercials and emphasizing that the purpose of commercials is to sell a product.

SUMMARY

Nutrition education is any activity which tells a person something about food. The basic concepts of nutrition education are (1) nutrition is the way the body uses food, (2) food is made up of chemical substances called nutrients, (3) all persons throughout life need the same nutrients but in varying amounts, and (4) the way food is handled influences the amount of nutrients in food, its safety, appearance, cost and taste.

The responsibility for teaching young children about nutrition rests with each member of the staff in an early childhood program, as well as with the parents of the children. Nutrition education in the early years should be based on some or all of the basic nutritional concepts and should promote children's skills in all developmental areas.

Nutrition education activities should be geared to the age and developmental level of the children within the group; nutrition activities should allow specific measurable goals to be attained. The primary goal of nutrition education in the early years is to teach children some simple basic principles of nutrition and to encourage them to eat and enjoy a variety of nutritious foods. The foods used in nutrition experiences should be nutritious, and the end product of a project should be edible. It is advisable to use actual foods whenever possible; however, books, games and puppets are good reinforcing materials.

Hands-on food experiences can effectively teach children basic principles of good nutrition and how these principles relate to health. Food experiences also promote language, cognitive, sensorimotor, and social/emotional development.

In planning nutrition activities for young children, safety factors must also be carefully considered. Lesson plans may be helpful, especially to a beginning teacher. Careful planning involved in developing lesson plans contributes to the success of the activity.

Care providers should also be aware of the other sources from which children receive information about nutrition—family members, peers, television. They should strive to reinforce the positive nutritional concepts presented by these sources and to counter any misinformation provided or implied by other sources.

LEARNING ACTIVITIES

1. Prepare lesson plans for a two-day nutrition education activity. Plans may be for two consecutive days or for any two days within one week. The lesson plan for each day should be in the format presented in this unit.

2. From the following list, choose three foods as the subjects of food experiences. Upon what criteria were the choices based? What was the primary basis for the decision to work with each food? What other considerations affected the choice of some foods and not others?
   a. raisin-oatmeal cookies
   b. granola
   c. brownies
   d. honey
   e. greens (lettuce, spinach) for salad
   f. pancakes

3. Outline an equipment list and safety plan for a food experience in which 4 and 5 year olds make pancakes in the classroom. Cooking will be done in an electric skillet on a table. What precautions should be taken? How should the room be safely arranged? What instructions should be given to the children?

4. Select 15–20 library books appropriate for young children. Note those instances where food is portrayed either in the story or pictures. What types

of foods are shown? Chart these foods according to the Basic Four Food Groups and the Other Foods Group, which includes foods high in sugar and calories. What percentage of foods were noted within each group? What was the general message about food presented in these books?

5. Watch one hour of children's television programs on Saturday morning.
   a. Determine the percent of observed advertisements that were for "sweets" (gum, candy, soft drinks, snack cakes and pre-sweetened cereals).
   b. Which Food Groups were least represented in these commercials?
   c. Discuss with your classmates the possible consequences of food and beverage advertisements on children's food preferences.

6. Review an article about nutrition from a popular magazine. Apply the suggested criteria for a good nutrition resource. Is this a good article? Why or why not?

UNIT REVIEW

A. Multiple Choice. Select the best answer.

1. One basic concept upon which nutrition education is based is
   a. the amounts of nutrients needed by a child are the same as needed by adults
   b. the way food is handled does not influence the amount of nutrients in food
   c. nutrition is the way the body uses the nutrients in food
   d. some foods contain all the nutrients needed for health

2. The *primary* goal of preschool nutrition education is that children learn
   a. the Basic Four Food Groups
   b. to choose a variety of nutritious foods
   c. to identify nutrients in foods
   d. various ways that food is processed

3. Objectives are behaviors the children
   a. already know before the activity
   b. should learn from the activity
   c. both a and b
   d. none of the above

4. An activity that illustrates that all living things need food is
   a. growing plants in the classroom
   b. caring for animals
   c. weighing and measuring children
   d. all of these

5. Important safety concepts for children to learn include
   a. all cooking must be supervised by an adult
   b. hands must be washed before eating
   c. all cooking utensils must be kept clean
   d. all of these

6. Effectiveness of a nutrition education activity can be assessed by
   a. lesson plans
   b. activities
   c. evaluation
   d. basic guidelines

7. Nutrition education activities can be a method of teaching
   a. math concepts
   b. team work
   c. basic nutrition
   d. all of these

8. Important sources of nutrition information for children are
   a. nutrition activities
   b. television
   c. parents and teachers
   d. all of these

9. Which of the following would be the best nutrition education project?
   a. Construction of a carrot puppet.
   b. A trip to the store on Monday to buy food for Thursday lunch.
   c. Stuffing celery with peanut butter for snacks served later that day.
   d. Necklaces made from macaroni.

10. Appropriate foods to use for a nutrition education activity include
    a. apples and oranges
    b. brownies
    c. frosted sugar cookies
    d. uncooked macaroni

B. Briefly answer the following questions.

1. List six guidelines for planning nutrition education activities.

2. What is the teacher's role in providing nutrition education activities for the young child?

3. List four ways that nutrition education activities aid child development.

4. What is the criteria used for choosing appropriate nutrition education concepts for young children?

REFERENCES

Alford, B. B., and Bogle, M. L. *Nutrition During the Life Cycle.* Englewood Cliffs, NJ: Prentice-Hall, Inc., 1982.

Birch, L. L. "Dimensions of Preschool Children's Food Preferences." *Journal of Nutrition Education* 11:77, November 1979.

Gahagan, G. *East Central Kansas Community Action Program Head Start Comprehensive Nutrition Education Program.* Ottawa, KS: CCFP Nutrition Education and Training Project, not dated.

Gussow, J. "Counternutritional Messages of TV Ads Aimed at Children." *Journal of Nutrition Education,* Spring 1972.

Williams, S. R. *Nutrition and Diet Therapy.* St. Louis: The C.V. Mosby Company, 1981.

Additional Reading

Baker, M. J. "Influence of Nutrition Education on Fourth and Fifth Graders." *Journal of Nutrition Education,* Winter 1972.

Holmes, C. L., and Bunda, M. A. "Comparative Ratings of Printed Materials Developed by Industry and Governmental Producers." *Journal of School Health* 53:320, May 1983.

National Dairy Council. *Nutrition Education Research: Directions for the Future.* Chicago: National Dairy Council, 1979.

Whitney, E. M., and Hamilton, E. N. "Books Not Recommended." In *Understanding Nutrition.* 3rd ed. St. Paul: West Publishing Company, 1984.

Instructional Aids

ACE Child Care Food Program Correspondence Course. Littleton, CO: Arapahoe County Extension Service.

Endres, J., and Rockwell, R. *Food, Nutrition, and the Young Child.* St. Louis: C.V. Mosby Company, 1980.

Feeding Your Child (1–5). Oklahoma City, OK: Nutrition Division, Oklahoma State Department of Health.

Feeding Your Preschooler. Corvallis, OR: Nutrition Graphics, 1981. (poster)

Food Before Six. Rosemont, IL: National Dairy Council, 1982.

Food for the Preschooler; Volumes I, II, and III. Olympia, WA: Department of Social and Health Services, 1981.

Food for Your Child Ages 1–5: A Guide for Parents. Raleigh, NC: North Carolina Agricultural Extension Service and North Carolina Department of Human Resources, 1980.

Food Models and Food Models Guide for Teachers and Other Leaders. Rosemont, IL: National Dairy Council.

Goodwin, M. T., and Pollen, G. *Creative Food Experiences for Children.* Washington, DC: Center for Science in the Public Interest, 1981.

Hinton, S., and Mann, B. *Foods for Toddlers and Preschoolers.* Raleigh, NC: North Carolina Agricultural Extension Service, A & T and North Carolina State Universities, 1981.

Hutchins, B. *Child Nutrition and Health.* Hightown, NJ: McGraw-Hill Book Company, 1979.

Ikeda, J. *To Mom and Dad—A Primer on Feeding the Preschooler.* Richmond, CA: Agricultural Sciences Publications, 1980.

Make Eating a Pleasure. Rochester, MN: Child Care Resource and Referral, Inc.

Making Mealtime a Happy Time for Preschoolers—A Guide for Teachers. Sacramento, CA: California State Department of Education, 1982.

Pipes, P. *Nutrition in Infancy and Childhood.* St. Louis: C.V. Mosby Co., 1981.

Pugliese, M. *Nutrition and All That Jazz: A Nutrition Handbook for Preschool Teachers.* Boston, MA: Simmons College.

Randell, Jill, and Olson, C. *Parents and Preschoolers—A Recipe for Good Nutrition.* Ithaca, NY: Division of Nutritional Sciences, Cornell University, 1979.

Snack Facts. NIH Publication No. 81–1680. Bethesda, MD: National Institute of Dental Research, 1981.

APPENDIXES

APPENDIX A   NUTRITIVE VALUES OF THE EDIBLE PART OF FOODS

(Dashes (—) denote lack of reliable data for a constituent believed to be present in measurable amount)

NUTRIENTS IN INDICATED QUANTITY

Item No.	Foods, approximate measures, units, and weight (cubic part unless footnotes indicate otherwise)		Water	Food energy	Protein	Fat	Fatty Acids Saturated (total)	Unsaturated Oleic	Linoleic	Carbohydrate	Calcium	Phosphorus	Iron	Potassium	Vitamin A value	Thiamin	Riboflavin	Niacin	Ascorbic acid
(A)	(B)	Grams	(C) Per cent	(D) Calories	(E) Grams	(F) Grams	(G) Grams	(H) Grams	(I) Grams	(J) Grams	(K) Milligrams	(L) Milligrams	(M) Milligrams	(N) Milligrams	(O) International units	(P) Milligrams	(Q) Milligrams	(R) Milligrams	(S) Milligrams

DAIRY PRODUCTS (CHEESE, CREAM, IMITATION CREAM, MILK; RELATED PRODUCTS)

Butter. See Fats, oils; related products, items 103–108.

Item No.	Foods	Grams	Water	Food energy	Protein	Fat	Sat	Oleic	Lino	Carb	Calcium	Phos	Iron	Potas	Vit A	Thiamin	Ribo	Niacin	Ascorbic
	Cheese:																		
	Natural:																		
1	Blue — 1 oz	28	42	100	6	8	5.3	1.9	0.2	1	150	110	0.1	73	200	0.01	0.11	0.3	0
2	Camembert (3 wedges per 4-oz container) — 1 wedge	38	52	115	8	9	5.8	2.2	.2	Trace	147	132	.1	71	350	.01	.19	.2	0
	Cheddar:																		
3	Cut pieces — 1 oz	28	37	115	7	9	6.1	2.1	.2	Trace	204	145	.2	28	300	.01	.11	Trace	0
4	1 cu in	17.2	37	70	4	6	3.7	1.3	.1	Trace	124	88	.1	17	180	Trace	.06	Trace	0
5	Shredded — 1 cup	113	37	455	28	37	24.2	8.5	.7	1	815	579	.8	111	1,200	.03	.42	.1	0
	Cottage (curd not pressed down):																		
	Creamed (cottage cheese, 4% fat):																		
6	Large curd — 1 cup	225	79	235	28	10	6.4	2.4	.2	6	135	297	.3	190	370	.05	.37	.3	Trace
7	Small curd — 1 cup	210	79	220	26	9	6.0	2.2	.2	6	126	277	.3	177	340	.04	.34	.3	Trace
8	Low fat (2%) — 1 cup	226	79	205	31	4	2.8	1.0	.1	8	155	340	.4	217	160	.05	.42	.3	Trace
9	Low fat (1%) — 1 cup	226	82	165	28	2	1.5	.5	.1	6	138	302	.3	193	80	.05	.37	.3	Trace
10	Uncreamed (cottage cheese dry curd, less than 1/2% fat) — 1 cup	145	80	125	25	1	.4	.1	Trace	3	46	151	.3	47	40	.04	.21	.2	0
11	Cream — 1 oz	28	54	100	2	10	6.2	2.4	.2	1	23	30	.3	34	400	Trace	.06	Trace	0
	Mozzarella, made with—																		
12	Whole milk — 1 oz	28	48	90	6	7	4.4	1.7	.2	1	163	117	.1	21	260	Trace	.08	Trace	0
13	Part skim milk — 1 oz	28	49	80	8	5	3.1	1.2	.1	1	207	149	.1	27	180	.01	.10	Trace	0
	Parmesan, grated:																		
14	Cup, not pressed down — 1 cup	100	18	455	42	30	19.1	7.7	.3	4	1,376	807	1.0	107	700	.05	.39	.3	0
15	Tablespoon — 1 tbsp	5	18	25	2	2	1.0	.4	Trace	Trace	69	40	Trace	5	40	Trace	.02	Trace	0
16	Ounce — 1 oz	28	18	130	12	9	5.4	2.2	.1	1	390	229	.3	30	200	.01	.11	.1	0
17	Provolone — 1 oz	28	41	100	7	8	4.8	1.7	.1	1	214	141	.1	39	230	.01	.09	Trace	0
	Ricotta, made with—																		
18	Whole milk — 1 cup	246	72	428	28	32	20.4	7.1	.7	7	509	389	.9	257	1,210	.03	.48	.3	0
19	Part skim milk — 1 cup	246	74	340	28	19	12.1	4.7	.5	13	669	449	1.1	308	1,060	.05	.46	.2	0
20	Romano — 1 oz	28	31	110	9	8	5.0	—	—	1	302	215	—	—	160	—	.11	—	0
21	Swiss — 1 oz	28	37	105	8	8	5.0	1.7	.2	1	272	171	Trace	31	240	.01	.10	Trace	0
	Pasteurized process cheese:																		
22	American — 1 oz	28	39	105	6	9	5.6	2.1	.2	Trace	174	211	.1	46	340	.01	.10	Trace	0
23	Swiss — 1 oz	28	42	95	7	7	4.5	1.7	.1	1	219	216	.2	61	230	Trace	.08	Trace	0
24	Pasteurized process cheese food, American — 1 oz	28	43	95	6	7	4.4	1.7	.1	2	163	130	.2	79	260	.01	.13	Trace	0
25	Pasteurized process cheese spread, American — 1 oz	28	48	82	5	6	3.8	1.5	.1	2	159	202	.1	69	220	.01	.12	Trace	0
	Cream, sweet:																		
26	Half-and-half (cream and milk) — 1 cup	242	81	315	7	28	17.3	7.0	.6	10	254	230	.2	314	260	.08	.36	.2	2
27	1 tbsp	15	81	20	Trace	2	1.1	.4	Trace	1	16	14	Trace	19	20	.01	.02	Trace	Trace
28	Light, coffee, or table — 1 cup	240	74	470	6	46	28.8	11.7	1.0	9	231	192	.1	292	1,730	.08	.36	.1	2
29	1 tbsp	15	74	30	Trace	3	1.8	.7	.1	1	14	12	Trace	18	110	Trace	.02	Trace	Trace

(A)	(B)	(g)	(C)	(D)	(E)	(F)	(G)	(H)	(I)	(J)	(K)	(L)	(M)	(N)	(O)	(P)	(Q)	(R)	(S)
	Whipping, unwhipped (volume about double when whipped):																		
30	Light---- 1 cup	239	64	700	5	74	46.2	18.3	1.5	7	166	146	0.1	231	2,690	0.06	0.30	0.1	1
31	---- 1 tbsp	15	64	45	Trace	5	2.9	1.1	Trace	Trace	10	9	Trace	15	170	Trace	.02	Trace	Trace
32	Heavy---- 1 cup	238	58	820	5	88	54.8	22.2	2.0	7	154	149	Trace	179	3,500	.05	.26	.1	1
33	---- 1 tbsp	15	58	80	Trace	6	3.5	1.4	.1	Trace	10	9	Trace	11	220	.02	.02	Trace	Trace
34	Whipped topping, (pressurized)- 1 cup	60	61	155	2	13	8.3	3.4	.3	7	61	54	Trace	88	550	.02	.04	Trace	0
35	---- 1 tbsp	3	61	10	Trace	1	.3	.2	Trace	Trace	3	3	Trace	4	30	Trace	Trace	Trace	0
36	Cream, sour---- 1 cup	230	71	495	7	48	30.0	12.1	1.1	10	268	195	.1	331	1,820	.08	.34	.2	2
37	---- 1 tbsp	12	71	25	Trace	3	1.6	.6	.1	1	14	10	Trace	17	90	Trace	.02	Trace	Trace
	Cream products, imitation (made with vegetable fat):																		
	Sweet:																		
	Creamers:																		
38	Liquid (frozen)---- 1 cup	245	77	335	2	24	22.8	.3	0	28	23	157	.1	467	[1]220	0	0	0	0
39	---- 1 tbsp	15	77	20	Trace	1	1.4	Trace	0	2	1	10	Trace	29	[1]10	0	0	0	0
40	Powdered---- 1 cup	94	2	515	5	33	30.6	.9	Trace	52	21	397	Trace	763	[1]190	0	[1].16	0	0
41	---- 1 tsp	2	2	10	Trace	1	.7	Trace	0	1	Trace	8	Trace	16	[1]Trace	0	[1]Trace	Trace	0
	Whipped topping:																		
42	Frozen---- 1 cup	75	50	240	1	19	16.3	1.0	.2	17	5	6	.1	14	[1]650	0	0	0	0
43	---- 1 tbsp	4	50	15	Trace	1	.9	.1	Trace	1	Trace	Trace	Trace	1	[1]30	0	0	0	0
44	Powdered, made with whole milk. 1 cup	80	67	150	3	10	8.5	.6	.1	13	72	69	Trace	121	[1]290	.02	.09	Trace	1
45	---- 1 tbsp	4	67	10	Trace	Trace	.4	Trace	Trace	1	4	3	Trace	6	[1]10	Trace	Trace	Trace	Trace
46	Pressurized---- 1 cup	70	60	185	1	16	13.2	1.4	.2	11	4	13	Trace	13	[1]330	0	0	0	0
47	---- 1 tbsp	4	60	10	Trace	1	.8	.1	Trace	1	Trace	1	Trace	1	[1]20	0	0	0	0
48	Sour dressing (imitation sour cream) made with nonfat dry milk. 1 cup	235	75	415	8	39	31.2	4.4	1.1	11	266	205	.1	380	[1]120	.09	.38	.2	2
	---- 1 tbsp	12	75	20	Trace	2	1.6	.2	.1	1	14	10	Trace	19	[1]Trace	.01	.02	Trace	Trace
49	Ice cream. See Milk desserts, frozen (items 75-80).																		
	Ice milk. See Milk desserts, frozen (items 81-83).																		
	Milk:																		
	Fluid:																		
50	Whole (3.3% fat)---- 1 cup	244	88	150	8	8	5.1	2.1	.2	11	291	228	.1	370	[2]310	.09	.40	.2	2
	Lowfat (2%):																		
51	No milk solids added---- 1 cup	244	89	120	8	5	2.9	1.2	.1	12	297	232	.1	377	500	.10	.40	.2	2
	Milk solids added:																		
52	Label claim less than 10 g of protein per cup. 1 cup	245	89	125	9	5	2.9	1.2	.1	12	313	245	.1	397	500	.10	.42	.2	2
53	Label claim 10 or more grams of protein per cup (protein fortified). 1 cup	246	88	135	10	5	3.0	1.2	.1	14	352	276	.1	447	500	.11	.48	.2	3
	Lowfat (1%):																		
54	No milk solids added---- 1 cup	244	90	100	8	3	1.6	.7	.1	12	300	235	.1	381	500	.10	.41	.2	2
	Milk solids added:																		
55	Label claim less than 10 g of protein per cup. 1 cup	245	90	105	9	2	1.5	.6	.1	12	313	245	.1	397	500	.10	.42	.2	2
56	Label claim 10 or more grams of protein per cup (protein fortified). 1 cup	246	89	120	10	3	1.8	.7	.1	14	349	273	.1	444	500	.11	.47	.2	3
	Nonfat (skim):																		
57	No milk solids added---- 1 cup	245	91	85	8	Trace	.3	.1	Trace	12	302	247	.1	406	500	.09	.37	.2	2

[1] Vitamin A value is largely from beta-carotene used for coloring. Riboflavin value for items 40-41 apply to products with added riboflavin.

[2] Applies to product without added vitamin A. With added vitamin A, value is 500 International Units (I.U.).

(Dashes (—) denote lack of reliable data for a constituent believed to be present in measurable amount)

NUTRIENTS IN INDICATED QUANTITY

Item No. (A)	Food, approximate measure, units, and weight (edible part unless footnotes indicate otherwise) (B)	Grams	Water (C) Percent	Food energy (D) Calories	Protein (E) Grams	Fat (F) Grams	Fatty Acids Saturated (total) (G) Grams	Unsaturated Oleic (H) Grams	Unsaturated Linoleic (I) Grams	Carbohydrate (J) Grams	Calcium (K) Milligrams	Phosphorus (L) Milligrams	Iron (M) Milligrams	Potassium (N) Milligrams	Vitamin A value (O) International units	Thiamin (P) Milligrams	Riboflavin (Q) Milligrams	Niacin (R) Milligrams	Ascorbic acid (S) Milligrams
	DAIRY PRODUCTS (CHEESE, CREAM, IMITATION CREAM, MILK; RELATED PRODUCTS)—Con.																		
	Milk—Continued																		
	Fluid—Continued																		
	Nonfat (skim)—Continued																		
	Milk solids added:																		
58	Label claim less than 10 g of protein per cup. 1 cup	245	90	90	9	1	0.4	0.1	Trace	12	316	255	0.1	416	500	0.10	0.43	0.2	2
59	Label claim 10 or more grams of protein per cup (protein fortified). 1 cup	246	89	100	10	1	.4	.1	Trace	14	352	275	.1	446	500	.11	.48	.2	3
60	Buttermilk. 1 cup	245	90	100	8	2	1.3	.5	Trace	12	285	219	.1	371	[8]80	.08	.38	.1	2
	Canned:																		
	Evaporated, unsweetened:																		
61	Whole milk. 1 cup	252	74	340	17	19	11.6	5.3	.4	25	657	510	.5	764	[9]610	.12	.80	.5	5
62	Skim milk. 1 cup	255	79	200	19	1				29	738	497	.7	845	[9]1,000	.11	.79	.4	3
63	Sweetened, condensed. 1 cup	306	27	980	24	27	16.8	6.7	.7	166	868	775	.6	1,136	[9]1,000	.28	1.27	.6	8
	Dried:																		
64	Buttermilk. 1 cup	120	3	465	41	7	4.3	1.7	.2	59	1,421	1,119	.4	1,910	[10]260	.47	1.90	1.1	7
	Nonfat instant:																		
65	Envelope, net wt., 3.2 oz[5]. 1 envelope	91	4	325	32	1	.4	.1	Trace	47	1,120	896	.3	1,552	[11]2,160	.38	1.59	.8	5
66	Cup. 1 cup	68	4	245	24	Trace	.3	.1	Trace	35	837	670	.2	1,160	[11]1,610	.28	1.19	.6	4
	Milk beverages:																		
	Chocolate milk (commercial):																		
67	Regular. 1 cup	250	82	210	8	8	5.3	2.2	.2	26	280	251	.6	417	300	.09	.41	.3	2
68	Lowfat (2%). 1 cup	250	84	180	8	5	3.1	1.3	.1	26	284	254	.6	422	500	.10	.42	.3	2
69	Lowfat (1%). 1 cup	250	85	160	8	3	1.5	.7	.1	26	287	257	.6	426	500	.10	.40	.2	2
70	Eggnog (commercial). 1 cup	254	74	340	10	19	11.3	5.0	.6	34	330	278	.5	420	890	.09	.48	.3	4
	Malted milk, home-prepared with 1 cup of whole milk and 2 to 3 heaping tsp of malted milk powder (about 3/4 oz):																		
71	Chocolate. 1 cup of milk plus 3/4 oz of powder.	265	81	235	9	9	5.5	—	—	29	304	265	.5	500	330	.14	.43	.7	2
72	Natural. 1 cup of milk plus 3/4 oz of powder.	265	81	235	11	10	6.0	—	—	27	347	307	.3	529	380	.20	.54	1.3	2
	Shakes, thick:[8]																		
73	Chocolate, container, net wt., 10.6 oz. 1 container	300	72	355	9	8	5.0	2.0	.2	63	396	378	.9	672	260	.14	.67	.4	0
74	Vanilla, container, net wt., 11 oz. 1 container	313	74	350	12	9	5.9	2.4	.2	56	457	361	.3	572	360	.09	.61	.5	0
	Milk desserts, frozen:																		
	Ice cream:																		
	Regular (about 11% fat):																		
	Hardened:																		
75	1/2 gal	1,064	61	2,155	38	115	71.3	28.8	2.6	254	1,406	1,075	1.0	2,052	4,340	.42	2.63	1.1	6
76	1 cup	133	61	270	5	14	8.9	3.6	.3	32	176	134	.1	257	540	.05	.33	.1	1
77	3-fl oz container	50	61	100	2	5	3.4	1.4	.1	12	66	51	Trace	96	200	.02	.12	.1	Trace
78	Soft serve (frozen custard). 1 cup	173	60	375	7	23	13.5	5.9	.6	38	236	199	.4	338	790	.08	.45	.2	1
	Rich (about 16% fat):																		
79	hardened. 1/2 gal	1,188	59	2,805	33	190	118.3	47.8	4.3	256	1,213	927	.8	1,771	7,200	.36	2.27	2.9	5
80	1 cup	148	59	350	4	24	14.7	6.0	.5	32	151	115	.1	221	900	.04	.28	.1	1
	Ice milk:																		
81	Hardened (about 4.3% fat). 1/2 gal	1,048	69	1,470	41	45	28.1	11.3	1.0	232	1,409	1,035	1.5	2,117	1,710	.61	2.78	.9	6
82	1 cup	131	69	185	5	6	3.5	1.4	.1	29	176	129	.1	265	210	.08	.35	.1	1

(A)	(B)	(C)	(D)	(E)	(F)	(G)	(H)	(I)	(J)	(K)	(L)	(M)	(N)	(O)	(P)	(Q)	(R)	(S)
83	Soft serve (about 2.6% fat)— 1 cup	175	70	225	8	5	2.9	1.2	0.1	38	274	202	0.3	412	180	0.12	0.54	0.2	1
84	Sherbet (about 2% fat)— 1/2 gal	1,542	66	2,160	17	31	19.0	7.7	.7	469	827	594	2.5	1,585	1,480	.26	.71	1.0	31
85	— 1 cup	193	66	270	2	4	2.4	1.0	.1	59	103	74	.3	198	190	.03	.09	.1	4
	Milk desserts, other:																		
	Custard, baked:																		
86	— 1 cup	265	77	305	14	15	6.8	5.4	.7	29	297	310	1.1	387	930	.11	.50	.3	1
	Puddings:																		
	From home recipe:																		
	Starch base:																		
87	Chocolate— 1 cup	260	66	385	8	12	7.6	3.3	.3	67	250	255	1.3	445	390	.05	.36	.3	1
88	Vanilla (blancmange)— 1 cup	255	76	285	9	10	6.2	2.5	.2	41	298	232	Trace	352	410	.08	.41	.3	2
89	Tapioca cream— 1 cup	165	72	220	8	8	4.1	2.5	.5	28	173	180	.7	223	480	.07	.30	.2	2
	From mix (chocolate) and milk:																		
90	Regular (cooked)— 1 cup	260	70	320	9	8	4.3	2.6	.2	59	265	247	.8	354	340	.05	.39	.3	2
91	Instant— 1 cup	260	69	325	8	7	3.6	2.2	.3	63	374	237	1.3	335	340	.08	.39	.3	2
	Yogurt:																		
	With added milk solids:																		
	Made with lowfat milk:																		
92	Fruit-flavored³— 1 container, net wt., 8 oz	227	75	230	10	3	1.8	.6	.1	42	343	269	.2	439	[10]120	.08	.40	.2	1
93	Plain— 1 container, net wt., 8 oz	227	85	145	12	4	2.3	.8	.1	16	415	326	.2	531	[10]150	.10	.49	.3	2
94	Made with nonfat milk— 1 container, net wt., 8 oz	227	85	125	13	Trace	.3	.3	Trace	17	452	355	.2	579	[10]20	.11	.53	.3	2
	Without added milk solids:																		
95	Made with whole milk— 1 container, net wt., 8 oz	227	88	140	8	7	4.8	1.7	.1	11	274	215	.1	351	280	.07	.32	.2	1

EGGS

(A)	(B)	(C)	(D)	(E)	(F)	(G)	(H)	(I)	(J)	(K)	(L)	(M)	(N)	(O)	(P)	(Q)	(R)	(S)
	Eggs, large (24 oz per dozen):																		
	Raw:																		
96	Whole, without shell— 1 egg	50	75	80	6	6	1.7	2.0	.6	1	28	90	1.0	65	260	.04	.15	Trace	0
97	White— 1 white	33	88	15	3	Trace	.7	0	0	Trace	4	4	Trace	45	0	Trace	.09	Trace	0
98	Yolk— 1 yolk	17	49	65	3	6	1.7	2.1	.6	1	26	86	.9	15	310	.04	.07	Trace	0
	Cooked:																		
99	Fried in butter— 1 egg	46	72	85	5	6	2.4	2.2	.6	1	26	80	.9	58	290	.03	.13	Trace	0
100	Hard-cooked, shell removed— 1 egg	50	75	80	6	6	1.7	2.0	.6	1	28	90	1.0	65	260	.04	.14	Trace	0
101	Poached— 1 egg	50	74	80	6	6	1.7	2.0	.6	1	28	90	1.0	65	260	.04	.13	Trace	0
102	Scrambled (milk added) in butter. Also omelet— 1 egg	64	76	95	6	7	2.8	2.3	.6	1	47	97	.9	85	310	.04	.16	Trace	0

FATS, OILS; RELATED PRODUCTS

(A)	(B)	(C)	(D)	(E)	(F)	(G)	(H)	(I)	(J)	(K)	(L)	(M)	(N)	(O)	(P)	(Q)	(R)	(S)
	Butter:																		
	Regular (1 brick or 4 sticks per lb):																		
103	Stick (1/2 cup)— 1 stick	113	16	815	1	92	57.3	23.1	2.1	Trace	27	26	.2	29	[11]3,470	.01	.04	Trace	0
104	Tablespoon (about 1/8 stick)— 1 tbsp	14	16	100	Trace	12	7.2	2.9	.3	Trace	3	3	Trace	4	[11]430	Trace	Trace	Trace	0
105	Pat (1 in square, 1/3 in high; 90 per lb)— 1 pat	5	16	35	Trace	4	2.5	1.0	.1	Trace	1	1	Trace	1	[11]150	Trace	Trace	Trace	0
	Whipped (6 sticks or two 8-oz containers per lb):																		
106	Stick (1/2 cup)— 1 stick	76	16	540	1	61	38.2	15.4	1.4	Trace	18	17	.1	20	[11]2,310	Trace	.03	Trace	0
107	Tablespoon (about 1/8 stick)— 1 tbsp	9	16	65	Trace	8	4.7	1.9	.2	Trace	2	2	Trace	2	[11]290	Trace	Trace	Trace	0
108	Pat (1 1/4 in square, 1/3 in high; 120 per lb)— 1 pat	4	16	25	Trace	3	1.9	.8	.1	Trace	1	1	Trace	1	[11]120	0	Trace	Trace	0

³Applies to product without vitamin A added.
⁴Applies to product with added vitamin A. Without added vitamin A, value is 20 International Units (I.U.).
⁵Yields 1 qt of fluid milk when reconstituted according to package directions.
⁶Applies to product with added vitamin A.
⁷Weight applies to product with label claim of 1 1/3 cups equal 3.2 oz.
⁸Applies to product with added vitamin A.
⁹Content of fat, vitamin A, and carbohydrate varies. Consult the label when precise values are needed for special diets.
[10]Applies to products made from thick shake mixes and that do not contain added ice cream. Products made from milk shake mixes are higher in fat and usually contain added ice cream.
[11]Based on year-round average.

(Dashes (–) denote lack of reliable data for a constituent believed to be present in measurable amount)

NUTRIENTS IN INDICATED QUANTITY

Item No. (A)	Foods, approximate measure, units, and weight (edible part unless footnotes indicate otherwise) (B)	(grams)	Water (C) Percent	Food energy (D) Calories	Protein (E) Grams	Fat (F) Grams	Fatty Acids — Saturated (total) (G) Grams	Fatty Acids — Oleic (H) Grams	Fatty Acids — Linoleic (I) Grams	Carbohydrate (J) Grams	Calcium (K) Milligrams	Phosphorus (L) Milligrams	Iron (M) Milligrams	Potassium (N) Milligrams	Vitamin A value (O) International units	Thiamin (P) Milligrams	Riboflavin (Q) Milligrams	Niacin (R) Milligrams	Ascorbic acid (S) Milligrams
	FATS, OILS; RELATED PRODUCTS—Con.																		
109	Fats, cooking (vegetable shortenings). 1 cup	200	0	1,770	0	200	48.8	88.2	48.4	0	0	0	0	0	—	0	0	0	0
110	1 tbsp	13	0	110	0	13	3.2	5.7	3.1	0	0	0	0	0	0	0	0	0	0
111	Lard— 1 cup	205	0	1,850	0	205	81.0	83.8	20.5	0	0	0	0	0	0	0	0	0	0
112	1 tbsp	13	0	115	0	13	5.1	5.3	1.3	0	0	0	0	0	0	0	0	0	0
	Margarine: Regular (1 brick or 4 sticks per lb):																		
113	Stick (1/2 cup)— 1 stick	113	16	815	1	92	16.7	42.9	24.9	Trace	27	26	.2	29	[12]3,750	.01	.04	Trace	0
114	Tablespoon (about 1/8 stick)— 1 tbsp	14	16	100	Trace	12	2.1	5.3	3.1	Trace	3	3	Trace	4	[12]470	Trace	Trace	Trace	0
115	Pat (1 in square, 1/3 in high; 90 per lb). 1 pat	5	16	35	Trace	4	.7	1.9	1.1	Trace	1	1	Trace	1	[12]170	Trace	Trace	Trace	0
116	Soft, two 8-oz containers per lb. 1 container	227	16	1,635	1	184	32.5	71.5	65.4	Trace	53	52	.4	59	[12]7,500	.01	.08	.1	0
117	1 tbsp	14	16	100	Trace	12	2.0	4.5	4.1	Trace	3	3	Trace	4	[12]470	Trace	Trace	Trace	0
	Whipped (6 sticks per lb):																		
118	Stick (1/2 cup)— 1 stick	76	16	545	Trace	61	11.2	28.7	16.7	Trace	18	17	.1	20	[12]2,500	Trace	.03	Trace	0
119	Tablespoon (about 1/8 stick)— 1 tbsp	9	16	70	Trace	8	1.4	3.6	2.1	Trace	2	2	Trace	2	[17]310	Trace	Trace	Trace	0
	Oils, salad or cooking:																		
120	Corn— 1 cup	218	0	1,925	0	218	27.7	53.6	125.1	0	0	0	0	0	—	0	0	0	0
121	1 tbsp	14	0	120	0	14	1.7	3.3	7.8	0	0	0	0	0	—	0	0	0	0
122	Olive— 1 cup	216	0	1,910	0	216	30.7	154.4	17.7	0	0	0	0	0	—	0	0	0	0
123	1 tbsp	14	0	120	0	14	1.9	9.7	1.1	0	0	0	0	0	—	0	0	0	0
124	Peanut— 1 cup	216	0	1,910	0	216	37.4	98.5	67.0	0	0	0	0	0	—	0	0	0	0
125	1 tbsp	14	0	120	0	14	2.3	6.2	4.2	0	0	0	0	0	—	0	0	0	0
126	Safflower— 1 cup	218	0	1,925	0	218	20.5	25.9	159.8	0	0	0	0	0	—	0	0	0	0
127	1 tbsp	14	0	120	0	14	1.3	1.6	10.0	0	0	0	0	0	—	0	0	0	0
128	Soybean oil, hydrogenated (partially hardened). 1 cup	218	0	1,925	0	218	31.8	93.1	75.6	0	0	0	0	0	—	0	0	0	0
129	1 tbsp	14	0	120	0	14	2.0	5.8	4.7	0	0	0	0	0	—	0	0	0	0
130	Soybean-cottonseed oil blend, hydrogenated. 1 cup	218	0	1,925	0	218	38.2	63.0	99.6	0	0	0	0	0	—	0	0	0	0
131	1 tbsp	14	0	120	0	14	2.4	3.9	6.2	0	0	0	0	0	—	0	0	0	0
	Salad dressings: Commercial: Blue cheese:																		
132	Regular. 1 tbsp	15	32	75	1	8	1.6	1.7	3.8	1	12	11	Trace	6	30	Trace	.02	Trace	Trace
133	Low calorie (5 Cal per tsp). 1 tbsp	16	84	10	Trace	1	.5	.3	Trace	1	10	8	Trace	5	30	Trace	.01	Trace	Trace
	French:																		
134	Regular. 1 tbsp	16	39	65	Trace	6	1.1	1.3	3.2	3	2	2	.1	13	—	—	—	—	—
135	Low calorie (5 Cal per tsp). 1 tbsp	16	77	15	Trace	Trace	.1	.1	.4	2	2	2	.1	13	—	—	—	—	—
	Italian:																		
136	Regular. 1 tbsp	15	28	85	Trace	9	1.6	1.9	4.7	1	2	1	Trace	2	Trace	Trace	Trace	Trace	—
137	Low calorie (2 Cal per tsp). 1 tbsp	15	90	10	Trace	1	.1	.1	.4	Trace	2	1	Trace	2	Trace	Trace	Trace	Trace	—
138	Mayonnaise. 1 tbsp	14	15	100	Trace	11	2.0	2.4	5.6	Trace	3	4	.1	5	40	Trace	.01	Trace	—
	Mayonnaise type:																		
139	Regular. 1 tbsp	15	41	65	Trace	6	1.1	1.4	3.2	2	2	4	Trace	1	30	Trace	Trace	Trace	—
140	Low calorie (8 Cal per tsp). 1 tbsp	16	81	20	Trace	2	.4	.4	1.0	2	3	4	Trace	1	40	Trace	Trace	Trace	—
141	Tartar sauce, regular. 1 tbsp	14	34	75	Trace	8	1.5	1.8	4.1	1	3	4	.1	11	30	Trace	Trace	Trace	Trace
	Thousand Island:																		
142	Regular. 1 tbsp	16	32	80	Trace	8	1.4	1.7	4.0	2	2	3	.1	18	50	Trace	Trace	Trace	Trace
143	Low calorie (10 Cal per tsp). 1 tbsp	15	68	25	Trace	2	.4	.4	1.0	2	2	3	.1	17	50	Trace	Trace	Trace	Trace
	From home recipe:																		
144	Cooked type[13]. 1 tbsp	16	68	25	1	2	.5	.6	.3	2	14	15	.1	19	80	.01	.03	Trace	Trace

FISH, SHELLFISH, MEAT, POULTRY; RELATED PRODUCTS

(A)	(B)	(C)	(D)	(E)	(F)	(G)	(H)	(I)	(J)	(K)	(L)	(M)	(N)	(O)	(P)	(Q)	(R)	(S)
145	Fish and shellfish: Bluefish, baked with butter or margarine. 3 oz	85	68	135	22	4	—	—	—	0	—	244	0.6	—	40	0.09	0.08	1.6	—
	Clams:																		
146	Raw, meat only. 3 oz	85	82	65	11	1	—	—	—	2	59	138	5.2	154	90	.08	.15	1.1	8
147	Canned, solids and liquid. 3 oz	85	86	45	7	1	0.2	Trace	Trace	2	47	116	3.5	119	—	.11	.09	.9	—
148	Crabmeat (white or king), canned. 1 cup	135	77	135	24	3	.6	0.4	0.1	1	61	246	1.1	149	—	.11	.11	2.6	—
149	Fish sticks, breaded, cooked, frozen (stick, 4 by 1 by 1/2 in). 1 fish stick or 1 oz	28	66	50	5	3	—	—	—	2	3	47	.1	—	0	.01	.02	.5	—
150	Haddock, breaded, fried[14]. 3 oz	85	66	140	17	5	1.4	2.2	1.2	5	34	210	1.0	296	—	.03	.06	2.7	2
151	Ocean perch, breaded, fried[14]. 1 fillet	85	59	195	16	11	2.7	4.4	2.3	6	28	192	1.1	242	—	.10	.10	1.6	—
152	Oysters, raw, meat only (13-19 medium Selects). 1 cup	240	85	160	20	4	1.3	.2	.1	8	226	343	13.2	290	740	.34	.43	6.0	—
153	Salmon, pink, canned, solids and liquid. 3 oz	85	71	120	17	5	.9	.8	.1	0	[15]167	243	.7	307	60	.03	.16	6.8	—
154	Sardines, Atlantic, canned in oil, drained solids. 3 oz	85	62	175	20	9	3.0	2.5	.5	0	372	424	2.5	502	190	.02	.17	4.6	—
155	Scallops, frozen, breaded, fried, reheated. 6 scallops	90	60	175	16	8	—	—	—	9	—	—	—	—	30	—	—	—	—
156	Shad, baked with butter or margarine, bacon. 3 oz	85	64	170	20	10	—	—	—	0	20	266	.5	320	30	.11	.22	7.3	—
	Shrimp:																		
157	Canned meat. 3 oz	85	70	100	21	9	.1	.1	Trace	0	98	224	2.6	104	50	.01	.03	1.5	—
158	French fried[16]. 3 oz	85	57	190	17	9	2.3	3.7	2.0	9	61	162	1.7	195	—	.03	.07	2.3	—
159	Tuna, canned in oil, drained solids. 3 oz	85	61	170	24	7	1.7	1.7	.7	0	7	199	1.6	—	70	.04	.10	10.1	—
160	Tuna salad[17]. 1 cup	205	70	350	30	22	4.3	6.3	6.7	7	41	291	2.7	—	590	.08	.23	10.3	2
161	Meat and meat products: Bacon, (20 slices per lb, raw), broiled or fried, crisp. 2 slices	15	8	85	4	8	2.5	3.7	.7	Trace	2	34	.5	35	0	.08	.05	.8	—
	Beef[18] cooked: Cuts braised, simmered or pot roasted:																		
162	Lean and fat (piece, 2 1/2 by 2 1/2 by 3/4 in). 3 oz	85	53	245	23	16	6.8	6.5	.4	0	10	114	2.9	184	30	.04	.18	3.6	—
163	Lean only from item 162. 2.5 oz	72	62	140	22	5	2.1	1.8	.2	0	10	108	2.7	176	10	.04	.17	3.3	—
	Ground beef, broiled:																		
164	Lean with 10% fat. 3 oz or patty 3 by 5/8 in	85	60	185	23	10	4.0	3.9	.3	0	10	196	3.0	261	20	.08	.20	5.1	—
165	Lean with 21% fat. 2.9 oz or patty 3 by 5/8 in	82	54	235	20	17	7.0	6.7	.4	0	9	159	2.6	221	30	.07	.17	4.4	—
166	Roast, oven cooked, no liquid added: Relatively fat, such as rib: Lean and fat (2 pieces, 4 1/8 by 2 1/4 by 1/4 in). 3 oz	85	40	375	17	33	14.0	13.6	.8	0	8	158	2.2	189	70	.05	.13	3.1	—
167	Relatively lean, such as heel of round: Lean only from item 166. 1.8 oz	51	57	125	14	7	3.0	2.5	.3	0	6	131	1.8	161	10	.04	.11	2.6	—
168	Lean and fat (2 pieces, 4 1/8 by 2 1/4 by 1/4 in). 3 oz	85	62	165	25	7	2.8	2.7	.2	0	11	208	3.2	279	10	.06	.19	4.5	—

[12] Based on average vitamin A content of fortified margarine. Federal specifications for fortified margarine require a minimum of 15,000 International Units (I.U.) of vitamin A per pound.
[13] Fatty acid values apply to product made with regular-type margarine.
[14] Dipped in egg, milk or water, and breadcrumbs; fried in vegetable shortening.
[15] If bones are discarded, value for calcium will be greatly reduced.
[16] Dipped in egg, breadcrumbs, and flour or batter.
[17] Prepared with tuna, celery, salad dressing (mayonnaise type), pickle, onion, and egg.
[18] Outer layer of fat on the cut was removed to within approximately 1/2 in of the lean. Deposits of fat within the cut were not removed.

[Dashes (—) denote lack of reliable data for a constituent believed to be present in measurable amount]

FISH, SHELLFISH, MEAT, POULTRY; RELATED PRODUCTS—Con.

Item No. (A)	Foods, approximate measure, units, and weight (edible part unless footnotes indicate otherwise) (B)	Grams	Water (C) Percent	Food energy (D) Calories	Protein (E) Grams	Fat (F) Grams	Fatty Acids Saturated (total) (G) Grams	Oleic (H) Grams	Linoleic (I) Grams	Carbohydrate (J) Grams	Calcium (K) Milligrams	Phosphorus (L) Milligrams	Iron (M) Milligrams	Potassium (N) Milligrams	Vitamin A value (O) International units	Thiamin (P) Milligrams	Riboflavin (Q) Milligrams	Niacin (R) Milligrams	Ascorbic acid (S) Milligrams
	Meat and meat products—Continued																		
	Beef[1] cooked—Continued																		
	Roast, oven cooked, no liquid added—Continued																		
	Relatively lean such as heel of round—Continued																		
169	Lean only from item 168—— 2.8 oz	78	65	125	24	3	1.2	1.0	0.1	0	10	199	3.0	268	Trace	0.06	0.18	4.3	—
	Steak:																		
	Relatively fat-sirloin, broiled:																		
170	Lean and fat (piece, 2 1/2 by 2 1/2 by 3/4 in). 3 oz	85	44	330	20	27	11.3	11.1	.6	0	9	162	2.5	220	50	.05	.15	4.0	—
171	Lean only from item 170—— 2.0 oz	56	59	115	18	4	1.8	1.6	.2	0	7	146	2.2	202	10	.05	.14	3.6	—
	Relatively lean-round, braised:																		
172	Lean and fat (piece, 4 1/8 by 2 1/4 by 1/2 in). 3 oz	85	55	220	24	13	5.5	5.2	.4	0	10	213	3.0	272	20	.07	.19	4.8	—
173	Lean only from item 172—— 2.4 oz	68	61	130	21	4	1.7	1.5	.2	0	9	182	2.5	238	10	.05	.16	4.1	—
	Beef, canned:																		
174	Corned beef—— 3 oz	85	59	185	22	10	4.9	4.5	.2	0	17	90	3.7		—	.01	.20	2.9	—
175	Corned beef hash—— 1 cup	220	67	400	19	25	11.9	10.9	.5	24	29	147	4.4	440	—	.02	.20	4.6	—
176	Beef, dried, chipped—— 2 1/2-oz jar	71	48	145	24	4	2.1	2.0	.1	0	14	287	3.6	142	—	.05	.23	2.7	0
177	Beef and vegetable stew—— 1 cup	245	82	220	16	11	4.9	4.5	.2	15	29	184	2.9	613	2,400	.15	.17	4.7	17
178	Beef potpie (home recipe), baked[19] (piece, 1/3 of 9-in diam. pie). 1 piece	210	55	515	21	30	7.9	12.8	6.7	39	29	149	3.8	334	1,720	.30	.30	5.5	6
179	Chili con carne with beans, canned. 1 cup	255	72	340	19	16	7.5	6.8	.3	31	82	321	4.3	594	150	.08	.18	3.3	—
180	Chop suey with beef and pork (home recipe). 1 cup	250	75	300	26	17	8.5	6.2	.7	13	60	248	4.8	425	600	.28	.38	5.0	33
181	Heart, beef, lean, braised—— 3 oz	85	61	160	27	5	1.5	1.1	.6	1	5	154	5.0	197	20	.21	1.04	6.5	1
	Lamb, cooked:																		
	Chop, rib (cut 3 per lb with bone), broiled:																		
182	Lean and fat—— 3.1 oz	89	43	360	18	32	14.8	12.1	1.2	0	8	139	1.0	200	—	.11	.19	4.1	—
183	Lean only from item 182—— 2 oz	57	60	120	16	6	2.5	2.1	.2	0	6	121	1.1	174	—	.09	.15	3.4	—
	Leg, roasted:																		
184	Lean and fat (2 pieces, 4 1/8 by 2 1/4 by 1/4 in). 3 oz	85	54	235	22	16	7.3	6.0	.6	0	9	177	1.4	241	—	.13	.23	4.7	—
185	Lean only from item 184—— 2.5 oz	71	62	130	20	5	2.1	1.8	.2	0	9	169	1.4	227	—	.12	.21	4.4	—
	Shoulder, roasted:																		
186	Lean and fat (3 pieces, 2 1/2 by 2 1/2 by 1/4 in). 3 oz	85	50	285	18	23	10.8	8.8	.9	0	9	146	1.0	206	—	.11	.20	4.0	—
187	Lean only from item 186—— 2.3 oz	64	61	130	17	6	3.6	2.3	.2	0	8	140	1.0	193	—	.10	.18	3.7	—
188	Liver, beef, fried[20] (slice, 6 1/2 by 2 3/8 by 3/8 in). 3 oz	85	56	195	22	9	2.5	3.5	.9	5	9	405	7.5	323	[2]45,390	.22	3.56	14.0	23
	Pork, cured, cooked:																		
189	Ham, light cure, lean and fat, roasted (2 pieces, 4 1/8 by 2 1/4 by 1/4 in).[22] 3 oz	85	54	245	18	19	6.8	7.9	1.7	0	8	146	2.2	199	0	.40	.15	3.1	—
	Luncheon meat:																		
190	Boiled ham, slice (8 per 8-oz pkg.). 1 oz	28	59	65	5	5	1.7	2.0	.4	0	3	47	.8	—	0	.12	.04	.7	—
191	Canned, spiced or unspiced: Slice, approx. 3 by 2 by 1/2 in. 1 slice	60	55	175	9	15	5.4	6.7	1.0	1	5	65	1.3	133	0	.19	.13	1.8	—

(A)	(B)	grams	(C)	(D)	(E)	(F)	(G)	(H)	(I)	(J)	(K)	(L)	(M)	(N)	(O)	(P)	(Q)	(R)	(S)
	Pork, fresh,[18] cooked:																		
	Chop, loin (cut 3 per lb with bone), broiled:																		
192	Lean and fat, broiled------ 2.7 oz	78	42	305	19	25	8.9	10.4	2.2	0	9	209	2.7	216	0	0.75	0.22	4.5	—
193	Lean only from item 192---- 2 oz	56	53	150	17	9	3.1	3.6	.8	0	7	181	2.2	192	0	.63	.18	3.8	—
	Roast, oven cooked, no liquid added:																		
194	Lean and fat (piece, 2 1/2 by 2 1/2 by 3/4 in.)-- 3 oz	85	46	310	21	24	8.7	10.2	2.2	0	9	218	2.7	233	0	.78	.22	4.8	—
195	Lean only from item 194---- 2.4 oz	68	55	175	20	10	3.5	4.1	.8	0	9	211	2.6	224	0	.73	.21	4.4	—
	Shoulder cut, simmered:																		
196	Lean and fat (3 pieces, 2 1/2 by 2 1/2 by 1/4 in.)-- 3 oz	85	46	320	20	26	9.3	10.9	2.3	0	9	118	2.6	158	0	.46	.21	4.1	—
197	Lean only from item 196--- 2.2 oz	63	60	135	18	6	2.2	2.6	.6	0	8	111	2.3	146	0	.42	.19	3.7	—
	Sausages (see also Luncheon meat (items 190-191)):																		
198	Bologna, slice (8 per 8-oz pkg.)-- 1 slice	28	56	85	3	8	3.0	3.4	.5	Trace	2	36	.5	65	—	.05	.06	.7	—
199	Braunschweiger, slice (6 per 6-oz pkg.)-- 1 slice	28	53	90	4	8	2.6	3.4	.8	1	3	69	1.7	—	1,850	.05	.41	2.3	—
200	Brown and serve (10-11 per 8-oz pkg.), browned-- 1 link	17	40	70	3	6	2.3	2.8	.7	Trace	—	—	—	—	—	—	—	—	—
201	Deviled ham, canned------- 1 tbsp	13	51	45	2	4	1.5	1.8	.4	0	1	12	.3	—	0	.02	.01	.2	—
202	Frankfurter (8 per 1-lb pkg.), cooked (reheated)-- 1 frankfurter	56	57	170	7	15	5.6	6.5	1.2	1	3	57	.8	—	—	.08	.11	1.4	—
203	Meat, potted (beef, chicken, turkey), canned-- 1 tbsp	13	61	30	2	2	—	—	—	0	—	—	—	—	—	Trace	.03	.2	—
204	Pork link (16 per 1-lb pkg.), cooked-- 1 link	13	35	60	2	6	2.1	2.4	.5	Trace	1	21	.3	35	0	.10	.04	.5	—
	Salami:																		
205	Dry type, slice (12 per 4-oz pkg.)-- 1 slice	10	30	45	2	4	1.6	1.6	.1	Trace	1	28	.4	—	—	.04	.03	.5	—
206	Cooked type, slice (8 per 8-oz pkg.)-- 1 slice	28	51	90	5	7	3.1	3.0	.2	Trace	3	57	.7	—	—	.07	.07	1.2	—
207	Vienna sausage (7 per 4-oz can)-- 1 sausage	16	63	40	2	3	1.2	1.4	.2	Trace	1	24	.3	—	—	.01	.02	.4	—
	Veal, medium fat, cooked, bone removed:																		
208	Cutlet (4 1/8 by 2 1/4 by 1/2 in.), braised or broiled-- 3 oz	85	60	185	23	9	4.0	3.4	.4	0	9	196	2.7	258	—	.06	.21	4.6	—
209	Rib (2 pieces, 4 1/8 by 2 1/4 by 1/4 in.), roasted-- 3 oz	85	55	230	23	14	6.1	5.1	.6	0	10	211	2.9	259	—	.11	.26	6.6	—
	Poultry and poultry products:																		
	Chicken, cooked:																		
210	Breast, fried,[23] bones removed, 1/2 breast (3.3 oz with bones)-- 2.8 oz	79	58	160	26	5	1.4	1.8	1.1	1	9	218	1.3	—	70	.04	.17	11.6	—
211	Drumstick, fried,[23] bones removed (2 oz with bones)-- 1.3 oz	38	55	90	12	4	1.1	1.3	.9	Trace	6	89	.9	—	50	.03	.15	2.7	—
212	Half broiler, broiled, bones removed (10.4 oz with bones)-- 6.2 oz	176	71	240	42	7	2.2	2.5	1.3	1	16	355	3.0	483	160	.09	.34	15.5	—
213	Chicken, canned, boneless----- 3 oz	85	65	170	18	10	3.2	3.8	2.0	0	18	210	1.3	117	200	.03	.11	3.7	3
214	Chicken a la king, cooked (home recipe)-- 1 cup	245	68	470	27	34	2.7	14.3	3.3	12	127	358	2.5	404	1,130	.10	.42	5.4	12
215	Chicken and noodles, cooked (home recipe)-- 1 cup	240	71	365	22	18	5.9	7.1	3.5	26	26	247	2.2	149	430	.05	.17	4.3	Trace

[18] Outer layer of fat on the cut was removed to within approximately 1/2 in. of the lean. Deposits of fat within the cut were not removed.

[19] Crust made with vegetable shortening and enriched flour.

[20] Regular-type margarine used.

[21] Value varies widely.

[22] About one-fourth of the outer layer of fat on the cut was removed. Deposits of fat within the cut were not removed.

[23] Vegetable shortening used.

(Dashes (—) denote lack of reliable data for a constituent believed to be present in measurable amount)

Item No. (A)	Foods, approximate measures, units, and weight (edible part unless footnotes indicate otherwise) (B)		Grams	Water (C) Per cent	Food energy (D) Calories	Protein (E) Grams	Fat (F) Grams	Fatty Acids Saturated (total) (G) Grams	Unsaturated Oleic (H) Grams	Unsaturated Linoleic (I) Grams	Carbohydrate (J) Grams	Calcium (K) Milligrams	Phosphorus (L) Milligrams	Iron (M) Milligrams	Potassium (N) Milligrams	Vitamin A value (O) International units	Thiamin (P) Milligrams	Riboflavin (Q) Milligrams	Niacin (R) Milligrams	Ascorbic acid (S) Milligrams
	FISH, SHELLFISH, MEAT, POULTRY; RELATED PRODUCTS—Con.																			
	Poultry and poultry products—Continued																			
	Chicken chow mein:																			
216	Canned-----	1 cup	250	89	95	7	Trace	—	—	—	18	45	85	1.3	418	150	0.05	0.10	1.0	13
217	From home recipe-----	1 cup	250	78	255	31	10	2.4	3.4	3.1	10	58	293	2.5	473	280	.08	.23	4.3	10
218	Chicken potpie (home recipe), baked,[13] piece (1/3 or 9-in diam. pie).	1 piece	232	57	545	23	31	11.3	10.9	5.6	42	70	232	3.0	343	3,090	.34	.31	5.5	5
	Turkey, roasted, flesh without skin:																			
219	Dark meat, piece, 2 1/2 by 1 5/8 by 1/4 in.	4 pieces	85	61	175	26	7	2.1	1.5	1.5	0	—	—	2.0	338	—	.03	.20	3.6	—
220	Light meat, piece, 4 by 2 by 1/4 in.	2 pieces	85	62	150	28	3	.9	.6	.7	0	—	—	1.0	349	—	.04	.12	9.4	—
	Light and dark meat:																			
221	Chopped or diced-----	1 cup	140	61	265	44	9	2.5	1.7	1.8	0	11	351	2.5	514	—	.07	.25	10.8	—
222	Pieces (1 slice white meat, 4 by 2 by 1/4 in with 2 slices dark meat, 2 1/2 by 1 5/8 by 1/4 in).	3 pieces	85	61	160	27	5	1.5	1.0	1.1	0	7	213	1.5	312	—	.04	.15	6.5	—
	FRUITS AND FRUIT PRODUCTS																			
	Apples, raw, unpeeled, without cores:																			
223	2 3/4-in diam. (about 3 per lb with cores).	1 apple	138	84	80	Trace	1	—	—	—	20	10	14	.4	152	120	.04	.03	.1	6
224	3 1/4 in diam (about 2 per lb with cores).	1 apple	212	84	125	Trace	1	—	—	—	31	15	21	.6	233	190	.06	.04	.2	8
225	Applejuice, bottled or canned[2]---	1 cup	248	88	120	Trace	Trace	—	—	—	30	15	22	1.5	250	—	.02	.05	.2	[2]2
	Applesauce, canned:																			
226	Sweetened-----	1 cup	255	76	230	1	Trace	—	—	—	61	10	13	1.3	166	100	.05	.03	.1	[2]3
227	Unsweetened-----	1 cup	244	89	100	Trace	Trace	—	—	—	26	10	12	1.2	190	100	.05	.02	.1	[2]2
	Apricots:																			
228	Raw, without pits (about 12 per lb with pits).	3 apricots	107	85	55	1	Trace	—	—	—	14	18	25	.5	301	2,890	.03	.04	.6	11
229	Canned in heavy sirup (halves and sirup).	1 cup	258	77	220	2	Trace	—	—	—	57	28	39	.8	604	4,490	.05	.05	1.0	10
	Dried:																			
230	Uncooked (28 large or 37 medium halves per cup).	1 cup	130	25	340	7	1	—	—	—	86	87	140	7.2	1,273	14,170	.01	.21	4.3	16
231	Cooked, unsweetened, fruit and liquid.	1 cup	250	76	215	4	1	—	—	—	54	55	88	4.5	795	7,500	.01	.13	2.5	8
232	Apricot nectar, canned-----	1 cup	251	85	145	1	Trace	—	—	—	37	23	30	.5	379	2,380	.03	.03	.5	[2]36
	Avocados, raw, whole, without skins and seeds:																			
233	California, mid- and late-winter (with skin and seed, 3 1/8-in diam.; wt. 10 oz).	1 avocado	216	74	370	5	37	5.5	22.0	3.7	13	22	91	1.3	1,303	630	.24	.43	3.5	30
234	Florida, late summer and fall (with skin and seed, 3 5/8-in diam.; wt. 1 lb).	1 avocado	304	78	390	4	33	6.7	15.7	5.3	27	30	128	1.8	1,836	880	.33	.61	4.9	43
235	Banana without peel (about 2.6 per lb with peel).	1 banana	119	76	100	1	Trace	—	—	—	26	10	31	.8	440	230	.06	.07	.8	12
236	Banana flakes-----	1 tbsp	6	3	20	Trace	Trace	—	—	—	5	2	6	.2	92	50	.01	.01	.2	Trace

(A)	(B)	(C)	(D)	(E)	(F)	(G)	(H)	(I)	(J)	(K)	(L)	(M)	(N)	(O)	(P)	(Q)	(R)	(S)
237	Blackberries, raw — 1 cup	85	85	2	1	—	—	—	19	46	27	1.3	245	290	0.04	0.06	0.6	30
238	Blueberries, raw — 1 cup	83	90	1	1	—	—	—	22	22	19	1.5	117	150	.04	.09	.7	20
	Cantaloup. See Muskmelons (item 271).																	
	Cherries:																	
239	Sour (tart), red, pitted, canned, water pack. 1 cup	88	105	2	Trace	—	—	—	26	37	32	.7	317	1,660	.07	.05	.5	12
240	Sweet, raw, without pits and stems. 10 cherries	80	45	1	Trace	—	—	—	12	15	13	.3	129	70	.03	.04	.3	7
241	Cranberry juice cocktail, bottled, sweetened. 1 cup	83	165	Trace	Trace	—	—	—	42	13	8	.8	25	Trace	.03	.03	.1	[26]81
242	Cranberry sauce, sweetened, canned, strained. 1 cup	62	405	Trace	1	—	—	—	104	17	11	.6	83	60	.03	.03	.1	6
	Dates:																	
243	Whole, without pits. 10 dates	23	220	2	Trace	—	—	—	58	47	50	2.4	518	40	.07	.08	1.8	0
244	Chopped. 1 cup	23	490	4	1	—	—	—	130	105	112	5.3	1,153	90	.16	.18	3.9	0
245	Fruit cocktail, canned, in heavy sirup. 1 cup	80	195	1	Trace	—	—	—	50	23	31	1.0	411	360	.05	.03	1.0	5
	Grapefruit:																	
	Raw, medium, 3 3/4-in diam. (about 1 lb 1 oz):																	
246	Pink or red. 1/2 grapefruit with peel[28]	89	50	1	Trace	—	—	—	13	20	20	.5	166	540	.05	.02	.2	44
247	White. 1/2 grapefruit with peel[28]	89	45	1	Trace	—	—	—	12	19	19	.5	159	10	.05	.02	.2	44
248	Canned, sections with sirup. 1 cup	81	180	2	Trace	—	—	—	45	33	36	.8	343	30	.08	.05	.5	76
	Grapefruit juice:																	
249	Raw, pink, red, or white. 1 cup	90	95	1	Trace	—	—	—	23	22	37	.5	399	(29)	.10	.05	.5	93
	Canned, white:																	
250	Unsweetened. 1 cup	89	100	1	Trace	—	—	—	24	20	35	1.0	400	20	.07	.05	.5	84
251	Sweetened. 1 cup	86	135	1	Trace	—	—	—	32	20	35	1.0	405	30	.08	.05	.5	78
	Frozen, concentrate, unsweetened:																	
252	Undiluted, 6-fl oz can. 1 can	62	300	4	1	—	—	—	72	70	124	.8	1,250	60	.29	.12	1.4	286
253	Diluted with 3 parts water by volume. 1 cup	89	100	1	Trace	—	—	—	24	25	42	.2	420	20	.10	.04	.5	96
254	Dehydrated crystals, prepared with water (1 lb yields about 1 gal). 1 cup	90	100	1	Trace	—	—	—	24	22	40	.2	412	20	.10	.05	.5	91
	Grapes, European type (adherent skin), raw:																	
255	Thompson Seedless. 10 grapes[30]	81	35	Trace	Trace	—	—	—	9	6	10	.2	87	50	.03	.02	.2	2
256	Tokay and Emperor, seeded types. 10 grapes[30]	81	40	Trace	Trace	—	—	—	10	7	11	.2	99	60	.03	.02	.2	2
	Grapejuice:																	
257	Canned or bottled. 1 cup	83	165	1	Trace	—	—	—	42	28	30	.8	293	—	.10	.05	.5	[25]Trace
	Frozen concentrate, sweetened:																	
258	Undiluted, 6-fl oz can. 1 can	53	395	1	Trace	—	—	—	100	22	32	.9	255	40	.13	.22	1.5	[31]32
259	Diluted with 3 parts water by volume. 1 cup	86	135	1	Trace	—	—	—	33	8	10	.3	85	10	.05	.08	.5	[31]10
260	Grape drink, canned. 1 cup	86	135	Trace	Trace	—	—	—	35	8	10	.3	88	10	[32].03	.03	.3	(32)
261	Lemon, raw, size 165, without peel and seeds (about 4 per lb with peels and seeds). 1 lemon	90	20	1	Trace	—	—	—	6	19	12	.4	102	10	.03	.01	.1	39
	Lemon juice:																	
262	Raw. 1 cup	91	60	1	Trace	—	—	—	20	17	24	.5	344	50	.07	.02	.2	112
263	Canned, or bottled, unsweetened. 1 cup	92	55	1	Trace	—	—	—	19	17	24	.5	344	50	.07	.02	.2	102
264	Frozen, single strength, unsweetened, 6-fl oz can. 1 can	92	40	1	Trace	—	—	—	13	13	16	.5	258	40	.05	.02	.2	81
	Lemonade concentrate, frozen:																	
265	Undiluted, 6-fl oz can. 1 can	49	425	Trace	Trace	—	—	—	112	9	13	.4	153	40	.05	.06	.7	66
266	Diluted with 4 1/3 parts water by volume. 1 cup	89	105	Trace	Trace	—	—	—	28	2	3	.1	40	10	.01	.02	.2	17

[19] Crust made with vegetable shortening and enriched flour.

[24] Also applies to pasteurized apple cider.

[25] Applies to product without added ascorbic acid. For value of product with added ascorbic acid, refer to label.

[26] Based on product with label claim of 45% of U.S. RDA in 6 fl oz.

[27] Based on product with label claim of 100% of U.S. RDA in 6 fl oz.

[28] Weight includes peel and membranes between sections. Without these parts, the weight of the edible portion is 123 g for item 246 and 118 g for item 247.

[29] For white-fleshed varieties, value is about 20 International Units (I.U.) per cup; for red-fleshed varieties, 1,080 I.U.

[30] Weight includes seeds. Without seeds, weight of the edible portion is 57 g.

[31] Applies to product without added ascorbic acid. With added ascorbic acid, based on claim that 6 fl oz of reconstituted juice contain 45% or 50% of the U.S. RDA, value in milligrams is 108 or 120 for a 6-fl oz can (item 258), 36 or 40 for 1 cup of diluted juice (item 259).

[32] For products with added thiamin and riboflavin but without added ascorbic acid, values in milligrams would be 0.60 for thiamin, 0.80 for riboflavin, and trace for ascorbic acid. For products with only ascorbic acid added, value varies with the brand. Consult the label.

(Dashes (—) denote lack of reliable data for a constituent believed to be present in measurable amount)

NUTRIENTS IN INDICATED QUANTITY

Item No. (A)	Foods, approximate measures, units, and weight (edible part unless footnotes indicate otherwise) (B)	(Grams)	Water (C) Per cent	Food energy (D) Cal- ories	Pro- tein (E) Grams	Fat (F) Grams	Fatty Acids Satu- rated (total) (G) Grams	Unsaturated Oleic (H) Grams	Lino- leic (I) Grams	Carbo- hydrate (J) Grams	Calcium (K) Milli- grams	Phos- phorus (L) Milli- grams	Iron (M) Milli- grams	Potas- sium (N) Milli- grams	Vitamin A value (O) Inter- national units	Thiamin (P) Milli- grams	Ribo- flavin (Q) Milli- grams	Niacin (R) Milli- grams	Ascorbic acid (S) Milli- grams
	FRUITS AND FRUIT PRODUCTS—Con.																		
	Limeade concentrate, frozen:																		
267	Undiluted, 6-fl oz can---------- 1 can--------	218	50	410	Trace	Trace	—	—	—	108	11	13	0.2	129	Trace	0.02	0.02	0.2	26
268	Diluted with 4 1/3 parts water by volume. 1 cup--------	247	89	100	Trace	Trace	—	—	—	27	3	3	Trace	32	Trace	Trace	Trace	Trace	6
	Limejuice:																		
269	Raw------------ 1 cup--------	246	90	65	1	Trace	—	—	—	22	22	27	.5	256	20	.05	.02	.2	79
270	Canned, unsweetened---- 1 cup--------	246	90	65	1	Trace	—	—	—	22	22	27	.5	256	20	.05	.02	.2	52
	Muskmelons, raw, with rind, with- out seed cavity:																		
271	Cantaloup, orange-fleshed (with rind and seed cavity, 5-in diam., 2 1/3 lb). 1/2 melon with rind[33]	477	91	80	2	Trace	—	—	—	20	38	44	1.1	682	9,240	.11	.08	1.6	90
272	Honeydew (with rind and seed cavity, 6 1/2-in diam., 5 1/4 lb). 1/10 melon with rind[33]	226	91	50	1	Trace	—	—	—	11	21	24	.6	374	60	.06	.04	.9	34
	Oranges, all commercial varieties, raw:																		
273	Whole, 2 5/8-in diam., without peel and seeds (about 2 1/2 per lb with peel and seeds). 1 orange-----	131	86	65	1	Trace	—	—	—	16	54	26	.5	263	260	.13	.05	.5	66
274	Sections without membranes--- 1 cup--------	180	86	90	2	Trace	—	—	—	22	74	36	.7	360	360	.18	.07	.7	90
	Orange juice:																		
275	Raw, all varieties------- 1 cup--------	248	88	110	2	Trace	—	—	—	26	27	42	.5	496	500	.22	.07	1.0	124
276	Canned, unsweetened------ 1 cup--------	249	87	120	2	Trace	—	—	—	28	25	45	1.0	496	500	.17	.05	.7	100
	Frozen concentrate:																		
277	Undiluted, 6-fl oz can---- 1 can--------	213	55	360	5	Trace	—	—	—	87	75	126	.9	1,500	1,620	.68	.11	2.8	360
278	Diluted with 3 parts water by volume. 1 cup--------	249	87	120	2	Trace	—	—	—	29	25	42	.2	503	540	.23	.03	.9	120
279	Dehydrated crystals, prepared with water (1 lb yields about 1 gal). 1 cup--------	248	88	115	1	Trace	—	—	—	27	25	40	.5	518	500	.20	.07	1.0	109
	Orange and grapefruit juice:																		
	Frozen concentrate:																		
280	Undiluted, 6-fl oz can---- 1 can--------	210	59	330	4	1	—	—	—	78	61	99	.8	1,308	800	.48	.06	2.3	302
281	Diluted with 3 parts water by volume. 1 cup--------	248	88	110	1	Trace	—	—	—	26	20	32	.2	439	270	.15	.02	.7	102
282	Papayas, raw, 1/2-in cubes------- 1 cup--------	140	89	55	1	Trace	—	—	—	14	28	22	.4	328	2,450	.06	.06	.4	78
	Peaches:																		
	Raw:																		
283	Whole, 2 1/2-in diam., peeled, pitted (about 4 per lb with peels and pits). 1 peach---	100	89	40	1	Trace	—	—	—	10	9	19	.5	202	[34]1,330	.02	.05	1.0	7
284	Sliced------------ 1 cup--------	170	89	65	1	Trace	—	—	—	16	15	32	.9	343	[34]2,260	.03	.09	1.7	12
	Canned, yellow-fleshed, solids and liquid (halves or slices):																		
285	Sirup pack----------- 1 cup--------	256	79	200	1	Trace	—	—	—	51	10	31	.8	333	1,100	.03	.05	1.5	8
286	Water pack----------- 1 cup--------	244	91	75	1	Trace	—	—	—	20	10	32	.7	334	1,100	.02	.07	1.5	7
	Dried:																		
287	Uncooked------------ 1 cup--------	160	25	420	5	1	—	—	—	109	77	187	9.6	1,520	6,240	.02	.30	8.5	8
288	Cooked, unsweetened, halves and juice. 1 cup--------	250	77	205	3	1	—	—	—	54	38	93	4.8	743	3,050	.01	.15	3.8	5

(A)	(B)		(C)	(D)	(E)	(F)	(G)	(H)	(I)	(J)	(K)	(L)	(M)	(N)	(O)	(P)	(Q)	(R)	(S)
	Frozen, sliced, sweetened:																		
289	10-oz container	1 container	77	250	1	Trace	—	—	—	64	11	37	1.4	352	1,850	0.03	0.11	2.0	[35]116
290	Cup	1 cup	77	220	1	Trace	—	—	—	57	10	33	1.3	310	1,630	.03	.10	1.8	[35]103
	Pears:																		
291	Raw, with skin, cored: Bartlett, 2 1/2-in diam. (about 2 1/2 per lb with cores and stems).	1 pear	83	100	1	1	—	—	—	25	13	18	.5	213	30	.03	.07	.2	7
292	Bosc, 2 1/2-in diam. (about 3 per lb with cores and stems).	1 pear	83	85	1	1	—	—	—	22	11	16	.4	83	30	.03	.06	.1	6
293	D'Anjou, 3-in diam. (about 2 per lb with cores and stems).	1 pear	83	120	1	1	—	—	—	31	16	22	.6	260	40	.04	.08	.2	8
294	Canned, solids and liquid, sirup pack, heavy (halves or slices).	1 cup	80	195	1	1	—	—	—	50	13	18	.5	214	10	.03	.05	.3	3
	Pineapple:																		
295	Raw, diced	1 cup	85	80	1	Trace	—	—	—	21	26	12	.8	226	110	.14	.05	.3	26
296	Canned, heavy sirup pack, solids and liquid: Crushed, chunks, tidbits	1 cup	80	190	1	Trace	—	—	—	49	28	13	.8	245	130	.20	.05	.5	18
297	Slices and liquid: Large	1 slice; 2 1/4 tbsp liquid.	80	80	Trace	Trace	—	—	—	20	12	5	.3	101	50	.08	.02	.2	7
298	Medium	1 slice; 1 1/4 tbsp liquid.	80	45	Trace	Trace	—	—	—	11	6	3	.2	56	30	.05	.01	.1	4
299	Pineapple juice, unsweetened, canned.	1 cup	86	140	1	Trace	—	—	—	34	38	23	.8	373	130	.13	.05	.5	[27]80
	Plums:																		
300	Raw, without pits: Japanese and hybrid (2 1/8-in diam., about 6 1/2 per lb with pits).	1 plum	87	30	Trace	Trace	—	—	—	8	8	12	.3	112	160	.02	.02	.3	4
301	Prune-type (1 1/2-in diam., about 15 per lb with pits).	1 plum	79	20	Trace	Trace	—	—	—	6	3	5	.1	48	80	.01	.01	.1	1
	Canned, heavy sirup pack (Italian prunes), with pits and liquid:																		
302	Cup[36]	1 cup[36]	77	215	1	1	—	—	—	56	23	26	2.3	367	3,130	.05	.05	1.0	5
303	Portion	3 plums; 2 3/4 tbsp liquid.[36]	77	110	1	1	—	—	—	29	12	13	1.2	189	1,610	.03	.03	.5	3
304	Prunes, dried, "softenized," with pits: Uncooked	4 extra large or 5 large prunes.[36]	28	110	1	Trace	—	—	—	29	22	34	1.7	298	690	.04	.07	.7	1
305	Cooked, unsweetened, all sizes, fruit and liquid.	1 cup[36]	66	255	2	1	—	—	—	67	51	79	3.8	695	1,590	.07	.15	1.5	2
306	Prune juice, canned or bottled	1 cup	80	195	1	Trace	—	—	—	49	36	51	1.8	602	—	.03	.03	1.0	5
	Raisins, seedless:																		
307	Cup, not pressed down	1 cup	18	420	4	Trace	—	—	—	112	90	146	5.1	1,106	30	.16	.12	.7	1
308	Packet, 1/2 oz (1 1/2 tbsp)	1 packet	18	40	Trace	Trace	—	—	—	11	9	14	.5	107	Trace	.02	.01	.1	Trace
	Raspberries, red:																		
309	Raw, capped, whole	1 cup	84	70	1	1	—	—	—	17	27	27	1.1	207	160	.04	.11	1.1	31
310	Frozen, sweetened, 10-oz container	1 container	74	280	2	1	—	—	—	70	37	48	1.7	284	200	.06	.17	1.7	60
	Rhubarb, cooked, added sugar:																		
311	From raw	1 cup	63	380	1	Trace	—	—	—	97	211	41	1.6	548	220	.05	.14	.8	16
312	From frozen, sweetened	1 cup	63	385	1	1	—	—	—	93	211	32	1.9	475	190	.05	.11	.5	16

[27]Based on product with label claim of 100% of U.S. RDA for item 271 and 149 g for item 272.
[33]Weight includes rind. Without rind, the weight of the edible portion is 272 g for item 272.
[34]Represents yellow-fleshed varieties. For white-fleshed varieties, value is 50 International Units (I.U.) for 1 peach, 90 I.U. for 1 cup of slices.
[35]Value represents products without added ascorbic acid. For products with added ascorbic acid, value in milligrams is 116 for a 10-oz container, 103 for 1 cup.
[36]Weight includes pits. After removal of the pits, the weight of the edible portion is 258 g for item 302, 133 g for item 303, 43 g for item 304, and 213 g for item 305.

(Dashes (—) denote lack of reliable data for a constituent believed to be present in measurable amount)

NUTRIENTS IN INDICATED QUANTITY

Item No. (A)	Foods, approximate measures, units, and weight (edible part unless footnotes indicate otherwise) (B)	Grams	Water (C) Per cent	Food energy (D) Calories	Protein (E) Grams	Fat (F) Grams	Saturated (total) (G) Grams	Unsaturated Oleic (H) Grams	Linoleic (J) Grams	Carbohydrate (I) Grams	Calcium (K) Milligrams	Phosphorus (L) Milligrams	Iron (M) Milligrams	Potassium (N) Milligrams	Vitamin A value (O) International units	Thiamin (P) Milligrams	Riboflavin (Q) Milligrams	Niacin (R) Milligrams	Ascorbic acid (S) Milligrams
	FRUITS AND FRUIT PRODUCTS—Con.																		
	Strawberries:																		
313	Raw, whole berries, capped — 1 cup	149	90	55	1	1	—	—	—	13	31	31	1.5	244	90	0.04	0.10	0.9	88
	Frozen, sweetened:																		
314	Sliced, 10-oz container — 1 container	284	71	310	1	1	—	—	—	79	40	48	2.0	318	90	.06	.17	1.4	151
315	Whole, 1-lb container (about 1 3/4 cups) — 1 container	454	76	415	2	1	—	—	—	107	59	73	2.7	472	140	.09	.27	2.3	249
316	Tangerine, raw, 2 3/8-in diam., size 176, without peel (about 4 per lb with peels and seeds) — 1 tangerine	86	87	40	1	Trace	—	—	—	10	34	15	.3	108	360	.05	.02	.1	27
317	Tangerine juice, canned, sweetened — 1 cup	249	87	125	1	Trace	—	—	—	30	44	35	.5	440	1,040	.15	.05	.2	54
318	Watermelon, raw, 4 by 8 in wedge with rind and seeds[37] (1/16 of 32 2/3-lb melon, 10 by 16 in) — 1 wedge with rind and seeds[37]	926	93	110	2	1	—	—	—	27	30	43	2.1	426	2,510	.13	.13	.9	30
	GRAIN PRODUCTS																		
	Bagel, 3-in diam.:																		
319	Egg — 1 bagel	55	32	165	6	2	0.5	0.9	0.8	28	9	43	1.2	41	30	.14	.10	1.2	0
320	Water — 1 bagel	55	29	165	6	1	.2	.4	.6	30	8	41	1.2	42	0	.15	.11	1.4	0
321	Barley, pearled, light, uncooked — 1 cup	200	11	700	16	2	.3	.2	.8	158	32	378	4.0	320	0	.24	.10	6.2	0
	Biscuits, baking powder, 2-in diam. (enriched flour, vegetable shortening):																		
322	From home recipe — 1 biscuit	28	27	105	2	5	1.2	2.0	1.2	13	34	49	.4	33	Trace	.08	.08	.7	Trace
323	From mix — 1 biscuit	28	29	90	2	3	.6	1.1	.7	15	19	65	.6	32	Trace	.09	.08	.8	Trace
324	Breadcrumbs (enriched):[38] Dry, grated — 1 cup	100	7	390	13	5	1.0	1.6	1.4	73	122	141	3.6	152	Trace	.35	.35	4.8	Trace
325	Soft. See White bread (items 349-350). Breads: Boston brown bread, canned, slice, 3 1/4 by 1/2 in.[38] — 1 slice	45	45	95	2	1	.1	.2	.2	21	41	72	.9	131	[39]0	.06	.04	.7	0
	Cracked-wheat bread (3/4 enriched wheat flour, 1/4 cracked wheat):[38]																		
326	Loaf, 1-lb — 1 loaf	454	35	1,195	39	10	2.2	3.0	3.9	236	399	581	9.5	608	Trace	1.52	1.13	14.4	Trace
327	Slice (18 per loaf) — 1 slice	25	35	65	2	1	.1	.2	.2	13	22	32	.5	34	Trace	.08	.06	.8	Trace
	French or vienna bread, enriched:[38]																		
328	Loaf, 1-lb — 1 loaf	454	31	1,315	41	14	3.2	4.7	4.6	251	195	386	10.0	408	Trace	1.80	1.10	15.0	Trace
	Slice:																		
329	French (5 by 2 1/2 by 1 in) — 1 slice	35	31	100	3	1	.2	.4	.4	19	15	30	.8	32	Trace	.14	.08	1.2	Trace
330	Vienna (4 3/4 by 4 by 1/2 in) — 1 slice	25	31	75	2	1	.1	.3	.3	14	11	21	.6	23	Trace	.10	.06	.8	Trace
	Italian bread, enriched:																		
331	Loaf, 1-lb — 1 loaf	454	32	1,250	41	4	.6	.3	1.5	256	77	349	10.0	336	0	1.80	1.10	15.0	0
332	Slice, 4 1/2 by 3 1/4 by 3/4 in. — 1 slice	30	32	85	3	Trace	Trace	Trace	.1	17	5	23	.7	22	0	.12	.07	1.0	0
	Raisin bread, enriched:[38]																		
333	Loaf, 1-lb — 1 loaf	454	35	1,190	30	13	3.0	4.7	3.9	243	322	395	10.0	1,057	Trace	1.70	1.07	10.7	Trace
334	Slice (18 per loaf) — 1 slice	25	35	65	2	1	.2	.3	.2	13	18	22	.6	58	Trace	.09	.06	.6	Trace

(A)	(B)	(C)	(D)	(E)	(F)	(G)	(H)	(I)	(J)	(K)	(L)	(M)	(N)	(O)	(P)	(Q)	(R)	(S)
	Rye Bread:																	
	American, light (2/3 enriched wheat flour, 1/3 rye flour):																	
335	Loaf, 1 lb	1 loaf	454	36	41	5	0.7	0.5	2.2	236	340	667	9.1	658	0	1.35	0.98	12.9	0
336	Slice (4 3/4 by 3 3/4 by 7/16 in).	1 slice	25	36	2	Trace	Trace	Trace	.1	13	19	37	.5	36	0	.07	.05	.7	0
	Pumpernickel (2/3 rye flour, 1/3 enriched wheat flour):																	
337	Loaf, 1 lb	1 loaf	454	34	41	5	.7	.5	2.4	241	381	1,039	11.8	2,059	0	1.30	.93	8.5	0
338	Slice (5 by 4 by 3/8 in)	1 slice	32	34	3	Trace	.1	Trace	.2	17	27	73	.8	145	0	.09	.07	.6	0
	White bread, enriched:[38]																	
	Soft-crumb type:																	
339	Loaf, 1 lb	1 loaf	454	36	39	15	3.4	5.3	4.6	229	381	440	11.3	476	Trace	1.80	1.10	15.0	Trace
340	Slice (18 per loaf)	1 slice	25	36	2	1	.2	.3	.3	13	21	24	.6	26	Trace	.10	.06	.8	Trace
341	Slice, toasted		22	25	2	1	.2	.3	.3	13	21	24	.6	26	Trace	.08	.06	.8	Trace
342	Slice (22 per loaf)	1 slice	20	36	2	1	.2	.2	.2	10	17	19	.5	21	Trace	.08	.05	.7	Trace
343	Slice, toasted		17	36	2	1	.2	.2	.2	10	17	19	.5	21	Trace	.06	.05	.7	Trace
344	Loaf, 1 1/2 lb	1 loaf	680	36	59	22	5.2	7.9	6.9	343	571	660	17.0	714	Trace	2.70	1.65	22.5	Trace
345	Slice (24 per loaf)	1 slice	28	36	2	1	.2	.3	.3	14	24	27	.7	29	Trace	.11	.07	.9	Trace
346	Slice, toasted		24	36	2	1	.2	.3	.3	14	24	27	.7	29	Trace	.09	.07	.9	Trace
347	Slice (28 per loaf)	1 slice	24	25	2	1	.2	.3	.3	12	20	23	.6	25	Trace	.10	.06	.8	Trace
348	Slice, toasted		21	25	2	1	.2	.3	.3	12	20	23	.6	25	Trace	.08	.06	.8	Trace
349	Cubes	1 cup	30	36	3	1	.3	.3	.5	15	25	29	.8	32	Trace	.12	.07	1.0	Trace
350	Crumbs	1 cup	45	36	4	1	.3	.5	.5	23	38	44	1.1	47	Trace	.18	.11	1.5	Trace
	Firm-crumb type:																	
351	Loaf, 1 lb	1 loaf	454	35	41	17	3.9	5.9	5.2	228	435	463	11.3	549	Trace	1.80	1.10	15.0	Trace
352	Slice (20 per loaf)	1 slice	23	35	2	1	.2	.3	.3	12	22	23	.6	28	Trace	.09	.06	.8	Trace
353	Slice, toasted		20	24	2	1	.2	.3	.3	12	22	23	.6	28	Trace	.07	.06	.8	Trace
354	Loaf, 2 lb	1 loaf	907	35	82	34	7.7	11.8	10.4	455	871	925	22.7	1,097	Trace	3.60	2.20	30.0	Trace
355	Slice (34 per loaf)	1 slice	27	35	2	1	.2	.3	.3	14	26	28	.7	33	Trace	.11	.06	.9	Trace
356	Slice, toasted		23	24	2	1	.2	.3	.3	14	26	28	.7	33	Trace	.09	.06	.9	Trace
	Whole-wheat bread:																	
	Soft-crumb type:[38]																	
357	Loaf, 1 lb	1 loaf	454	36	41	12	2.2	2.9	4.2	224	381	1,152	13.6	1,161	Trace	1.37	.45	12.7	Trace
357P	Slice (16 per loaf)	1 slice	28	36	3	1	.1	.2	.2	14	24	71	.8	72	Trace	.09	.03	.8	Trace
359	Slice, toasted		24	24	3	1	.1	.2	.2	14	24	71	.8	72	Trace	.07	.03	.8	Trace
	Firm-crumb type:[38]																	
360	Loaf, 1 lb	1 loaf	454	36	48	14	2.5	3.3	4.9	216	449	1,034	13.6	1,238	Trace	1.17	.54	12.7	Trace
361	Slice (18 per loaf)	1 slice	25	36	3	1	.1	.2	.2	12	25	57	.8	68	Trace	.06	.03	.7	Trace
362	Slice, toasted		21	24	3	1	.1	.2	.2	12	25	57	.8	68	Trace	.05	.03	.7	Trace
	Breakfast cereals:																	
	Hot type, cooked:																	
	Corn (hominy) grits, degermed:																	
363	Enriched	1 cup	245	87	3	Trace	Trace	Trace	.1	27	2	25	.7	27	[40]Trace	.10	.07	1.0	0
364	Unenriched	1 cup	245	87	3	Trace	Trace	Trace	.1	27	2	25	[42].2	27	[40]Trace	.05	.02	.5	0
365	Farina, quick-cooking, enriched	1 cup	245	89	3	Trace	Trace	Trace	.1	22	147	[41]113	[42]	25	0	.12	.07	1.0	0
366	Oatmeal or rolled oats	1 cup	240	87	5	2	.4	.8	.9	23	22	137	1.4	146	0	.19	.05	.2	0
367	Wheat, rolled	1 cup	240	80	5	1	—	—	—	41	19	182	1.7	202	0	.17	.07	2.2	0
368	Wheat, whole-meal	1 cup	245	88	4	1	—	—	—	23	17	127	1.2	118	0	.15	.05	1.5	0
	Ready-to-eat:																	
369	Bran flakes (40% bran), added sugar, salt, iron, vitamins.	1 cup	35	3	4	1	—	—	—	28	19	125	15.6	137	1,650	.41	.49	4.1	12
370	Bran flakes with raisins, added sugar, salt, iron, vitamins.	1 cup	50	7	4	1	—	—	—	40	28	146	16.9	154	2,350	.58	.71	5.8	18

[3] Weight includes rind and seeds. Without rind and seeds, weight of the edible portion is 426 g.
[38] Made with vegetable shortening.
[39] Applies to product made with white cornmeal. With yellow cornmeal, value is 30 International Units (I.U.).
[40] Applies to white varieties. For yellow varieties, value is 150 International Units (I.U.).
[41] Applies to products that do not contain di-sodium phosphate. If di-sodium phosphate is an ingredient, value is 162 mg.
[42] Value may range from less than 1 mg to about 8 mg depending on the brand. Consult the label.

(Dashes (–) denote lack of reliable data for a constituent believed to be present in measurable amount)

							Fatty Acids												
								Unsaturated											
Item No.	Foods, approximate measures, units, and weight (edible part unless footnotes indicate otherwise)		Water	Food energy	Protein	Fat	Saturated (total)	Oleic	Linoleic	Carbohydrate	Calcium	Phosphorus	Iron	Potassium	Vitamin A value	Thiamin	Riboflavin	Niacin	Ascorbic acid
(A)	(B)		(C)	(D)	(E)	(F)	(G)	(H)	(I)	(J)	(K)	(L)	(M)	(N)	(O)	(P)	(Q)	(R)	(S)
		Grams	Per cent	Cal- ories	Grams	Grams	Grams	Grams	Grams	Grams	Milli- grams	Milli- grams	Milli- grams	Milli- grams	Inter- national units	Milli- grams	Milli- grams	Milli- grams	Milli- grams
	GRAIN PRODUCTS—Con.																		
	Breakfast cereals—Continued																		
	Ready-to-eat—Continued																		
	Corn flakes:																		
371	Plain, added sugar, salt, iron, vitamins. 1 cup	25	4	95	2	Trace	—	—	—	21	(²)	9	0.6	30	1,180	0.29	0.35	2.9	9
372	Sugar-coated, added salt, iron, vitamins. 1 cup	40	2	155	2	Trace	—	—	—	37	1	10	1.0	27	1,880	.46	.56	4.6	14
373	Corn, puffed, plain, added sugar, salt, iron, vita- mins. 1 cup	20	4	80	2	1	—	—	—	16	4	18	2.3	—	940	.23	.28	2.3	7
374	Corn, shredded, added sugar, salt, iron, thiamin, niacin. 1 cup	25	3	95	2	Trace	—	—	—	22	1	10	.6	—	0	.11	.05	.5	0
375	Oats, puffed, added sugar, salt, minerals, vitamins. 1 cup	25	3	100	3	1	—	—	—	19	44	102	2.9	—	1,180	.29	.35	2.9	9
	Rice, puffed:																		
376	Plain, added iron, thiamin, niacin. 1 cup	15	4	60	1	Trace	—	—	—	13	3	14	.3	15	0	.07	.01	.7	0
377	Presweetened, added salt, iron, vitamins. 1 cup	28	3	115	1	0	—	—	—	26	3	14	⁴⁴1.1	43	1,250	.38	.43	5.0	⁴515
378	Wheat flakes, added sugar, salt, iron, vitamins. 1 cup	30	4	105	3	Trace	—	—	—	24	12	83	(⁴⁴)	81	1,410	.35	.42	3.5	11
	Wheat, puffed:																		
379	Plain, added iron, thiamin, niacin. 1 cup	15	3	55	2	Trace	—	—	—	12	4	48	.6	51	0	.08	.03	1.2	0
380	Presweetened, added salt, iron, vitamins. 1 cup	38	3	140	3	Trace	—	—	—	33	7	52	⁴1.6	63	1,680	.50	.57	6.7	⁴520
381	Wheat, shredded, plain. 1 oblong biscuit or 1/2 cup spoon-size biscuits.	25	7	90	2	1	—	—	—	20	11	97	.9	87	0	.06	.03	1.1	0
382	Wheat germ, without salt and sugar, toasted. 1 tbsp.	6	4	25	2	1	—	—	—	3	3	70	.5	57	10	.11	.05	.3	1
383	Buckwheat flour, light, sifted. 1 cup	98	12	340	6	1	0.2	0.4	0.4	78	11	86	1.0	314	0	.08	.04	.4	0
384	Bulgur, canned, seasoned. 1 cup	135	56	245	8	4	—	—	—	44	27	263	1.9	151	0	.08	.05	4.1	0
	Cake icings. See Sugars and Sweets (items 532-536).																		
	Cakes made from cake mixes with enriched flour:⁴⁶																		
	Angelfood:																		
385	Whole cake (9 3/4-in diam. tube cake). 1 cake	635	34	1,645	36	1	—	—	—	377	603	756	2.5	381	0	.37	.95	3.6	0
386	Piece, 1/12 of cake. 1 piece	53	34	135	3	Trace	—	—	—	32	50	63	.2	32	0	.03	.08	.3	0
	Coffeecake:																		
387	Whole cake (7 3/4 by 5 5/8 by 1 1/4 in). 1 cake	430	30	1,385	27	41	11.7	16.3	8.8	225	262	748	6.9	469	690	.82	.91	7.7	1
388	Piece, 1/6 of cake. 1 piece	72	30	230	5	7	2.0	2.7	1.5	38	44	125	1.2	78	120	.14	.15	1.3	Trace
	Cupcakes, made with egg, milk, 2 1/2-in diam.:																		
389	Without icing. 1 cupcake	25	26	90	1	3	.8	1.2	.7	14	40	59	.3	21	40	.05	.05	.4	Trace
390	With chocolate icing. 1 cupcake	36	22	130	2	5	2.0	1.6	.6	21	47	71	.4	42	60	.05	.06	.4	Trace
	Devil's food cake with chocolate icing:																		
391	Whole, 2 layer cake (8- or 9-in diam.). 1 cake	1,107	24	3,755	49	136	50.0	44.9	17.0	645	653	1,162	16.6	1,439	1,660	1.06	1.65	10.1	1
392	Piece, 1/16 of cake. 1 piece	69	24	235	3	8	3.1	2.8	1.1	40	41	72	1.0	90	100	.07	.10	.6	Trace
393	Cupcake, 2 1/2-in diam. 1 cupcake	35	24	120	2	4	1.6	1.4	.5	20	21	37	.5	46	50	.03	.05	.3	Trace

(A)	(B)	(C)	(D)	(E)	(F)	(G)	(H)	(I)	(J)	(K)	(L)	(M)	(N)	(O)	(P)	(Q)	(R)	(S)
	Gingerbread:																	
394	Whole cake (8-in square)------ 1 cake------	570	1,575	18	39	9.7	16.6	10.0	291	513	570	8.6	1,562	Trace	0.84	1.00	7.4	Trace
395	Piece, 1/9 of cake----- 1 piece----	63	175	2	4	1.1	1.8	1.1	32	57	63	.9	173	Trace	.09	.11	.8	Trace
	White, 2 layer with chocolate icing:																	
396	Whole cake (8- or 9-in diam.)-- 1 cake------	1,140	4,000	44	122	48.2	46.4	20.0	716	1,129	2,041	11.4	1,322	680	1.50	1.77	12.5	2
397	Piece, 1/16 of cake--------- 1 piece----	71	250	3	8	3.0	2.9	1.2	45	70	127	.7	82	40	.09	.11	.8	Trace
	Yellow, 2 layer with chocolate icing:																	
398	Whole cake (8- or 9-in diam.)-- 1 cake------	1,108	3,735	45	125	47.8	47.8	20.3	638	1,008	2,017	12.2	1,208	1,550	1.24	1.67	10.6	2
399	Piece, 1/16 of cake-------- 1 piece----	69	235	3	8	3.0	3.0	1.3	40	63	126	.8	75	100	.08	.10	.7	Trace
	Cakes made from home recipes using enriched flour:[47]																	
	Boston cream pie with custard filling:																	
400	Whole cake (8-in diam.)------ 1 cake------	825	2,490	41	78	23.0	30.1	15.2	412	553	833	8.2	[48]734	1,730	1.04	1.27	9.6	2
401	Piece, 1/12 of cake--------- 1 piece----	69	210	3	6	1.9	2.5	1.3	34	46	70	.7	[48]61	140	.09	.11	.8	Trace
	Fruitcake, dark:																	
402	Loaf, 1-lb (7 1/2 by 2 by 1 1/2 in). 1 loaf------	454	1,720	22	69	14.4	33.5	14.8	271	327	513	11.8	2,250	540	.72	.73	4.9	2
	Plain, sheet cake:																	
403	Slice, 1/30 of loaf----- 1 slice----	15	55	1	2	.5	1.1	.5	9	11	17	.4	74	20	.02	.02	.2	Trace
	Without icing:																	
404	Whole cake (9-in square)----- 1 cake------	777	2,830	35	108	29.5	44.4	23.9	434	497	793	8.5	[48]614	1,320	1.21	1.40	10.2	2
405	Piece, 1/9 of cake---------- 1 piece----	86	315	4	12	3.3	4.9	2.6	48	55	88	.9	[48]68	150	.13	.15	1.1	Trace
	With uncooked white icing:																	
406	Whole cake (9-in square)----- 1 cake------	1,096	4,020	37	129	42.2	49.5	24.4	694	548	822	8.2	[48]669	2,190	1.22	1.47	10.2	2
407	Piece, 1/9 of cake---------- 1 piece----	121	445	4	14	4.7	5.5	2.7	77	61	91	.8	[48]74	240	.14	.16	1.1	Trace
	Pound:[49]																	
408	Loaf, 8 1/2 by 3 1/2 by 3 1/4 in. 1 loaf------	565	2,725	31	170	42.9	73.1	39.6	273	107	418	7.9	345	1,410	.90	.99	7.3	0
409	Slice, 1/17 of loaf----- 1 slice----	33	160	2	10	2.5	4.3	2.3	16	6	24	.5	20	80	.05	.06	.4	0
	Spongecake:																	
410	Whole cake (9 3/4-in diam. tube cake). 1 cake------	790	2,345	60	45	13.1	15.8	5.7	427	237	885	13.4	687	3,560	1.10	1.64	7.4	Trace
411	Piece, 1/12 of cake--------- 1 piece----	66	195	5	4	1.1	1.3	.5	36	20	74	1.1	57	300	.09	.14	.6	Trace
	Cookies made with enriched flour:[50][51]																	
	Brownies with nuts:																	
	Home-prepared, 1 3/4 by 1 3/4 by 7/8 in:																	
412	From home recipe------ 1 brownie----	20	95	1	6	1.5	3.0	1.2	10	8	30	.4	38	40	.04	.03	.2	Trace
413	From commercial recipe----- 1 brownie----	20	85	1	4	.9	1.4	1.3	13	9	27	.4	34	20	.03	.02	.2	Trace
414	Frozen, with chocolate icing,[52] 1 1/2 by 1 3/4 by 7/8 in. 1 brownie----	25	105	1	5	2.0	2.2	.7	15	10	31	.4	44	50	.03	.03	.2	Trace
	Chocolate chip:																	
415	Commercial, 2 1/4-in diam., 3/8 in thick. 4 cookies----	42	200	2	9	2.8	2.9	2.2	29	16	48	1.0	56	50	.10	.17	.9	Trace
416	From home recipe, 2 1/3-in diam. 4 cookies----	40	205	2	12	3.5	4.5	2.9	24	14	40	.8	47	40	.06	.06	.5	Trace
417	Fig bars, square (1 5/8 by 1 5/8 by 3/8 in) or rectangular (1 1/2 by 1 3/4 by 1/2 in). 4 cookies----	56	200	2	3	.8	1.2	.7	42	44	34	1.0	111	60	.04	.14	.9	Trace
418	Gingersnaps, 2-in diam., 1/4 in thick. 4 cookies----	28	90	2	2	.7	1.0	.6	22	20	13	.7	129	20	.08	.06	.7	0
419	Macaroons, 2 3/4-in diam., 1/4 in thick. 2 cookies----	38	180	2	9	—	—	—	25	10	32	.3	176	0	.02	.06	.2	0
420	Oatmeal with raisins, 2 5/8-in diam., 1/4 in thick. 4 cookies----	52	235	3	8	2.0	3.3	2.0	38	11	53	1.4	192	30	.15	.10	1.0	Trace

[43]Value varies with the brand. Consult the label.
[44]Value varies with the brand. Consult the label.
[45]Applies to product with added ascorbic acid. Without added ascorbic acid, value is trace.
[46]Excepting angelfood cake, cakes were made from mixes containing vegetable shortening; icings, with butter.
[47]Excepting spongecake, vegetable shortening used for cake portion; butter, for icing. If butter or margarine used for cake portion, vitamin A values would be higher.
[48]Applies to product made with a sodium aluminum-sulfate type baking powder. With a low-sodium type baking powder containing potassium, value would be about twice the amount shown.
[49]Equal weights of flour, sugar, eggs, and vegetable shortening.
[50]Products are commercial unless otherwise specified.
[51]Made with enriched flour and vegetable shortening except for macaroons which do not contain flour or shortening.
[52]Icing made with butter.

(Dashes (—) denote lack of reliable data for a constituent believed to be present in measurable amount)

Item No. (A)	Foods, approximate measures, units, and weight (edible part unless footnotes indicate otherwise) (B)		Water (C)	Food energy (D)	Protein (E)	Fat (F)	Fatty Acids			Carbohydrate (J)	Calcium (K)	Phosphorus (L)	Iron (M)	Potassium (N)	Vitamin A value (O)	Thiamin (P)	Riboflavin (Q)	Niacin (R)	Ascorbic acid (S)
							Saturated (total) (G)	Unsaturated Oleic (H)	Linoleic (I)										
		Grams	Percent	Calories	Grams	Grams	Grams	Grams	Grams	Grams	Milligrams	Milligrams	Milligrams	Milligrams	International units	Milligrams	Milligrams	Milligrams	Milligrams

GRAIN PRODUCTS—Con.

Cookies made with enriched flour[50][51]—Continued

Item	Food	Measure	Grams	Water	Energy	Protein	Fat	Sat	Oleic	Lino	Carb	Ca	P	Fe	K	Vit A	Thiamin	Ribo	Niacin	Asc
421	Plain, prepared from commercial chilled dough, 2 1/2-in diam., 1/4 in thick.	4 cookies	48	5	240	2	12	3.0	5.2	2.9	31	17	35	0.6	23	30	0.10	0.08	0.9	0
422	Sandwich type (chocolate or vanilla), 1 3/4-in diam., 3/8 in thick.	4 cookies	40	2	200	2	9	2.2	3.9	2.2	28	10	96	.7	15	0	.06	.10	.7	0
423	Vanilla wafers, 1 3/4-in diam., 1/4 in thick.	10 cookies	40	3	185	2	6	—	—	—	30	16	25	.6	29	50	.10	.09	.8	0
	Cornmeal:																			
424	Whole-ground, unbolted, dry form.	1 cup	122	12	435	11	5	.5	1.0	2.5	90	24	312	2.9	346	[53]620	.46	.13	2.4	0
425	Bolted (nearly whole-grain), dry form.	1 cup	122	12	440	11	4	.5	.9	2.1	91	21	272	2.2	303	[53]590	.37	.10	2.3	0
	Degermed, enriched:																			
426	Dry form	1 cup	138	12	500	11	2	.2	.4	.9	108	8	137	4.0	166	[53]610	.61	.36	4.8	0
427	Cooked	1 cup	240	88	120	3	Trace	Trace	.1	.2	26	2	34	1.0	38	[53]140	.14	.10	1.2	0
	Degermed, unenriched:																			
428	Dry form	1 cup	138	12	500	11	2	.2	.4	.9	108	8	137	1.5	166	[53]610	.19	.07	1.4	0
429	Cooked	1 cup	240	88	120	3	Trace	Trace	.1	.2	26	2	34	.5	38	[53]140	.05	.02	.2	0
	Crackers:[38]																			
430	Graham, plain, 2 1/2-in square	2 crackers	14	6	55	1	1	.3	.5	.3	10	6	21	.5	55	0	.02	.08	.5	0
431	Rye wafers, whole-grain, 1 7/8 by 3 1/2 in.	2 wafers	13	6	45	2	Trace	—	—	—	10	7	50	.5	78	0	.04	.03	.2	0
432	Saltines, made with enriched flour.	4 crackers or 1 packet	11	4	50	1	1	.3	.5	.4	8	2	10	.5	13	0	.05	.05	.4	0
	Danish pastry (enriched flour), plain without fruit or nuts:[54]																			
433	Packaged ring, 12 oz	1 ring	340	22	1,435	25	80	24.3	31.7	16.5	155	170	371	6.1	381	1,050	.97	1.01	8.6	Trace
434	Round piece, about 4 1/4-in diam. by 1 in.	1 pastry	65	22	275	5	15	4.7	6.1	3.2	30	33	71	1.2	73	200	.18	.19	1.7	Trace
435	Ounce	1 oz	28	22	120	2	7	2.0	2.7	1.4	13	14	31	.5	32	90	.08	.08	.7	Trace
	Doughnuts, made with enriched flour:[38]																			
436	Cake type, plain, 2 1/2-in diam., 1 in high.	1 doughnut	25	24	100	1	5	1.2	2.0	1.1	13	10	48	.4	23	20	.05	.05	.4	Trace
437	Yeast-leavened, glazed, 3 3/4-in diam., 1 1/4 in high.	1 doughnut	50	26	205	3	11	3.3	5.8	3.3	22	16	33	.6	34	25	.10	.10	.8	0
	Macaroni, enriched, cooked (cut lengths, elbows, shells):																			
	Firm stage (hot):																			
438		1 cup	130	64	190	7	1	—	—	—	39	14	85	1.4	103	0	.23	.13	1.8	0
	Tender stage:																			
439	Cold macaroni	1 cup	105	73	115	4	Trace	—	—	—	24	8	53	.9	64	0	.15	.08	1.2	0
440	Hot macaroni	1 cup	140	73	155	5	1	—	—	—	32	11	70	1.3	85	0	.20	.11	1.5	0
	Macaroni (enriched) and cheese:																			
441	Canned[55]	1 cup	240	80	230	9	10	4.2	3.1	1.4	26	199	182	1.0	139	260	.12	.24	1.0	Trace
442	From home recipe[56]	1 cup	200	58	430	17	22	8.9	8.8	2.9	40	362	322	1.8	240	860	.20	.40	1.8	Trace
	Muffins made with enriched flour:[38]																			
	From home recipe:																			
443	Blueberry, 2 3/8-in diam., 1 1/2 in high.	1 muffin	40	39	110	3	4	1.1	1.4	.7	17	34	53	.6	46	90	.09	.10	.7	Trace
444	Bran	1 muffin	40	35	105	3	4	1.2	1.4	.8	17	57	162	1.5	172	90	.07	.10	1.7	Trace
445	Corn (enriched degermed cornmeal and flour), 2 3/8-in diam., 1 1/2 in high.	1 muffin	40	33	125	3	4	1.2	1.6	.9	19	42	68	.7	54	[57]120	.10	.10	.7	Trace

(A)	(B)	Measure	Weight (g)	(C)	(D)	(E)	(F)	(G)	(H)	(I)	(J)	(K)	(L)	(M)	(N)	(O)	(P)	(Q)	(R)	(S)
446	Plain, 3-in diam., 1 1/2 in high.	1 muffin	40	38	120	3	4	1.0	1.7	1.0	17	42	60	0.6	50	40	0.09	0.12	0.9	Trace
447	From mix, egg, milk: Corn, 2 3/8-in diam., 1 1/2 in high.[56]	1 muffin	40	30	130	3	4	1.2	1.7	.9	20	96	152	.6	44	[57]100	.08	.09	.7	Trace
448	Noodles (egg noodles), enriched, cooked.	1 cup	160	71	200	7	2				37	16	94	1.4	70	110	.22	.13	1.9	0
449	Noodles, chow mein, canned	1 cup	45	1	220	6	11				26	—	—	—	—	—	—	—	—	—
450	Pancakes, (4-in diam.):[38] Buckwheat, made from mix (with buckwheat and enriched flours), egg and milk added.	1 cake	27	58	55	2	2	.8	.9	.4	6	59	91	.4	66	60	.04	.05	.2	Trace
451	Plain: Made from home recipe using enriched flour.	1 cake	27	50	60	2	2	.5	.8	.5	9	27	38	.4	33	30	.06	.07	.5	Trace
452	Made from mix with enriched flour, egg and milk added.	1 cake	27	51	60	2	2	.7	.7	.3	9	58	70	.3	42	70	.04	.06	.2	Trace
	Pies, piecrust made with enriched flour, vegetable shortening (9-in diam.):																			
	Apple:																			
453	Whole	1 pie	945	48	2,420	21	105	27.0	44.5	25.2	360	76	208	6.6	756	280	1.06	.79	9.3	9
454	Sector, 1/7 of pie	1 sector	135	48	345	3	15	3.9	6.4	3.6	51	11	30	.9	108	40	.15	.11	1.3	2
	Banana cream:																			
455	Whole	1 pie	910	54	2,010	41	85	26.7	33.2	16.2	279	601	746	7.3	1,847	2,280	.77	1.51	7.0	9
456	Sector, 1/7 of pie	1 sector	130	54	285	6	12	3.8	4.7	2.3	40	86	107	1.0	264	330	.11	.22	1.0	1
	Blueberry:																			
457	Whole	1 pie	945	51	2,285	23	102	24.8	43.7	25.1	330	104	217	9.5	614	280	1.03	.80	10.0	28
458	Sector, 1/7 of pie	1 sector	135	51	325	3	15	3.5	6.2	3.6	47	15	31	1.4	88	40	.15	.11	1.4	4
	Cherry:																			
459	Whole	1 pie	945	47	2,465	25	107	28.2	45.0	25.3	363	132	236	6.6	992	4,160	1.09	.84	9.8	Trace
460	Sector, 1/7 of pie	1 sector	135	47	350	4	15	4.0	6.4	3.6	52	19	34	.9	142	590	.16	.12	1.4	Trace
	Custard:																			
461	Whole	1 pie	910	58	1,985	56	101	33.9	38.5	17.5	213	874	1,028	8.2	1,247	2,090	.79	1.92	5.6	0
462	Sector, 1/7 of pie	1 sector	130	58	285	8	14	4.8	5.5	2.5	30	125	147	1.2	178	300	.11	.27	.8	0
	Lemon meringue:																			
463	Whole	1 pie	840	47	2,140	31	86	26.1	33.8	16.4	317	118	412	6.7	420	1,430	.61	.84	5.2	25
464	Sector, 1/7 of pie	1 sector	120	47	305	4	12	3.7	4.8	2.3	45	17	59	1.0	60	200	.09	.12	.7	4
	Mince:																			
465	Whole	1 pie	945	43	2,560	24	109	28.0	45.9	25.2	389	265	359	13.3	1,682	20	.96	.86	9.8	9
466	Sector, 1/7 of pie	1 sector	135	43	365	3	16	4.0	6.6	3.6	56	38	51	1.9	240	Trace	.14	.12	1.4	1
	Peach:																			
467	Whole	1 pie	945	48	2,410	24	101	24.8	43.7	25.1	361	95	274	8.5	1,408	6,900	1.04	.97	14.0	28
468	Sector, 1/7 of pie	1 sector	135	48	345	3	14	3.5	6.2	3.6	52	14	39	1.2	201	990	.15	.14	2.0	4
	Pecan:																			
469	Whole	1 pie	825	20	3,450	42	189	27.8	101.0	44.2	423	388	850	25.6	1,015	1,320	1.80	.95	6.9	Trace
470	Sector, 1/7 of pie	1 sector	118	20	495	6	27	4.0	14.4	6.3	61	55	122	3.7	145	190	.26	.14	1.0	Trace
	Pumpkin:																			
471	Whole	1 pie	910	59	1,920	36	102	37.4	37.5	16.6	223	464	628	7.3	1,456	22,480	.78	1.27	7.0	Trace
472	Sector, 1/7 of pie	1 sector	130	59	275	5	15	5.4	5.4	3.2	32	66	90	1.0	208	3,210	.11	.18	1.0	Trace
473	Piecrust (home recipe) made with enriched flour and vegetable shortening, baked.	1 pie shell, 9-in diam.	180	15	900	11	60	14.8	26.1	14.9	79	25	90	3.1	89	0	.47	.40	5.0	0
474	Piecrust mix with enriched flour and vegetable shortening, 10-oz pkg. prepared and baked.	Piecrust for 2-crust pie, 9-in diam.	320	19	1,485	20	93	22.7	39.7	23.4	141	131	272	6.1	179	0	1.07	.79	9.9	0

[38] Made with vegetable shortening.
[50] Products are commercial unless otherwise specified.
[51] Made with enriched flour and vegetable shortening except for macaroons which do not contain flour or shortening.
[53] Applies to yellow varieties; white varieties contain only a trace.
[54] Made with corn oil.
[55] Contains vegetable shortening and butter.
[56] Made with regular margarine.
[57] Applies to product made with yellow cornmeal.
[58] Made with enriched degermed cornmeal and enriched flour.

(Dashes (—) denote lack of reliable data for a constituent believed to be present in measurable amount)

NUTRIENTS IN INDICATED QUANTITY

Item No. (A)	Foods, approximate measures, units, and weight (edible part unless footnotes indicate otherwise) (B)	(Grams)	Water (C) Percent	Food energy (D) Calories	Protein (E) Grams	Fat (F) Grams	Fatty Acids Saturated (total) (G) Grams	Unsaturated Oleic (H) Grams	Unsaturated Linoleic (I) Grams	Carbohydrate (J) Grams	Calcium (K) Milligrams	Phosphorus (L) Milligrams	Iron (M) Milligrams	Potassium (N) Milligrams	Vitamin A value (O) International units	Thiamin (P) Milligrams	Riboflavin (Q) Milligrams	Niacin (R) Milligrams	Ascorbic acid (S) Milligrams
	GRAIN PRODUCTS—Con.																		
475	Pizza (cheese) baked, 4 3/4-in sector; 1/8 of 12-in diam. pie.[15] 1 sector	60	45	145	6	4	1.7	1.5	0.6	22	86	89	1.1	67	230	0.16	0.18	1.6	4
	Popcorn, popped:																		
476	Plain, large kernel 1 cup	6	4	25	1	Trace	Trace	.1	.2	5	1	17	.2	—	—	—	.01	.1	0
477	With oil (coconut) and salt added, large kernel. 1 cup	9	3	40	1	2	1.5	.2	.2	5	1	19	.2	—	—	—	.01	.2	0
478	Sugar coated 1 cup	35	4	135	2	1	.5	.2	.4	30	2	47	.5	—	—	—	.02	.4	0
	Pretzels, made with enriched flour:																		
479	Dutch, twisted, 2 3/4 by 2 5/8 in. 1 pretzel	16	5	60	2	1	—	—	—	12	4	21	.2	21	0	.05	.04	.7	0
480	Thin, twisted, 3 1/4 by 2 1/4 by 1/4 in. 10 pretzels	60	5	235	6	3	—	—	—	46	13	79	.9	78	0	.20	.15	2.5	0
481	Stick, 2 1/4 in long 10 pretzels	3	5	10	Trace	Trace	—	—	—	2	1	4	Trace	4	0	.01	.01	.1	0
	Rice, white, enriched:																		
482	Instant, ready-to-serve, hot 1 cup	165	73	180	4	Trace	Trace	Trace	Trace	40	5	31	1.3	—	0	.21	(59)	1.7	0
	Long grain:																		
483	Raw 1 cup	185	12	670	12	1	.2	.2	.2	149	44	174	5.4	170	0	.81	.06	6.5	0
484	Cooked, served hot 1 cup	205	73	225	4	Trace	.1	.1	.1	50	21	57	1.8	57	0	.23	.02	2.1	0
	Parboiled:																		
485	Raw 1 cup	185	10	685	14	1	.2	.1	.1	150	111	370	5.4	278	0	.81	.07	6.5	0
486	Cooked, served hot 1 cup	175	73	185	4	Trace	.1	.1	.1	41	33	100	1.4	75	0	.19	.02	2.1	0
	Rolls, enriched:[38] Commercial:																		
487	Brown-and-serve (12 per 12-oz pkg.), browned. 1 roll	26	27	85	2	2	.4	.7	.5	14	20	23	.5	25	Trace	.10	.06	.9	Trace
488	Cloverleaf or pan, 2 1/2-in diam., 2 in high. 1 roll	28	31	85	2	2	.4	.6	.4	15	21	24	.5	27	Trace	.11	.07	.9	Trace
489	Frankfurter and hamburger (8 per 11 1/2-oz pkg.). 1 roll	40	31	120	3	2	.5	.8	.6	21	30	34	.8	38	Trace	.16	.10	1.3	Trace
490	Hard, 3 3/4-in diam., 2 in high. 1 roll	50	25	155	5	2	.4	.6	.5	30	24	46	1.2	49	Trace	.20	.12	1.7	Trace
491	Hoagie or submarine, 11 1/2 by 3 by 2 1/2 in. 1 roll	135	31	390	12	4	.9	1.4	1.4	75	58	115	3.0	122	Trace	.54	.32	4.5	Trace
	From home recipe:																		
492	Cloverleaf, 2 1/2-in diam., 2 in high. 1 roll	35	26	120	3	3	.8	1.1	.7	20	16	36	.7	41	30	.12	.12	1.2	Trace
	Spaghetti, enriched, cooked:																		
493	Firm stage, "al dente," served hot. 1 cup	130	64	190	7	1	—	—	—	39	14	85	1.4	103	0	.23	.13	1.8	0
494	Tender stage, served hot. 1 cup	140	73	155	5	1	—	—	—	32	11	70	1.3	85	0	.20	.11	1.5	0
	Spaghetti (enriched) in tomato sauce with cheese:																		
495	From home recipe 1 cup	250	77	260	9	9	2.0	5.4	.7	37	80	135	2.3	408	1,080	.25	.18	2.3	13
496	Canned 1 cup	250	80	190	6	2	.5	.3	.4	39	40	88	2.8	303	930	.35	.28	4.5	10
	Spaghetti (enriched) with meat balls and tomato sauce:																		
497	From home recipe 1 cup	248	70	330	19	12	3.3	6.3	3.3	39	124	236	3.7	665	1,590	.25	.30	4.0	22
498	Canned 1 cup	250	78	260	12	10	2.2	3.3	3.9	29	53	113	3.3	245	1,000	.15	.18	2.3	5
499	Toaster pastries 1 pastry	50	12	200	3	6	—	—	—	36	[6]54	[6]67	1.9	[6]74	500	.16	.17	2.1	(60)
	Waffles, made with enriched flour, 7-in diam.:[38]																		
500	From home recipe 1 waffle	75	41	210	7	7	2.3	2.8	1.4	28	85	130	1.3	109	250	.17	.23	1.4	Trace
501	From mix, egg and milk added. 1 waffle	75	42	205	7	8	2.8	2.9	1.2	27	179	257	1.0	146	170	.14	.22	.9	Trace

(A)	(B)	(C)	(D)	(E)	(F)	(G)	(H)	(I)	(J)	(K)	(L)	(M)	(N)	(O)	(P)	(Q)	(R)	(S)
	Wheat flours:																	
	All-purpose or family flour, enriched:																	
502	Sifted, spooned — 1 cup	12	420	12	1	0.2	0.1	0.5	88	18	100	3.3	109	0	0.74	0.46	6.1	0
503	Unsifted, spooned — 1 cup	12	455	13	1	.2	.1	.5	95	20	109	3.6	119	0	.80	.50	6.6	0
504	Cake or pastry flour, enriched, sifted, spooned. — 1 cup	12	350	7	1	.1	.1	.3	76	16	70	2.8	91	0	.61	.38	5.1	0
505	Self-rising, enriched, unsifted, spooned. — 1 cup	12	440	12	1	.2	.1	.5	93	331	583	3.6	—	0	.80	.50	6.6	0
506	Whole-wheat, from hard wheats, stirred. — 1 cup	12	400	16	2	.4	.2	1.0	85	49	446	4.0	444	0	.66	.14	5.2	0
	LEGUMES (DRY), NUTS, SEEDS; RELATED PRODUCTS																	
	Almonds, shelled:																	
507	Chopped (about 130 almonds) — 1 cup	5	775	24	70	5.6	47.7	12.8	25	304	655	6.1	1,005	0	.31	1.20	4.6	Trace
508	Slivered, not pressed down (about 115 almonds). — 1 cup	5	690	21	62	5.0	42.2	11.3	22	269	580	5.4	889	0	.28	1.06	4.0	Trace
	Beans, dry:																	
	Common varieties as Great Northern, navy, and others:																	
	Cooked, drained:																	
509	Great Northern — 1 cup	69	210	14	1	—	—	—	38	90	266	4.9	749	0	.25	.13	1.3	0
510	Pea (navy) — 1 cup	69	225	15	1	—	—	—	40	95	281	5.1	790	0	.27	.13	1.3	0
	Canned, solids and liquid:																	
	White with—																	
511	Frankfurters (sliced) — 1 cup	71	365	19	18	2.4	2.8	.6	32	94	303	4.8	668	330	.18	.15	3.3	Trace
512	Pork and tomato sauce — 1 cup	71	310	16	7	4.3	5.0	1.1	48	138	235	4.6	536	330	.20	.08	1.5	5
513	Pork and sweet sauce — 1 cup	66	385	15	12	—	—	—	54	161	291	5.9	—	—	.15	—	1.3	—
514	Red kidney — 1 cup	76	230	15	1	—	—	—	42	74	278	4.6	673	10	.13	.10	1.5	—
515	Lima, cooked, drained — 1 cup	64	260	16	1	—	—	—	49	55	293	5.9	1,163	—	.25	.11	1.3	—
516	Blackeye peas, dry, cooked (with residual cooking liquid). — 1 cup	80	190	13	1	—	—	—	35	43	238	3.3	573	30	.40	.10	1.0	—
517	Brazil nuts, shelled (6-8 large kernels). — 1 oz	5	185	4	19	4.8	6.2	7.1	3	53	196	1.0	203	Trace	.27	.03	.5	—
518	Cashew nuts, roasted in oil — 1 cup	5	785	24	64	12.9	36.8	10.2	41	53	522	5.3	650	140	.60	.35	2.5	—
	Coconut meat, fresh:																	
519	Piece, about 2 by 2 in — 1 piece	51	155	2	16	14.0	.9	.3	4	6	43	.8	115	0	.02	.01	.2	1
520	Shredded or grated, not pressed down. — 1 cup	51	275	3	28	24.8	1.6	.5	8	10	76	1.4	205	0	.04	.02	.4	2
521	Filberts (hazelnuts), chopped (about 80 kernels). — 1 cup	6	730	14	72	5.1	55.2	7.3	19	240	388	3.9	810	—	.53	—	1.0	Trace
522	Lentils, whole, cooked — 1 cup	72	210	16	Trace	13.7	33.0	20.7	39	50	238	4.2	498	40	.14	.12	1.2	0
523	Peanuts, roasted in oil, salted (whole, halves, chopped). — 1 cup	2	840	37	72	13.7	33.0	20.7	27	107	577	3.0	971	—	.46	.19	24.8	0
524	Peanut butter — 1 tbsp	2	95	4	8	1.5	3.7	2.3	3	9	61	.3	100	—	.02	.02	2.4	0
525	Peas, split, dry, cooked — 1 cup	70	230	16	1	—	—	—	42	22	178	3.4	592	80	.30	.18	1.8	—
526	Pecans, chopped or pieces (about 120 large halves). — 1 cup	3	810	11	84	7.2	50.5	20.0	17	86	341	2.8	712	150	1.01	.15	1.1	2
527	Pumpkin and squash kernels, dry, hulled. — 1 cup	4	775	41	65	11.8	23.5	27.5	21	71	1,602	15.7	1,386	100	.34	.27	3.4	—
528	Sunflower seeds, dry, hulled — 1 cup	5	810	35	69	8.2	13.7	43.2	29	174	1,214	10.3	1,334	70	2.84	.33	7.8	—
	Walnuts:																	
	Black:																	
529	Chopped or broken kernels — 1 cup	3	785	26	74	6.3	13.3	45.7	19	Trace	713	7.5	575	380	.28	.14	.9	—
530	Ground (finely) — 1 cup	3	500	16	47	4.0	8.5	29.2	12	Trace	456	4.8	368	240	.18	.09	.6	—
531	Persian or English, chopped (about 60 halves). — 1 cup	4	780	18	77	8.4	11.8	42.2	19	119	456	3.7	540	40	.40	.16	1.1	2

19 Crust made with vegetable shortening and enriched flour.
38 Made with vegetable shortening.
55 Product may or may not be enriched with riboflavin. Consult the label.
59 Product may or may not be enriched with riboflavin. Consult the label.
6 Value varies with the brand. Consult the label.

(Dashes (—) denote lack of reliable data for a constituent believed to be present in measurable amount)

							Fatty Acids												
								Unsaturated											
Item No.	Foods, approximate measures, units, and weight (edible part unless footnotes indicate otherwise)		Water	Food energy	Protein	Fat	Saturated (total)	Oleic	Lino-leic	Carbo-hydrate	Calcium	Phos-phorus	Iron	Potas-sium	Vitamin A value	Thiamin	Ribo-flavin	Niacin	Ascorbic acid
(A)	(B)	Grams	Per cent (C)	Cal-ories (D)	Grams (E)	Grams (F)	Grams (G)	Grams (H)	Grams (I)	Grams (J)	Milli-grams (K)	Milli-grams (L)	Milli-grams (M)	Milli-grams (N)	Inter-national units (O)	Milli-grams (P)	Milli-grams (Q)	Milli-grams (R)	Milli-grams (S)

SUGARS AND SWEETS

Item No.	Food	Grams	Water	Food energy	Protein	Fat	Sat.	Oleic	Lino.	Carb.	Ca	P	Fe	K	Vit A	Thiamin	Ribo.	Niacin	Asc.
	Cake icings:																		
	Boiled, white:																		
532	Plain------- 1 cup-------	94	18	295	1	0	0	0	0	75	2	2	Trace	17	0	Trace	0.03	Trace	0
533	With coconut------- 1 cup-------	166	15	605	3	13	11.0	.9	Trace	124	10	50	0.8	277	0	0.02	.07	0.3	0
	Uncooked:																		
534	Chocolate made with milk and butter. 1 cup	275	14	1,035	9	38	23.4	11.7	1.0	185	165	305	3.3	536	580	.06	.28	.6	1
535	Creamy fudge from mix and water. 1 cup	245	15	830	7	16	5.1	6.7	3.1	183	96	218	2.7	238	Trace	.05	.20	.7	Trace
536	White------- 1 cup-------	319	11	1,200	2	21	12.7	5.1	.5	260	48	38	Trace	57	860	Trace	.06	Trace	Trace
	Candy:																		
537	Caramels, plain or chocolate--- 1 oz---	28	8	115	1	3	1.6	1.1	.1	22	42	35	.4	54	Trace	.01	.05	.1	Trace
	Chocolate:																		
538	Milk, plain------- 1 oz---	28	1	145	2	9	5.5	3.0	.3	16	65	65	.3	109	80	.02	.10	.1	Trace
539	Semisweet, small pieces (60 per oz). 1 cup or 6-oz pkg	170	1	860	7	61	36.2	19.8	1.7	97	51	255	4.4	553	30	.02	.14	.9	0
540	Chocolate-coated peanuts--- 1 oz---	28	1	160	5	12	4.0	4.7	2.1	11	33	84	.4	143	Trace	.10	.05	2.1	Trace
541	Fondant, uncoated (mints, candy corn, other). 1 oz	28	8	105	Trace	1	.1	.3	.1	25	4	2	.3	1	0	Trace	Trace	Trace	0
542	Fudge, chocolate, plain--- 1 oz---	28	8	115	1	3	1.3	1.4	.6	21	22	24	.3	42	Trace	.01	.03	.1	Trace
543	Gum drops------- 1 oz---	28	12	100	Trace	Trace	—	—	—	25	2	Trace	.1	1	0	0	Trace	Trace	0
544	Hard------- 1 oz---	28	1	110	0	Trace	—	—	—	28	6	2	.5	1	0	0	0	0	0
545	Marshmallows------- 1 oz---	28	17	90	1	Trace	—	—	—	23	5	2	.5	2	0	0	Trace	Trace	0
	Chocolate-flavored beverage powders (about 4 heaping tsp per oz):																		
546	With nonfat dry milk--- 1 oz---	28	2	100	5	1	.5	.3	Trace	20	167	155	.5	227	10	.04	.21	.2	1
547	Without milk--- 1 oz---	28	1	100	1	1	.4	.2	Trace	25	9	48	.6	142	—	.01	.03	.1	0
548	Honey, strained or extracted--- 1 tbsp---	21	17	65	Trace	0	0	0	0	17	1	1	.1	11	0	Trace	.01	.1	Trace
549	Jams and preserves--- 1 tbsp---	20	29	55	Trace	Trace	—	—	—	14	4	2	.2	18	Trace	Trace	.01	Trace	Trace
550	Jellies--- 1 tbsp---	18	29	50	Trace	Trace	—	—	—	13	4	1	.3	14	Trace	Trace	.01	Trace	1
551	--- 1 packet---	14	29	40	Trace	Trace	—	—	—	10	3	1	.1	12	Trace	Trace	Trace	Trace	Trace
552	--- 1 packet---	14	29	40	Trace	Trace	—	—	—	10	3	1	.2	11	Trace	Trace	.01	Trace	1
	Syrups:																		
	Chocolate-flavored syrup or topping:																		
553	Thin type--- 1 fl oz or 2 tbsp---	38	32	90	1	1	.5	.3	Trace	24	6	35	.6	106	Trace	.01	.03	.2	0
554	Fudge type--- 1 fl oz or 2 tbsp---	38	25	125	2	5	3.1	1.6	.1	20	48	60	.5	107	60	.02	.08	.2	Trace
	Molasses, cane:																		
555	Light (first extraction)--- 1 tbsp---	20	24	50	—	—	—	—	—	13	33	9	.9	183	—	.01	.01	Trace	—
556	Blackstrap (third extraction)- 1 tbsp---	20	24	45	—	—	—	—	—	11	137	17	3.2	585	—	.02	.04	.4	—
557	Sorghum--- 1 tbsp---	21	23	55	—	—	—	—	—	14	35	5	2.6	—	—	—	.02	Trace	—
558	Table blends, chiefly corn, light and dark. 1 tbsp---	21	24	60	0	0	0	0	0	15	9	3	.8	1	0	0	0	0	0
	Sugars:																		
559	Brown, pressed down--- 1 cup---	220	2	820	0	0	0	0	0	212	187	42	7.5	757	0	.02	.07	.4	0
	White:																		
560	Granulated--- 1 cup---	200	1	770	0	0	0	0	0	199	0	0	.2	6	0	0	0	0	0
561	--- 1 tbsp---	12	1	45	0	0	0	0	0	12	0	0	Trace	Trace	0	0	0	0	0
562	--- 1 packet---	6	1	23	0	0	0	0	0	6	0	0	Trace	Trace	0	0	0	0	0
563	Powdered, sifted, spooned into cup. 1 cup---	100	1	385	0	0	0	0	0	100	0	0	.1	3	0	0	0	0	0

VEGETABLE AND VEGETABLE PRODUCTS

(A)	(B)	grams	(C)	(D)	(E)	(F)	(G)	(H)	(I)	(J)	(K)	(L)	(M)	(N)	(O)	(P)	(Q)	(R)	(S)
	Asparagus, green: Cooked, drained: Cuts and tips, 1 1/2- to 2-in lengths:																		
564	From raw——— 1 cup	145	94	30	3	Trace	—	—	—	5	30	73	0.9	265	1,310	0.23	0.26	2.0	38
565	From frozen—— 1 cup	180	93	40	6	Trace	—	—	—	6	40	115	2.2	396	1,530	.25	.23	1.8	41
	Spears, 1/2-in diam. at base:																		
566	From raw——— 4 spears	60	94	10	1	Trace	—	—	—	2	13	30	.4	110	540	.10	.11	.8	16
567	From frozen—— 4 spears	60	92	15	2	Trace	—	—	—	2	13	40	.7	143	470	.10	.08	.7	16
568	Canned, spears, 1/2-in diam. at base. 4 spears	80	93	15	2	Trace	—	—	—	3	15	42	1.5	133	640	.05	.08	.6	12
	Beans: Lima, immature seeds, frozen, cooked, drained:																		
569	Thick-seeded types (Fordhooks) 1 cup	170	74	170	10	Trace	—	—	—	32	34	153	2.9	724	390	.12	.09	1.7	29
570	Thin-seeded types (baby limas) 1 cup	180	69	210	13	Trace	—	—	—	40	63	227	4.7	709	400	.16	.09	2.2	22
	Snap: Green: Cooked, drained:																		
571	From raw (cuts and French style). 1 cup	125	92	30	2	Trace	—	—	—	7	63	46	.8	189	680	.09	.11	.6	15
	From frozen:																		
572	Cuts——— 1 cup	135	92	35	2	Trace	—	—	—	8	54	43	.9	205	780	.09	.12	.5	7
573	French style—— 1 cup	130	92	35	2	Trace	—	—	—	8	49	39	1.2	177	690	.08	.10	.4	9
574	Canned, drained solids (cuts). 1 cup	135	92	30	2	Trace	—	—	—	7	61	34	2.0	128	630	.04	.07	.4	5
	Yellow or wax: Cooked, drained:																		
575	From raw (cuts and French style). 1 cup	125	93	30	2	Trace	—	—	—	6	63	46	.8	189	290	.09	.11	.6	16
576	From frozen (cuts)—— 1 cup	135	92	35	2	Trace	—	—	—	8	47	42	.9	221	140	.09	.11	.5	8
577	Canned, drained solids (cuts). 1 cup	135	92	30	2	Trace	—	—	—	7	61	34	2.0	128	140	.04	.07	.4	7
	Beans, mature. See Beans, dry (items 509-515) and Blackeye peas, dry (item 516).																		
	Bean sprouts (mung):																		
578	Raw——— 1 cup	105	89	35	4	Trace	—	—	—	7	20	67	1.4	234	20	.14	.14	.8	20
579	Cooked, drained—— 1 cup	125	91	35	4	Trace	—	—	—	7	21	60	1.1	195	30	.11	.13	.9	8
	Beets: Cooked, drained, peeled:																		
580	Whole beets, 2-in diam.— 2 beets	100	91	30	1	Trace	—	—	—	7	14	23	.5	208	20	.03	.04	.3	6
581	Diced or sliced——— 1 cup	170	91	55	2	Trace	—	—	—	12	24	39	.9	354	30	.05	.07	.5	10
	Canned, drained solids:																		
582	Whole beets, small—— 1 cup	160	89	60	2	Trace	—	—	—	14	30	29	1.1	267	30	.02	.05	.2	5
583	Diced or sliced—— 1 cup	170	89	65	2	Trace	—	—	—	15	32	31	1.2	284	30	.02	.05	.2	5
584	Beet greens, leaves and stems, cooked, drained. 1 cup	145	94	25	2	Trace	—	—	—	5	144	36	2.8	481	7,400	.10	.22	.4	22
	Blackeye peas, immature seeds, cooked and drained:																		
585	From raw——— 1 cup	165	72	180	13	1	—	—	—	30	40	241	3.5	625	580	.50	.18	2.3	28
586	From frozen—— 1 cup	170	66	220	15	1	—	—	—	40	43	286	4.8	573	290	.68	.19	2.4	15
	Broccoli, cooked, drained: From raw:																		
587	Stalk, medium size——— 1 stalk	180	91	45	6	1	—	—	—	8	158	112	1.4	481	4,500	.16	.36	1.4	162
588	Stalks cut into 1/2-in pieces- 1 cup	155	91	40	5	Trace	—	—	—	7	136	96	1.2	414	3,880	.14	.31	1.2	140
	From frozen:																		
589	Stalk, 4 1/2 to 5 in long——— 1 stalk	30	91	10	1	Trace	—	—	—	1	12	17	.2	66	570	.02	.03	.2	22
590	Chopped——— 1 cup	185	92	50	5	1	—	—	—	9	100	104	1.3	392	4,810	.11	.22	.9	105
591	Brussels sprouts, cooked, drained: From raw, 7-8 sprouts (1 1/4- to 1 1/2-in diam.). 1 cup	155	88	55	7	1	—	—	—	10	50	112	1.7	423	810	.12	.22	1.2	135
592	From frozen—— 1 cup	155	89	50	5	Trace	—	—	—	10	33	95	1.2	457	880	.12	.16	.9	126

(Dashes (—) denote lack of reliable data for a constituent believed to be present in measurable quantity)

Item No. (A)	Food, approximate measures, units, and weight (edible part unless footnotes indicate otherwise) (B)		Water (C) Per cent	Food energy (D) Cal-ories	Pro-tein (E) Grams	Fat (F) Grams	Satu-rated (total) (G) Grams	Unsaturated Oleic (H) Grams	Lino-leic (I) Grams	Carbo-hydrate (J) Grams	Calcium (K) Milli-grams	Phos-phorus (L) Milli-grams	Iron (M) Milli-grams	Potas-sium (N) Milli-grams	Vitamin A value (O) Inter-national units	Thiamin (P) Milli-grams	Ribo-flavin (Q) Milli-grams	Niacin (R) Milli-grams	Ascorbic acid (S) Milli-grams
		Grams																	
	VEGETABLE AND VEGETABLE PRODUCTS—Con.																		
	Cabbage:																		
	Common varieties:																		
	Raw:																		
593	Coarsely shredded or sliced - 1 cup	70	92	15	1	Trace	—	—	—	4	34	20	0.3	163	90	0.04	0.04	0.2	33
594	Finely shredded or chopped - 1 cup	90	92	20	1	Trace	—	—	—	5	44	26	.4	210	120	.05	.05	.3	42
595	Cooked, drained - 1 cup	145	94	30	2	Trace	—	—	—	6	64	29	.4	236	190	.06	.06	.4	48
596	Red, raw, coarsely shredded or - 1 cup	70	90	20	1	Trace	—	—	—	5	29	25	.6	188	30	.06	.04	.3	43
597	Savoy, raw, coarsely shredded or sliced - 1 cup	70	92	15	2	Trace	—	—	—	3	47	38	.6	188	140	.04	.06	.2	39
598	Cabbage, celery (also called pe-tsai or wongbok), raw, 1-in pieces - 1 cup	75	95	10	1	Trace	—	—	—	2	32	30	.5	190	110	.04	.03	.5	19
599	Cabbage, white mustard (also called bokchoy or pakchoy), cooked, drained - 1 cup	170	95	25	2	Trace	—	—	—	4	252	56	1.0	364	5,270	.07	.14	1.2	26
	Carrots:																		
	Raw, without crowns and tips, scraped:																		
600	Whole, 7 1/2 by 1 1/8 in, or strips, 2 1/2 to 3 in long - 1 carrot or 18 strips	72	88	30	1	Trace	—	—	—	7	27	26	.5	246	7,930	.04	.04	.4	6
601	Grated - 1 cup	110	88	45	1	Trace	—	—	—	11	41	40	.8	375	12,100	.07	.06	.7	9
602	Cooked (crosswise cuts), drained - 1 cup	155	91	50	1	Trace	—	—	—	11	51	43	.9	344	16,280	.08	.08	.8	9
	Canned:																		
603	Sliced, drained solids - 1 cup	155	91	45	1	Trace	—	—	—	10	47	34	1.1	186	23,250	.03	.05	.6	3
604	Strained or junior (baby food) - 1 oz (1 3/4 to 2 tbsp)	28	92	10	Trace	Trace	—	—	—	2	7	6	.1	51	3,690	.01	.01	.1	1
	Cauliflower:																		
605	Raw, chopped - 1 cup	115	91	31	3	Trace	—	—	—	6	29	64	1.3	339	70	.13	.12	.8	90
	Cooked, drained:																		
606	From raw (flower buds) - 1 cup	125	93	30	3	Trace	—	—	—	5	26	53	.9	258	80	.11	.10	.8	69
607	From frozen (flowerets) - 1 cup	180	94	30	3	Trace	—	—	—	6	31	68	.9	373	50	.07	.09	.7	74
	Celery, Pascal type, raw:																		
608	Stalk, large outer, 8 by 1 1/2 in, at root end - 1 stalk	40	94	5	Trace	Trace	—	—	—	2	16	11	.1	136	110	.01	.01	.1	4
609	Pieces, diced - 1 cup	120	94	20	1	Trace	—	—	—	5	47	34	.4	409	320	.04	.04	.4	11
	Collards, cooked, drained:																		
610	From raw (leaves without stems) - 1 cup	190	90	65	7	1	—	—	—	10	357	99	1.5	498	14,820	.21	.38	2.3	144
611	From frozen (chopped) - 1 cup	170	90	50	5	1	—	—	—	10	299	87	1.7	401	11,560	.10	.24	1.0	56
	Corn, sweet:																		
	Cooked, drained:																		
612	From raw, ear 5 by 1 3/4 in - 1 ear[61]	140	74	70	2	1	—	—	—	16	2	69	.5	151	[62]310	.09	.08	1.1	7
	From frozen:																		
613	Ear, 5 in long - 1 ear[61]	229	73	120	4	1	—	—	—	27	4	121	1.0	291	[62]440	.18	.10	2.1	9
614	Kernels - 1 cup	165	77	130	5	1	—	—	—	31	5	120	1.3	304	[62]580	.15	.10	2.5	8
	Canned:																		
615	Cream style - 1 cup	256	76	210	5	2	—	—	—	51	8	143	1.5	248	[62]840	.08	.13	2.6	13
	Whole kernel:																		
616	Vacuum pack - 1 cup	210	76	175	5	1	—	—	—	43	6	153	1.1	204	[62]740	.06	.13	2.3	11
617	Wet pack, drained solids - 1 cup	165	76	140	4	1	—	—	—	33	8	81	.8	160	[62]580	.05	.08	1.5	7
	Cowpeas. See Blackeye peas. (Items 585-586).																		
	Cucumber slices, 1/8 in thick (large, 2 1/8-in diam.; small, 1 3/4-in diam.):																		
618	With peel - 6 large or 8 small slices	28	95	5	Trace	Trace	—	—	—	1	7	8	.3	45	70	.01	.01	.1	3

NUTRIENTS IN INDICATED QUANTITY

(A)	(B)	(g)	(C)	(D)	(E)	(F)	(G)	(H)	(I)	(J)	(K)	(L)	(M)	(N)	(O)	(P)	(Q)	(R)	(S)
619	Without peel — 6 1/2 large or 9 small pieces.	28	96	5	Trace	Trace	—	—	—	1	5	5	0.1	45	Trace	0.01	0.01	0.1	3
620	Dandelion greens, cooked, drained — 1 cup	105	90	35	2	1	—	—	—	7	147	44	1.9	244	12,290	.14	.17	—	19
621	Endive, curly (including escarole), raw, small pieces — 1 cup	50	93	10	1	Trace	—	—	—	2	41	27	.9	147	1,650	.04	.07	.3	5
	Kale, cooked, drained:																		
622	From raw (leaves without stems and midribs) — 1 cup	110	88	45	5	1	—	—	—	7	206	64	1.8	243	9,130	.11	.20	1.8	102
623	From frozen (leaf style) — 1 cup	130	91	40	4	1	—	—	—	7	157	62	1.3	251	10,660	.08	.20	.9	49
	Lettuce, raw:																			
	Butterhead, as Boston types:																			
624	Head, 5-in diam. — 1 head	220	95	25	2	Trace	—	—	—	4	57	42	3.3	430	1,580	.10	.10	.5	13
625	Leaves — 1 outer or 2 inner or 3 heart leaves.	15	95	Trace	Trace	Trace	—	—	—	Trace	5	4	.3	40	150	.01	.01	Trace	1
	Crisphead, as Iceberg:																			
626	Head, 6-in diam. — 1 head	567	96	70	5	1	—	—	—	16	108	118	2.7	943	1,780	.32	.32	1.6	32
627	Wedge, 1/4 of head — 1 wedge	135	96	20	1	Trace	—	—	—	4	27	30	.7	236	450	.08	.08	.4	8
628	Pieces, chopped or shredded — 1 cup	55	96	5	1	Trace	—	—	—	2	11	12	.3	96	180	.03	.03	.2	3
629	Looseleaf (bunching varieties including romaine or cos), chopped or shredded pieces — 1 cup	55	94	10	1	Trace	—	—	—	2	37	14	.8	145	1,050	.03	.04	.2	10
630	Mushrooms, raw, sliced or chopped — 1 cup	70	90	20	2	Trace	—	—	—	3	4	81	.6	290	Trace	.07	.32	2.9	2
631	Mustard greens, without stems and midribs, cooked, drained — 1 cup	140	93	30	3	1	—	—	—	6	193	45	2.5	308	8,120	.11	.20	.8	67
632	Okra pods, 3 by 5/8 in, cooked — 10 pods	106	91	30	2	Trace	—	—	—	6	98	43	.5	184	520	.14	.19	1.0	21
	Onions:																			
	Mature:																			
	Raw:																			
633	Chopped — 1 cup	170	89	65	3	Trace	—	—	—	15	46	61	.9	267	[68][71]Trace	.05	.07	.3	17
634	Sliced — 1 cup	115	89	45	2	Trace	—	—	—	10	31	41	.6	181	[68][71]Trace	.03	.05	.2	12
635	Cooked (whole or sliced), drained — 1 cup	210	92	60	3	Trace	—	—	—	14	50	61	.8	231	[68][71]Trace	.06	.06	.4	15
636	Young green, bulb (3/8 in diam.) and white portion of top. — 6 onions	30	88	15	Trace	Trace	—	—	—	3	12	12	.2	69	Trace	.02	.01	.1	8
637	Parsley, raw, chopped — 1 tbsp	4	85	Trace	Trace	Trace	—	—	—	Trace	7	2	.2	25	300	Trace	.01	Trace	6
638	Parsnips, cooked (diced or 2-in lengths) — 1 cup	155	82	100	2	1	—	—	—	23	70	96	.9	587	50	.11	.12	.2	16
	Peas, green:																			
	Canned:																			
639	Whole, drained solids — 1 cup	170	77	150	8	1	—	—	—	29	44	129	3.2	163	1,170	.15	.10	1.4	14
640	Strained (baby food) — 1 oz (1 3/4 to 2 tbsp.)	28	86	15	1	Trace	—	—	—	3	3	18	.3	28	140	.02	.03	.4	3
641	Frozen, cooked, drained — 1 cup	160	82	110	8	Trace	—	—	—	19	30	138	3.0	216	960	.43	.14	2.7	21
642	Peppers, hot, red, without seeds, dried (ground chili powder, added seasonings). — 1 tsp	2	9	5	Trace	Trace	—	—	—	1	5	4	.3	20	1,300	Trace	.02	.2	Trace
	Peppers, sweet (about 5 per lb, whole), stem and seeds removed:																			
643	Raw — 1 pod	74	93	15	1	Trace	—	—	—	4	7	16	.5	157	310	.06	.06	.4	94
644	Cooked, boiled, drained — 1 pod	73	95	15	1	Trace	—	—	—	3	7	12	.4	109	310	.05	.05	.4	70
	Potatoes, cooked:																			
645	Baked, peeled after baking (about 2 per lb, raw) — 1 potato	156	75	145	4	Trace	—	—	—	33	14	101	1.1	782	Trace	.15	.07	2.7	31
	Boiled (about 3 per lb, raw):																			
646	Peeled after boiling — 1 potato	137	80	105	3	Trace	—	—	—	23	10	72	.8	556	Trace	.12	.05	2.0	22
647	Peeled before boiling — 1 potato	135	83	90	3	Trace	—	—	—	20	8	57	.7	385	Trace	.12	.05	1.6	22
	French-fried, strip, 2 to 3 1/2 in long:																			
648	Prepared from raw — 10 strips	50	45	135	2	7	1.7	1.2	3.3	18	8	56	.7	427	Trace	.07	.04	1.6	11
649	Frozen, oven heated — 10 strips	50	53	110	2	4	1.1	.8	2.1	17	5	43	.9	326	Trace	.07	.01	1.3	11
650	Hashed brown, prepared from frozen — 1 cup	155	56	345	3	18	4.6	3.2	9.0	45	28	78	1.9	439	Trace	.11	.03	1.6	12
	Mashed, prepared from—																			
	Raw:																			
651	Milk added — 1 cup	210	83	135	4	2	.7	.4	Trace	27	50	103	.8	548	40	.17	.11	2.1	21

[67] Weight includes cob. Without cob, weight is 77 g for item 612, 126 g for item 613.
[68] Based on yellow varieties. For white varieties, value is trace.
[69] Weight includes refuse of outer leaves and core. Without these parts, weight is 163 g.
[70] Weight includes core. Without core, weight is 539 g.
[71] Value based on white-fleshed varieties. For yellow-fleshed varieties, value in International Units (I.U.) is 70 for item 633, 50 for item 634, and 80 for item 635.

(Dashes (—) denote lack of reliable data for a constituent believed to be present in measurable amount)

NUTRIENTS IN INDICATED QUANTITY

Item No.	Foods, approximate measures, units, and weight (edible part unless footnotes indicate otherwise)		Grams	Water (Percent)	Food energy (Calories)	Protein (Grams)	Fat (Grams)	Fatty Acids Saturated (total) (Grams)	Unsaturated Oleic (Grams)	Unsaturated Linoleic (Grams)	Carbohydrate (Grams)	Calcium (Milligrams)	Phosphorus (Milligrams)	Iron (Milligrams)	Potassium (Milligrams)	Vitamin A value (International units)	Thiamin (Milligrams)	Riboflavin (Milligrams)	Niacin (Milligrams)	Ascorbic acid (Milligrams)
(A)	(B)			(C)	(D)	(E)	(F)	(G)	(H)	(I)	(J)	(K)	(L)	(M)	(N)	(O)	(P)	(Q)	(R)	(S)
	VEGETABLE AND VEGETABLE PRODUCTS—Con.																			
	Potatoes, cooked—Continued																			
	Mashed, prepared from—Continued																			
	Raw—Continued																			
652	Milk and butter added	1 cup	210	80	195	4	9	5.6	2.3	0.2	26	50	101	0.8	525	360	0.17	0.11	2.1	19
653	Dehydrated flakes (without milk), water, milk, butter, and salt added.	1 cup	210	79	195	4	7	3.6	2.1	.2	30	65	99	.6	601	270	.08	.08	1.9	11
654	Potato chips, 1 3/4 by 2 1/2 in oval cross section.	10 chips	20	2	115	1	8	2.1	1.4	4.0	10	8	28	.4	226	Trace	.04	.01	1.0	3
655	Potato salad, made with cooked salad dressing.	1 cup	250	76	250	7	7	2.0	2.7	1.3	41	80	160	1.5	798	350	.20	.18	2.8	28
656	Pumpkin, canned	1 cup	245	90	80	2	1	—	—	—	19	61	64	1.0	588	15,680	.07	.12	1.5	12
657	Radishes, raw (prepackaged) stem ends, rootlets cut off.	4 radishes	18	95	5	Trace	Trace	—	—	—	1	5	6	.2	58	Trace	.01	.01	.1	5
658	Sauerkraut, canned, solids and liquid.	1 cup	235	93	40	2	Trace	—	—	—	9	85	42	1.2	329	120	.07	.09	.5	33
	Southern peas. See Blackeye peas (items 585-586).																			
	Spinach:																			
659	Raw, chopped	1 cup	55	91	15	2	Trace	—	—	—	2	51	28	1.7	259	4,460	.06	.11	.3	28
	Cooked, drained:																			
660	From raw	1 cup	180	92	40	5	1	—	—	—	6	167	68	4.0	583	14,580	.13	.25	.9	50
	From frozen:																			
661	Chopped	1 cup	205	92	45	6	1	—	—	—	8	232	90	4.3	683	16,200	.14	.31	.8	39
662	Leaf	1 cup	190	92	45	6	1	—	—	—	7	200	84	4.8	688	15,390	.15	.27	1.0	53
663	Canned, drained solids	1 cup	205	91	50	6	1	—	—	—	7	242	53	5.3	513	16,400	.04	.25	.6	29
	Squash, cooked:																			
664	Summer (all varieties), diced, drained.	1 cup	210	96	30	2	Trace	—	—	—	7	53	53	.8	296	820	.11	.17	1.7	21
665	Winter (all varieties), baked, mashed.	1 cup	205	81	130	4	1	—	—	—	32	57	98	1.6	945	8,610	.10	.27	1.4	27
	Sweetpotatoes:																			
	Cooked (raw, 5 by 2 in; about 2 1/2 per lb):																			
666	Baked in skin, peeled	1 potato	114	64	160	2	1	—	—	—	37	46	66	1.0	342	9,230	.10	.08	.8	25
667	Boiled in skin, peeled	1 potato	151	71	170	3	1	—	—	—	40	48	71	1.1	367	11,940	.14	.09	.9	26
668	Candied, 2 1/2 by 2-in piece	1 piece	105	60	175	1	3	2.0	.8	.1	36	39	45	.9	200	6,620	.06	.04	.4	11
	Canned:																			
669	Solid pack (mashed)	1 cup	255	72	275	5	1	—	—	—	63	64	105	2.0	510	19,890	.13	.10	1.5	36
670	Vacuum pack, piece 2 3/4 by 1 in.	1 piece	40	72	45	1	Trace	—	—	—	10	10	16	.3	80	3,120	.02	.02	.2	6
	Tomatoes:																			
671	Raw, 2 3/5-in diam. (3 per 12 oz pkg.).	1 tomato[66]	135	94	25	1	Trace	—	—	—	6	16	33	.6	300	1,110	.07	.05	.9	[67]28
672	Canned, solids and liquid	1 cup	241	94	50	2	Trace	—	—	—	10	[68]14	46	1.2	523	2,170	.12	.07	1.7	41
673	Tomato catsup	1 cup	273	69	290	5	1	—	—	—	69	60	137	2.2	991	3,820	.25	.19	4.4	41
674		1 tbsp	15	69	15	Trace	Trace	—	—	—	4	3	8	.1	54	210	.01	.01	.2	2
	Tomato juice, canned:																			
675	Cup	1 cup	243	94	45	2	Trace	—	—	—	10	17	44	2.2	552	1,940	.12	.07	1.9	39
676	Glass (6 fl oz)	1 glass	182	94	35	2	Trace	—	—	—	8	13	33	1.6	413	1,460	.09	.05	1.5	29
677	Turnips, cooked, diced	1 cup	155	94	35	1	Trace	—	—	—	8	54	37	.6	291	Trace	.06	.08	.5	34
	Turnip greens, cooked, drained:																			
678	From raw (leaves and stems)	1 cup	145	94	30	3	Trace	—	—	—	5	252	49	1.5	246	8,270	.15	.33	.7	68
679	From frozen (chopped)	1 cup	165	93	40	4	Trace	—	—	—	6	195	64	2.6	—	11,390	.08	.15	.7	31
680	Vegetables, mixed, frozen, cooked	1 cup	182	83	115	6	1	—	—	—	24	46	115	2.4	348	9,010	.22	.13	2.0	15

MISCELLANEOUS ITEMS

(A)	(B)	(C)	(D)	(E)	(F)	(G)	(H)	(I)	(J)	(K)	(L)	(M)	(N)	(O)	(P)	(Q)	(R)	(S)
	Baking powders for home use:																	
	Sodium aluminum sulfate:																	
681	With monocalcium phosphate monohydrate — 1 tsp — 3.0	2	5	Trace	Trace	0	0	0	1	58	87	—	5	0	0	0	0	0
682	With monocalcium phosphate monohydrate, calcium sulfate — 1 tsp — 2.9	1	5	Trace	Trace	0	0	0	1	183	45	—	—	0	0	0	0	0
683	Straight phosphate — 1 tsp — 3.8	2	5	Trace	Trace	0	0	0	1	239	359	—	6	0	0	0	0	0
684	Low sodium — 1 tsp — 4.3	2	5	Trace	Trace	0	0	0	2	207	314	—	471	0	0	0	0	0
685	Barbecue sauce — 1 cup — 250	81	230	4	17	2.2	4.3	10.0	20	53	50	2.0	435	900	.03	.03	.8	13
686	Beverages, alcoholic: Beer — 12 fl oz — 360	92	150	1	0	0	0	0	14	18	108	Trace	90	—	.01	.11	2.2	—
	Gin, rum, vodka, whisky:																	
687	80-proof — 1 1/2-fl oz jigger — 42	67	95	—	—	0	0	0	Trace				1					
688	86-proof — 1 1/2-fl oz jigger — 42	64	105	—	—	0	0	0	Trace				1					
689	90-proof — 1 1/2-fl oz jigger — 42	62	110	—	—	0	0	0	Trace				1					
	Wines:																	
690	Dessert — 3 1/2-fl oz glass — 103	77	140	Trace	0	0	0	0	8	8	10	.4	77	—	.01	.02	.2	—
691	Table — 3 1/2-fl oz glass — 102	86	85	Trace	0	0	0	0	4	9			94	—	Trace	.01	.1	—
	Beverages, carbonated, sweetened, nonalcoholic:																	
692	Carbonated water — 12 fl oz — 366	92	115	0	0	0	0	0	25	—	—	—	—	0	0	0	0	0
693	Cola type — 12 fl oz — 369	90	145	0	0	0	0	0	37	—	—	—	—	0	0	0	0	0
694	Fruit-flavored sodas and Tom Collins mixer — 12 fl oz — 372	88	170	0	0	0	0	0	45	—	—	—	—	0	0	0	0	0
695	Ginger ale — 12 fl oz — 366	92	115	0	0	0	0	0	29	—	—	—	0	0	0	0	0	0
696	Root beer — 12 fl oz — 370	90	150	0	0	0	0	0	39	—	—	—	0	0	0	0	0	0
	Chili powder. See Peppers, hot, red (item 642).																	
	Chocolate:																	
697	Bitter or baking — 1 oz — 28	2	145	3	15	8.9	4.9	.4	8	22	109	1.9	235	20	.01	.07	.4	0
	Semisweet, see Candy, chocolate (item 539).																	
698	Gelatin, dry — 1 7-g envelope — 7	13	25	6	Trace	0	0	0	0	—	—	—	—	—	—	—	—	—
699	Gelatin dessert prepared with gelatin dessert powder and water — 1 cup — 240	84	140	4	0	0	0	0	34	—	—	—	—	—	—	—	—	—
700	Mustard, prepared, yellow — 1 tsp or individual serving pouch or cup — 5	80	5	Trace	Trace	—	—	—	Trace	4	4	.1	7	—	—	—	—	—
	Olives, pickled, canned:																	
701	Green — 4 medium or 3 extra large or 2 giant.[69] — 16	78	15	Trace	2	.2	1.2	.1	Trace	8	2	.2	7	40	—	—	—	—
702	Ripe, Mission — 3 small or 2 large[69] — 10	73	15	Trace	2	.2	1.2	.1	Trace	9	1	.1	2	10	Trace	Trace	—	—
	Pickles, cucumber:																	
703	Dill, medium, whole, 3 3/4 in long, 1 1/4-in diam — 1 pickle — 65	93	5	Trace	Trace	—	—	—	1	17	14	.7	130	70	Trace	.01	Trace	4
704	Fresh-pack, slices 1 1/2-in diam, 1/4-in thick — 2 slices — 15	79	10	Trace	Trace	—	—	—	3	5	4	.3		20	Trace	Trace	Trace	1
705	Sweet, gherkin, small, whole, about 2 1/2 in long, 3/4-in diam — 1 pickle — 15	61	20	Trace	Trace	—	—	—	5	2	2	.2		10	Trace	Trace	Trace	1
706	Relish, finely chopped, sweet — 1 tbsp — 15	63	20	Trace	Trace	—	—	—	5	3	2	.1		—	Trace	Trace	Trace	—
	Popcorn. See items 476-478.																	
707	Popsicle, 3-fl oz size — 1 popsicle — 95	80	70	0	0	0	0	0	18	0	—	Trace	—	0	0	0	0	0

[66] Weight includes cores and stem ends. Without these parts, weight is 123 g.

[67] Based on year-round average. For tomatoes marketed from November through May, value is about 12 mg; from June through October, 32 mg.

[68] Applies to product with calcium salts added. Value for products with calcium salts added may be as much as 63 mg for whole tomatoes, 241 mg for cut forms.

[69] Weight includes pits. Without pits, weight is 13 g for item 701, 9 g for item 702.

(Dashes (—) denote lack of reliable data for a constituent believed to be present in measurable amount)

						NUTRIENTS IN INDICATED QUANTITY												
							Fatty Acids											
						Satu-	Unsaturated											
Item No.	Foods, approximate measures, units, and weight (edible part unless footnotes indicate otherwise)	Water	Food energy	Protein	Fat	rated (total)	Oleic	Lino-leic	Carbo-hydrate	Calcium	Phos-phorus	Iron	Potas-sium	Vitamin A value	Thiamin	Ribo-flavin	Niacin	Ascorbic acid
(A)	(B)	(C) Per-cent	(D) Cal-ories	(E) Grams	(F) Grams	(G) Grams	(H) Grams	(I) Grams	(J) Grams	(K) Milli-grams	(L) Milli-grams	(M) Milli-grams	(N) Milli-grams	(O) Inter-national units	(P) Milli-grams	(Q) Milli-grams	(R) Milli-grams	(S) Milli-grams
		Grams																
	MISCELLANEOUS ITEMS—Con.																	
	Soups:																	
	Canned, condensed:																	
	Prepared with equal volume of milk:																	
708	Cream of chicken---- 1 cup---- 245	85	180	7	10	4.2	3.6	1.3	15	172	152	0.5	260	610	0.05	0.27	0.7	2
709	Cream of mushroom---- 1 cup---- 245	83	215	7	14	5.4	2.9	4.6	16	191	169	.5	279	250	.05	.34	.7	1
710	Tomato---- 1 cup---- 250	84	175	7	7	3.4	1.7	1.0	23	168	155	.8	418	1,200	.10	.25	1.3	15
	Prepared with equal volume of water:																	
711	Bean with pork---- 1 cup---- 250	84	170	8	6	1.2	1.8	2.4	22	63	128	2.3	395	650	.13	.08	1.0	3
712	Beef broth, bouillon, consomme 1 cup---- 240	96	30	5	0	0	0	0	3	Trace	31	.5	130	Trace	Trace	.02	1.2	—
713	Beef noodle---- 1 cup---- 240	93	65	4	3	.6	.7	.8	7	7	48	1.0	77	50	.05	.07	1.0	Trace
714	Clam chowder, Manhattan type (with tomatoes, without milk). 1 cup---- 245	92	80	2	3	.5	.4	1.3	12	34	47	1.0	184	880	.02	.02	1.0	—
715	Cream of chicken---- 1 cup---- 240	92	95	3	6	1.6	2.3	1.1	8	24	34	.5	79	410	.02	.05	.5	Trace
716	Cream of mushroom---- 1 cup---- 240	90	135	2	10	2.6	1.7	4.5	10	41	50	.5	98	70	.02	.12	.7	Trace
717	Minestrone---- 1 cup---- 245	90	105	5	3	.7	.9	1.3	14	37	59	1.0	314	2,350	.07	.05	1.0	—
718	Split pea---- 1 cup---- 245	85	145	9	3	1.1	1.2	.4	21	29	149	1.5	270	440	.25	.15	1.5	1
719	Tomato---- 1 cup---- 245	91	90	2	3	.5	.5	1.0	16	15	34	.7	230	1,000	.05	.05	1.2	12
720	Vegetable beef---- 1 cup---- 245	92	80	5	2	—	—	—	10	12	49	.7	162	2,700	.05	.05	1.0	—
721	Vegetarian---- 1 cup---- 245	92	80	2	2	—	—	—	13	20	39	1.0	172	2,940	.05	.05	1.0	—
	Dehydrated:																	
722	Bouillon cube, 1/2 in---- 1 cube---- 4	4	5	1	Trace	—	—	—	Trace	—	—	—	4	—	—	—	—	—
	Mixes:																	
	Unprepared:																	
723	Onion---- 1 1/2-oz pkg---- 43	3	150	6	5	1.1	2.3	1.0	23	42	49	.6	238	30	.05	.03	.3	6
	Prepared with water:																	
724	Chicken noodle---- 1 cup---- 240	95	55	2	1	—	—	—	8	7	19	.2	19	50	.07	.05	.5	Trace
725	Onion---- 1 cup---- 240	96	35	1	1	—	—	—	6	10	12	.2	58	Trace	Trace	Trace	Trace	2
726	Tomato vegetable with noodles. 1 cup---- 240	93	65	1	1	—	—	—	12	7	19	.2	29	480	.05	.02	.5	5
727	Vinegar, cider---- 1 tbsp---- 15	94	Trace	Trace	0	0	0	0	1	1	1	.1	15	—	—	—	—	—
728	White sauce, medium, with enriched flour. 1 cup---- 250	73	405	10	31	19.3	7.8	.8	22	288	233	.5	348	1,150	.12	.43	.7	2
	Yeast:																	
729	Baker's, dry, active---- 1 pkg---- 7	5	20	3	Trace	—	—	—	3	3	90	1.1	140	Trace	.16	.38	2.6	Trace
730	Brewer's, dry---- 1 tbsp---- 8	5	25	3	Trace	—	—	—	3	[70]17	140	1.4	152	Trace	1.25	.34	3.0	Trace

[70]Value may vary from 6 to 60 mg.

Source: *Nutritive Values of Foods*, United States Department of Agriculture, Home and Garden Bulletin No. 72.

APPENDIX B   ADMINISTRATION OF MEDICATION

The administration of medicine to young children is a responsibility that should always be taken seriously. Explicit policies and procedures pertaining to the administration of both prescription and nonprescription medication, including ointments and creams, eye, ear and nose drops, cough syrups, baby aspirin, vitamins or other tablets should be carefully developed for the protection of staff members and to safeguard the child. Descriptions of these policies and procedures should be in writing, familiar to all staff members, and filed in an accessible location.

Part-day care arrangements allow greater flexibility for parents to adjust medication schedules and administer prescribed medications at times when the child is at home. However, this option is not feasible for children enrolled in full-day care settings. In these instances parents will need to make prior arrangements with child care providers to administer prescribed medication in their absence.

Medication should never be administered by a care provider without the written consent of the child's parent and written direction of a licensed physician. The label on a prescription drug is an acceptable directive from the physician. In the case of nonprescription medicines, the parent should obtain a written note from the physician stating the child's name, the medication to be given, the dose, frequency it is to be administered and any special precautions that may be necessary. It is the professional and legal responsibility of the physician to determine the type and the exact amount of medication that is appropriate for an individual child.

Some additional points to remember include:

1. Be honest when giving young children medication! Do not use force or attempt to trick children into believing that medicines are candy. Instead, use the opportunity to help children understand the relationship between taking a medication and recovering from an illness or infection. Also, acknowledge the fact that the taste of a medicine may be disagreeable or a treatment may be somewhat unpleasant; offer a small sip of juice or cracker to eliminate an unpleasant taste or to read a favorite story as a reward for cooperating.

2. In care centers, designate one individual to be personally responsible for accepting medication from parents and administering it to children; this could be the director or the head teacher. This step will help minimize the opportunity for errors, such as omitting a dose or giving a dose twice.

3. When medication is accepted from a parent, it should be in the original container, labelled with the child's name, name of the drug and with directions for the exact amount and frequency the medication is to be given. NEVER give medicine from a container that has been prescribed for another individual.

4. Store all medicines in a locked cabinet. If it is necessary to refrigerate a particular medicine, place it in a locked box and store on a shelf in the refrigerator.

5. Be cautious during the process of administering medications to children. Concentrate on what you are doing and do not talk with anyone until you are finished.
   a. Read the label on the bottle or container three times:
      - when removing it from the locked cabinet
      - before pouring it from the container
      - after pouring it from the container

    b. Only give the *exact* amount of medication that is ordered and on time.

    c. Be sure you have the correct child! If the child is old enough to talk, ask ''What is your name?'' and let the child state his/her name.

6. Record and maintain a permanent record of each dose of medicine that is administered. Include the:

- date and time the medicine was given

- name of the care provider administering the medication

- dose of medication given

- any unusual physical changes or behaviors observed after the medicine was administered.

7. At the end of the session, inform the parent of the time and dose(s) of medication given and if anything unusual occurred.

ADMINISTRATION OF MEDICATION FORM

Child's name ⎯⎯⎯⎯⎯⎯⎯⎯⎯⎯⎯⎯⎯⎯⎯⎯⎯⎯⎯⎯⎯

Prescription Number ⎯⎯⎯⎯⎯⎯⎯⎯⎯⎯⎯⎯⎯⎯⎯⎯⎯

Date of Prescription ⎯⎯⎯⎯⎯⎯⎯⎯⎯⎯⎯⎯⎯⎯⎯⎯⎯

Doctor prescribing medicine ⎯⎯⎯⎯⎯⎯⎯⎯⎯⎯⎯⎯⎯⎯

Medication being given for ⎯⎯⎯⎯⎯⎯⎯⎯⎯⎯⎯⎯⎯⎯⎯

Time medication is to be given by staff ⎯⎯⎯⎯⎯⎯⎯⎯⎯

Time medication last given by parent ⎯⎯⎯⎯⎯⎯⎯⎯⎯⎯

Amount to be given at each time (dosage) ⎯⎯⎯⎯⎯⎯⎯⎯

· ·

I, ⎯⎯⎯⎯⎯⎯⎯⎯⎯⎯⎯⎯⎯⎯⎯⎯ give my permission for the staff to administer the above prescription medication (according to the above guidelines) to
⎯⎯⎯⎯⎯⎯⎯⎯⎯⎯⎯⎯⎯. I understand that the staff cannot be
       (child's name)
held responsible for allergic reactions or other complications resulting from administration of
the above medication given according to the directions.

signed ⎯⎯⎯⎯⎯⎯⎯⎯⎯⎯⎯⎯⎯⎯⎯
              (parent or guardian)

date ⎯⎯⎯⎯⎯⎯⎯⎯⎯⎯⎯⎯⎯⎯⎯⎯

· ·

Staff Record

Staff accepting medication and form ⎯⎯⎯⎯⎯⎯⎯⎯⎯⎯⎯

Is drug in original bottle, or in other container? ⎯⎯⎯⎯⎯⎯⎯

Is original label intact? ⎯⎯⎯⎯⎯⎯⎯⎯⎯⎯⎯⎯⎯⎯⎯

Is there written permission from the doctor attached (or the original prescription)? ⎯⎯⎯⎯

signature of accepting staff ⎯⎯⎯⎯⎯⎯⎯⎯⎯⎯⎯⎯⎯

· ·

Administration Record

DATE	TIME	AMOUNT GIVEN	STAFF ADMINISTERING	INITIAL

APPENDIX C   GROWTH CHARTS
FOR BOYS AND GIRLS

Source: National Center for Health Statistics, United States Department of Health, Education, and Welfare.

LENGTH BY AGE PERCENTILES FOR GIRLS AGED BIRTH-36 MONTHS

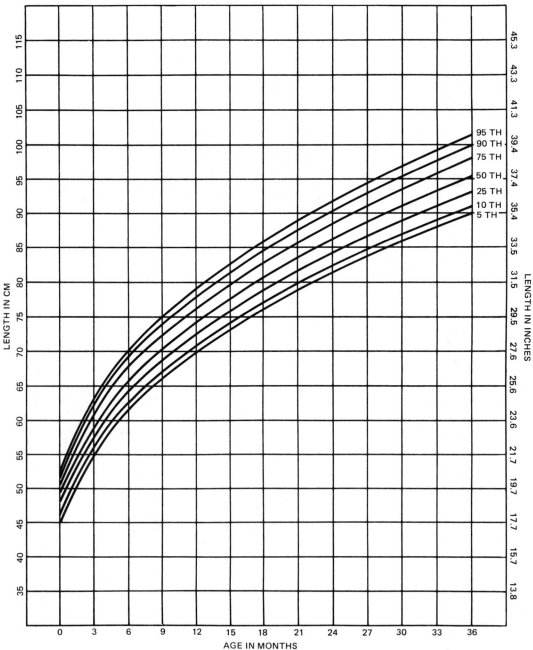

LENGTH BY AGE PERCENTILES FOR BOYS AGED BIRTH-36 MONTHS

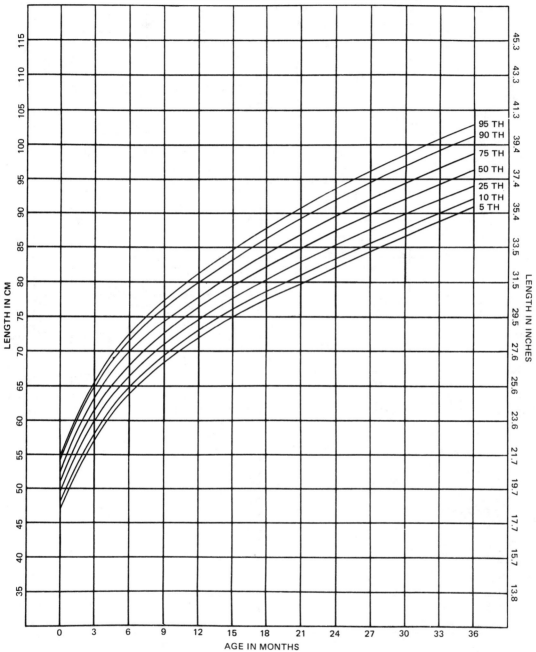

WEIGHT BY AGE PERCENTILES FOR GIRLS AGED BIRTH-36 MONTHS

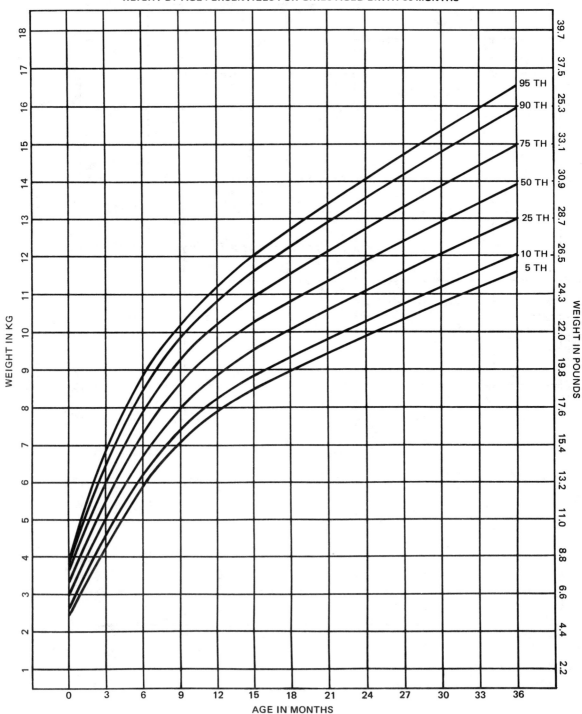

WEIGHT BY AGE PERCENTILES FOR BOYS AGED BIRTH-36 MONTHS

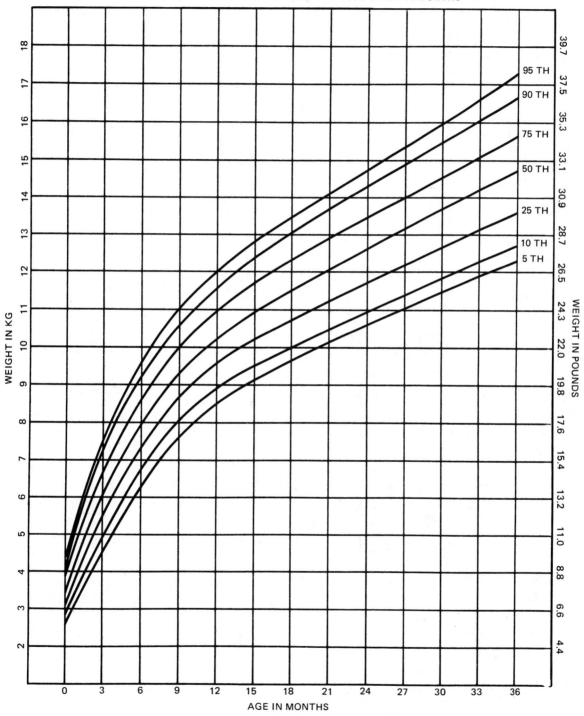

WEIGHT BY AGE PERCENTILES FOR GIRLS AGED 2 TO 18 YEARS

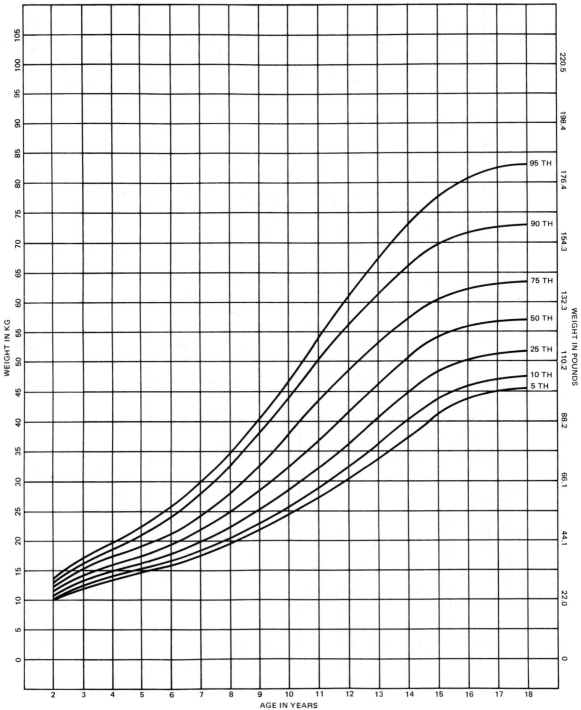

WEIGHT BY AGE PERCENTILES FOR BOYS AGED 2 TO 18 YEARS

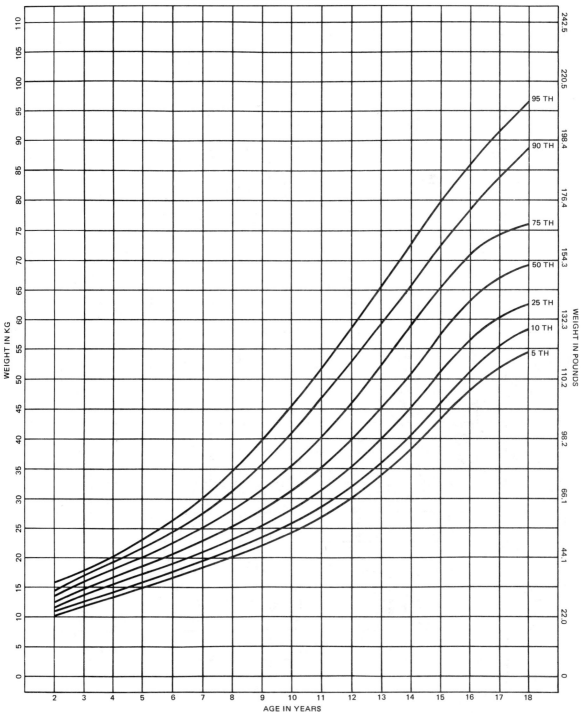

STATURE BY AGE PERCENTILES FOR GIRLS AGED 2 TO 18 YEARS

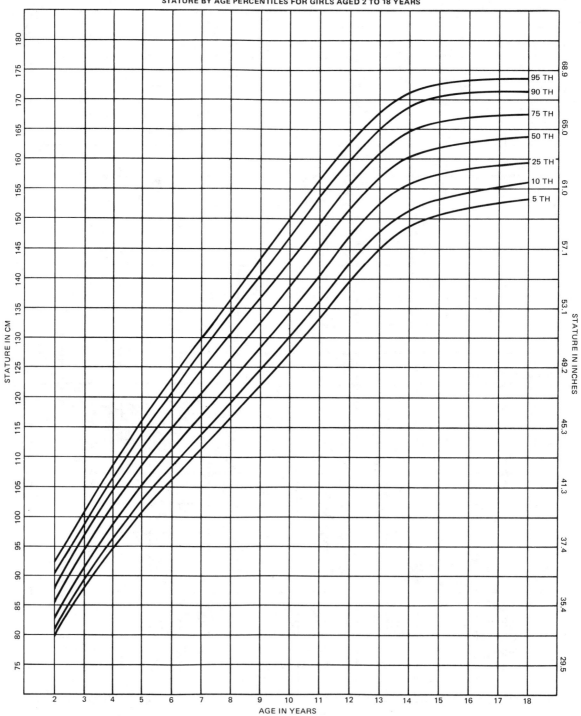

STATURE BY AGE PERCENTILES FOR BOYS AGED 2 TO 18 YEARS

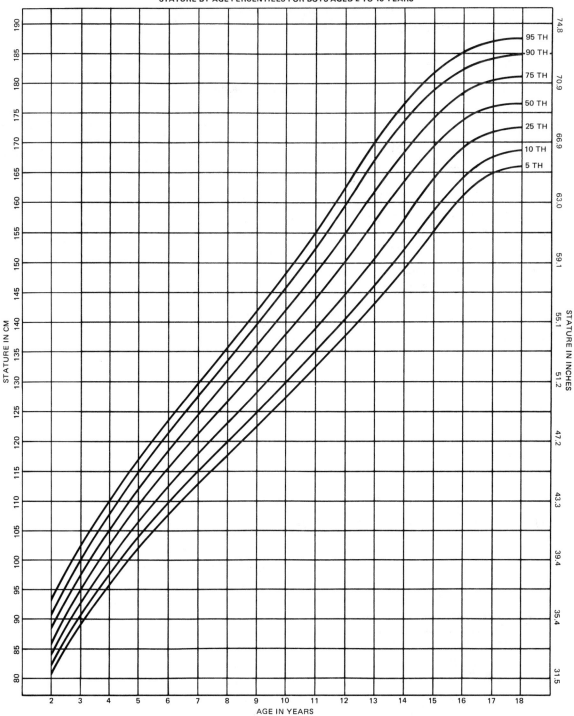

APPENDIX D   ADDITIONAL LESSON PLANS FOR NUTRITION EDUCATION ACTIVITIES

FOOD ACTIVITY (TITLE): **BUILDING A FOOD SHIELD**

DATE:_____ LENGTH OF TIME REQUIRED:10–15 minutes

TYPE OF GROUP: Individual_____ Small___x___ Large_____

NUTRITIONAL CONCEPTS TO BE REINFORCED:
Nutrition is how the body uses food. ___x___
Many kinds of food contribute to a balanced diet. _____
Food must be safe to be healthful. _____
Food handling influences the nutrients in food. _____

OBJECTIVES OF ACTIVITY (Reasons for choosing activity):
1. Children explore the various reasons for choosing foods.
2. Children learn that factors other than nutrition enter into food choices.

Motor Skills Involved:	mixing	dipping	pouring
	beating	peeling	spreading
	grinding	(measuring)	(cutting)
	grating	rolling	other _____

Sensory Experiences:	smelling	feeling	tasting
	(seeing)	hearing	

Related Concepts/Developmental Areas: Language: descriptions of feelings (happy, sad). Cognitive: introduction to "healthy" foods.

MATERIALS/EQUIPMENT:
1. Pieces of cardboard (pizza liners)
2. Scissors
3. Paste
4. Magazines
5. Pictures of shields and coats of arms

SETTING FOR ACTIVITY:
Child care center or small group with 2–3 children

PRE-LESSON PREPARATION NEEDED: ___x___yes _____no
Describe. Read stories about medieval times (armor, shields for protection).

PROCEDURE (step-by-step):
1. Divide cardboard into 4 parts.
2. Cut out and paste or draw in each section:
    food eaten when happy
    favorite food
    food for celebrations
    a "healthy" food

CAUTIONS:

DISCUSSION QUESTIONS/OPPORTUNITIES FOR EXTENDING LEARNING EXPERIENCE:

What is a shield? How does it protect us? Can foods protect us?
How do you think foods can protect us? Can foods make us feel happy?
Can foods that make us feel happy also protect us? How?
What is a "healthy" food? What makes a food "healthy"?

EVALUATION AND COMMENTS:

Children are able to describe their feelings and begin to relate them to some of their food choices.

SUGGESTIONS FOR FOLLOW-UP ACTIVITIES:

Further exploration of "healthy" foods through snack preparation.

FOOD ACTIVITY (TITLE): **WATCH ME GROW**

DATE: _____ LENGTH OF TIME REQUIRED: 10–15 minutes

TYPE OF GROUP: Individual_____ Small_____ Large___x___

NUTRITIONAL CONCEPTS TO BE REINFORCED:

Nutrition is how the body uses food. ___x___
Many kinds of food contribute to a balanced diet. _____
Food must be safe to be healthful. _____
Food handling influences the nutrients in food. _____

OBJECTIVES OF ACTIVITY (Reasons for choosing activity):

1. Children compare present size to that of infants.
2. Children discuss foods which produced changes in size.

Motor Skills Involved: mixing   dipping   pouring
                        beating   peeling   spreading
                        grinding   (measuring) cutting
                        grating   rolling   other _____

Sensory Experiences: smelling   feeling   tasting
                       (seeing)   (hearing)

Related Concepts/Developmental Areas: Language: comparison of sizes (small/large), types of food eaten by infants and older children.

MATERIALS/EQUIPMENT:

Each child bring:
   item of baby clothing
   item of clothing currently worn

SETTING FOR ACTIVITY:

Classroom, children on rug squares in circle.

PRE-LESSON PREPARATION NEEDED: ___x___yes   _____no

Describe. Prepare nursing bottle (or doll's bottle). Either use sample of that day's snack or use discussion as introduction to snack.

PROCEDURE (step-by-step):
1. Sit in circle.
2. Place current clothing on floor.
3. Place baby clothing on top of current clothing.
4. Compare and discuss differences in sizes.

CAUTIONS:

DISCUSSION QUESTIONS/OPPORTUNITIES FOR EXTENDING LEARNING EXPERIENCE:

What did you eat when you wore the baby clothing? Did you learn to eat other foods? Did you grow larger when you ate other foods in addition to milk?

EVALUATION AND COMMENTS:

Children should learn that variety in food contributes to growth by comparing foods eaten by infants to that eaten by young children.

SUGGESTIONS FOR FOLLOW-UP ACTIVITIES:

Have a mother bring her infant to the classroom.
Have the mother feed the infant.

FOOD ACTIVITY (TITLE): **SOME SEEDS ARE GOOD TO EAT**

DATE:_____ LENGTH OF TIME REQUIRED: 30 minutes

TYPE OF GROUP: Individual_____   Small_____   Large___x___

NUTRITIONAL CONCEPTS TO BE REINFORCED:

Nutrition is how the body uses food. _____
Many kinds of food contribute to a balanced diet. ___x___
Food must be safe to be healthful. _____
Food handling influences the nutrients in food. _____

OBJECTIVES OF ACTIVITY (Reasons for choosing activity):
1. The children will discover that some seeds are delicious.

Motor Skills Involved: mixing (dipping) pouring
beating peeling spreading
grinding measuring (cutting)
grating rolling other _____

Sensory Experiences: (smelling) (feeling) (tasting)
(seeing) hearing

Related Concepts/Developmental Areas: Math: counting seeds. Language: description of hard, soft, size, color, slick. Social: taking turns scooping out seeds. Cognitive: how to remove pulp from seeds.

MATERIALS/EQUIPMENT:
1. Pumpkin(s)
2. Large spoon(s)

3. Cookie sheet
4. Oven (or toaster oven) or electric skillet.

SETTING FOR ACTIVITY:
Classroom or kitchen (may want to use kitchen oven to roast seeds)

PRE-LESSON PREPARATION NEEDED: ____x____yes   _____no
Describe. Remove top from pumpkin(s).

PROCEDURE (step-by-step):
1. Wash hands.
2. Have children take turns scooping seeds from the pumpkin.
3. Place seeds in colander and rinse.
4. Spread seeds on cookie sheet.
5. Sprinkle lightly with corn oil.
6. Roast seeds in 350°F oven for 30 minutes.
7. Sprinkle lightly with salt.

CAUTIONS:
Instruction on use of knife (if children cut top from pumpkin). Place electric skillet on table next to wall to prevent children from tripping over cord.

DISCUSSION QUESTIONS/OPPORTUNITIES FOR EXTENDING LEARNING EXPERIENCE:
Are seeds useful? What can we do with seeds? What other seeds have you eaten?

EVALUATION AND COMMENTS:
Children taste the roasted seeds.

SUGGESTIONS FOR FOLLOW-UP ACTIVITIES:
Carve Jack-O-Lantern from pumpkin.
Make pumpkin bread for snack from pumpkin meat.

FOOD ACTIVITY (TITLE): **INTRODUCING SQUASH**

DATE:_____ LENGTH OF TIME REQUIRED: 8–10 minutes

TYPE OF GROUP: Individual_____   Small_____   Large____x____

NUTRITIONAL CONCEPTS TO BE REINFORCED:
Nutrition is how the body uses food. _____
Many kinds of food contribute to a balanced diet.____x____
Food must be safe to be healthful. ____x____
Food handling influences the nutrients in food. _____

OBJECTIVES OF ACTIVITY (Reasons for choosing activity):
1. To introduce a less familiar vegetable.

Motor Skills Involved: mixing   dipping   pouring
                         beating   peeling   spreading
                         grinding   measuring   (cutting)
                         grating   rolling   other spooning

Sensory Experiences: (smelling)   (feeling)   (tasting)
(seeing)   (hearing)

Related Concepts/Developmental Areas: Language: comparisons of size, shape, color. Social skills: cooperation with class members. Cognitive skills: how food can be prepared.

MATERIALS/EQUIPMENT:

1. Summer squash
2. Winter squash
3. Spaghetti squash
4. Cutting board
5. Sharp knife
6. Bowls
7. Spoons
8. Plate

SETTING FOR ACTIVITY: Classroom or child care center

PRE-LESSON PREPARATION NEEDED: ____x____yes   _____ no
Describe. Assemble equipment and materials.

PROCEDURE (step-by-step):

1. Wash hands.
2. Show varieties of squash.
3. Ask children to name varieties.
4. Ask children what they think squash looks like inside.
5. Pass squashes around for children to examine.
6. Teacher cuts squashes in half.
7. Spoon out seeds; save some for planting.
8. Have squash prepared for lunch.

CAUTIONS:
If children cut squash, review the proper use of the knife:
Use cutting board.
One hand should grip knife handle tightly.
Cut with knife away from body.
Keep other hand on top of knife.

DISCUSSION QUESTIONS/OPPORTUNITIES FOR EXTENDING LEARNING EXPERIENCE:
What color are squashes?
What does squash look like inside?
What part is eaten?
How do squash grow?
How are the various types of squash different from each other? How are they the same?

EVALUATION AND COMMENTS:
Children should identify this vegetable as squash.
Children should taste some of the squash that is prepared.

SUGGESTIONS FOR FOLLOW-UP ACTIVITIES:
Plant seeds and observe growth.
Save some seeds to put outside in winter for birds and squirrels.

FOOD ACTIVITY (TITLE): **WHAT IS FOOD? WHAT IS NOT?**

DATE:_____ LENGTH OF TIME REQUIRED: 5–10 minutes

TYPE OF GROUP: Individual_____   Small_____   Large___x___

NUTRITIONAL CONCEPTS TO BE REINFORCED:
   Nutrition is how the body uses food. _____
   Many kinds of food contribute to a balanced diet. _____
   Food must be safe to be healthful. ___x___
   Food handling influences the nutrients in food. _____

OBJECTIVES OF ACTIVITY (Reasons for choosing activity):
   1. Children will discriminate between food and nonfood items.
   2. Children will learn that only food items should be eaten.

Motor Skills Involved: mixing   dipping   pouring
                        beating   peeling   spreading
                        grinding   measuring   cutting
                        grating   rolling   other _____

Sensory Experiences: smelling   feeling   tasting
                       (seeing)   hearing

Related Concepts/Developmental Areas: Cognitive: recognition of food items. Language: names of food items. Self-help: appropriate uses for nonfood items.

MATERIALS/EQUIPMENT:
   1. Series of sets of 3–4 pictures or drawings
   2. 3 food items and 1 nonfood item in each series.

SETTING FOR ACTIVITY:
   Large group—circle

PRE-LESSON PREPARATION NEEDED: ___x___ yes   _____ no
   Describe. Draw or use magazine pictures for each set of food/nonfood items.

PROCEDURE (step-by-step):
   1. Show each set of 4 pictures.   3. Which ones are foods?
   2. Discuss what each item is.   4. Which ones are not?

CAUTIONS:
   Stress that nonfood items should never be put in the mouth.
   Point out positive uses for nonfood items.

DISCUSSION QUESTIONS/OPPORTUNITIES FOR EXTENDING LEARNING EXPERIENCE:
   Which of these pictures are foods? Which ones can you eat?
   What are the names of the foods? What do we do with the (nonfood item)?

EVALUATION AND COMMENTS:
   Children can name foods from each set of pictures and can discriminate foods from nonfoods.

SUGGESTIONS FOR FOLLOW-UP ACTIVITIES:
   Repeat activity with another set of foods and nonfoods.

FOOD ACTIVITY (TITLE): **STONE SOUP**

DATE:_____ LENGTH OF TIME REQUIRED: varies

TYPE OF GROUP: Individual_____ Small_____ Large___x___

NUTRITIONAL CONCEPTS TO BE REINFORCED:
Nutrition is how the body uses food. _____
Many kinds of food contribute to a balanced diet. ___x___
Food must be safe to be healthful. _____
Food handling influences the nutrients in food. ___x___

OBJECTIVES OF ACTIVITY (Reasons for choosing activity):
1. Children observe changes that occur when vegetables are cooked.
2. Children learn that many vegetables contribute to good soup.
3. This is an opportunity to share with class members (maybe parents).

Motor Skills Involved: mixing   dipping   (pouring)
                        beating   (peeling)   spreading
                        grinding   (measuring)   (cutting)
                        grating   rolling   other _____

Sensory Experiences: (smelling)   feeling   (tasting)
                       (seeing)   hearing

Related Concepts/Developmental Areas: Language: discussion of favorite terms such as crunchy, leafy, soft, hard; shapes/sizes/colors. Social: acceptance of other children's favorites, cooperation with others in group; interaction with other adults (especially if parents are invited). Cognitive: measuring, counting, changes brought about from heating.

MATERIALS/EQUIPMENT:
1. Vegetables brought by children   6. Colander
2. Salt   7. Large soup kettle
3. Pepper
4. Beef bouillon (or soup bone)
5. Paring knives and/or peelers

SETTING FOR ACTIVITY:
Kitchen

PRE-LESSON PREPARATION NEEDED: ___x___ yes   _____ no
Describe. Send notes home requesting each child bring his/her favorite vegetable for soup pot. Send invitations if parents are to be invited to share soup.

PROCEDURE (step-by-step):
1. Read *Stone Soup* by Marilyn Brown.   7. Cook until vegetables are tender.
2. Wash vegetables.   8. Season lightly with salt and pepper.
3. Peel vegetables.   9. Serve and enjoy.
4. Cut vegetables into pieces.
5. Heat 2 quarts of water.
6. Have each child drop vegetables
   into water.

CAUTIONS:
    Adults heat water and cook the soup.
    Carefully supervise children's use of knives and/or peelers.

DISCUSSION QUESTIONS/OPPORTUNITIES FOR EXTENDING LEARNING EXPERIENCE:
    How did cooking change the vegetables? texture? flavor? color? aroma?
    Did you taste any vegetable you had never tasted before?
    Is your favorite vegetable the same as your friend's favorite?

EVALUATION AND COMMENTS:
    Children participate in preparation of and taste the soup.

SUGGESTIONS FOR FOLLOW-UP ACTIVITIES:
    Teach the children the song, *Beautiful Soup,* by Lewis Carroll.
    This is a fun lunch to invite the parents to share. Make it a sharing party.

FOOD ACTIVITY (TITLE): **MAKING PEANUT BUTTER**

DATE:_____ LENGTH OF TIME REQUIRED: 10–15 minutes

TYPE OF GROUP: Individual_____   Small___x___   Large_____

NUTRITIONAL CONCEPTS TO BE REINFORCED:
    Nutrition is how the body uses food. _____
    Many kinds of food contribute to a balanced diet. _____
    Food must be safe to be healthful. _____
    Food handling influences the nutrients in food. ___x___

OBJECTIVES OF ACTIVITY (Reasons for choosing activity):
    1. Children can observe the change that occurs when peanuts are ground into peanut
       butter.

    Motor Skills Involved: mixing   dipping   pouring
                            beating   peeling   (spreading)
                            (grinding)   (measuring)   cutting
                            grating   rolling   other *shelling peanuts

    Sensory Experiences: (smelling)   feeling   (tasting)
                            (seeing)   (hearing)

    Related Concepts/Developmental Areas: Language: description of changes. Creativity: other uses for peanut butter. Social: taking turns.

MATERIALS/EQUIPMENT:
    1. Peanuts (roasted in shells)   6. Bowl
    2. Corn oil   7. Spoons
    3. Bread, crackers, or celery   8. Spreaders/blunt knives
    4. Small plates
    5. Blender (may use grinder)

SETTING FOR ACTIVITY:
   Kitchen or Center (blender on table next to wall)

PRE-LESSON PREPARATION NEEDED: ___x___ yes _____ no
   Describe.* Shell peanuts (may let children do it with supervision).

PROCEDURE (step-by-step):
   1. Put 1½ tablespoons corn oil in
      blender.
   2. Add about 1 cup of shelled peanuts.
   3. Blend peanuts and corn oil.
   4. Spread peanut butter on bread,
      crackers, or celery.

CAUTIONS:
   Adult operates blender. (If using hand grinder, children often enjoy turning the handle
   and may safely do so with instruction and supervision.)
   Check for allergies to nuts!

DISCUSSION QUESTIONS/OPPORTUNITIES FOR EXTENDING LEARNING
EXPERIENCE:
   Is this peanut butter like that we buy in the store? How is it the same? How is it
   different? Let some of the peanut butter stand for a period of time. What happens?
   Why?

EVALUATION AND COMMENTS:
   Children can describe differences between peanuts and peanut butter.
   Children have fun.
   Children realize that a common food can be homemade.

SUGGESTIONS FOR FOLLOW-UP ACTIVITIES:
   Sing "Found a Peanut" with this activity.
   Crush peanut shells for art projects.

APPENDIX E   SOURCES OF FREE AND INEXPENSIVE MATERIALS RELATED TO HEALTH, SAFETY, AND NUTRITION

Abbott Laboratories
14th and Sheridan Road
North Chicago, IL 60064
(pharmacy, nutrition, and drugs)

Aetna Life and Casualty Companies
Information and Public Relations
    Department
151 Farmington Avenue
Hartford, CT 06115
(health and safety)

Alexander Graham Bell Association for
    the Deaf, Inc.
The Volta Bureau for the Deaf
3417 Volta Place, NW
Washington, DC 20007

Allergy Foundation of America
801 Second Avenue
New York, NY 10017

Allstate Insurance Company
F–3
Northbrook, IL 60062

American Academy of Pediatrics
P.O. Box 1034
Evanston, IL 60204

American Association for Health,
    Physical Education and Recreation
1201 16th Street, NW
Washington, DC 20006
(school health, physical education and
    recreation)

American Association for Maternal and
    Child Health
116 South Michigan Avenue
Chicago, IL 60603

American Association on Mental
    Deficiency
5201 Connecticut Avenue, NW
Washington, DC 20015

American Automobile Association
1712 F Street, NW
Washington, DC 20006
(highway and pedestrian safety)

American Cancer Society, Inc.
219 East 42nd Street
New York, NY 10017

American Dental Association
Bureau of Dental Health Education
211 East Chicago Avenue
Chicago, IL 60611
(dental health)

American Diabetes Association, Inc.
2 Park Avenue
New York, NY 10016
(diabetes information)

American Dietetic Association
430 North Michigan Avenue
Chicago, IL 60611
(nutrition and diet)

American Dry Milk Institute, Inc.
130 North Franklin Street
Chicago, IL 60601
(nutrition)

American Fire Insurance Companies
Engineering Department
80 Maiden Lane
New York, NY 10007
(safety)

American Foundation for the Blind
15 West 16th Street
New York, NY 10011

American Hearing Society
919 18th Street, NW
Washington, DC 20006

American Heart Association
Inquiries Section
7320 Greenville Avenue
Dallas, TX 75231

American Hospital Association
840 North Lake Shore Drive
Chicago, IL 60611
(hospital care)

American Institute of Baking
Consumer Service Department
400 East Ontario Street
Chicago, IL 60611
(nutrition)

American Institute of Family Relations
5287 Sunset Boulevard
Los Angeles, CA 90027
(family living and mental health)

American Lung Association
1740 Broadway
New York, NY 10019

American Medical Association
Department of Community Health and
  Health Education
535 North Dearborn Street
Chicago, IL 60610
(health, safety and poison education)

American National Red Cross
17th and D Streets
Washington, DC 20006
(contact local chapter first)
(first aid, safety and nutrition)

American Optometric Association
Department of Public Information
243 North Lindbergh Boulevard
St. Louis, MO 63141
(eye health)

American Podiatry Association
3301 16th Street, NW
Washington, DC 20010
(foot health)

American Printing House for the Blind
P.O. Box 6085
Louisville, KY 40206

American Public Health Association
1015 Fifteenth Street, NW
Washington, DC 20005

American Social Health Association
1790 Broadway
New York, NY 10019
(sex education)

American Speech and Hearing
  Association
9030 Old Georgetown Road
Washington, DC 20014

The Arthritis Foundation
10 Columbus Circle
New York, NY 10019

Association for Children with Learning
  Disabilities
2200 Brownsville Road
Pittsburgh, PA 15210

Association for Education of the Visually
  Handicapped
1604 Spruce Street
Philadelphia, PA 19103

Association for Family Living
32 West Randolph, Suite 1818
Chicago, IL 60601
(family health)

Association for the Aid of Crippled
  Children
345 East 46th Street
New York, NY 10017

Association for the Visually Handicapped
1839 Frankfort Avenue
Louisville, KY 40206

Association of American Railroads
School and College Service
Transportation Building
Washington, DC 20006

Association of Casualty and Surety
  Companies
Accident Prevention Department
Publications Division
60 John Street
New York, NY 10038
(safety)

Asthma and Allergy Foundation of
  America
1302 18th Street NW
Suite 303
Washington, DC 20036

Better Vision Institute, Inc.
230 Park Avenue
New York, NY 10017
(glasses and eye health)

Bicycle Institute of America
122 East 42nd Street
New York, NY 10017
(bicycle safety)

The Borden Company
Consumer Services
350 Madison Avenue
New York, NY 10017
(nutrition, weight control and health
  inventory)

Carnation Milk Company
Home Service Department
5045 Wilshire Boulevard
Los Angeles, CA 90036

Center for Sickle Cell Anemia
College of Medicine
Howard University
520 W Street, NW
Washington, DC 20001

Cereal Institute, Inc.
Home Economics Department
135 South LaSalle Street
Chicago, IL 60603
(nutrition education)

Ciba Pharmaceutical Company
556 Morris Avenue
Summit, NJ 07901
(health service)

Colgate-Palmolive Company
300 Park Avenue
New York, NY 10010
(skin care and dental health)

Committee to Combat Huntington's
  Disease
200 West 57th Street
New York, NY 10019

Consumer Information Center
Pueblo, CO 81009
(An index of selected federal
  publications)

Council for Exceptional Children
1411 Jefferson Davis Highway
Arlington, VA 22202

DelMonte Teaching Aids
P.O. Box 9075
Clinton, IA 52736

Eli Lily and Company
Public Relations Department
Box 618
Indianapolis, IN 46206

Environmental Protection Agency
401 M Street, SW
Washington, DC 20406

Epilepsy Association of America
111 West 57th Street
New York, NY 10019

Epilepsy Foundation of America
1828 L Street, NW
Washington, DC 20036

Equitable Life Assurance Society of the
  United States
Office of Community Services and
  Health Education
1285 Avenue of the Americas
New York, NY 10019

Florida Citrus Commission
Institutional and School Marketing
  Department
P.O. Box 148
Lakeland, FL 33802

Ford Motor Company
Research and Information Department
The American Road
Dearborn, MI 48127
(traffic safety and seat belts)

Foundation for Research and Education
  in Sickle Cell Disease
421–431 West 120th Street
New York, NY 10027

General Mills
Public Relations Department
Educational Services
9200 Wayzata Boulevard
Minneapolis, MN 55426
(nutrition)

Health Information Foundation
Public Relations Director
420 Lexington Avenue
New York, NY 10017

Health Insurance Council
488 Madison Avenue
New York, NY 10022
(health education)

Heart Disease Control Program
Division of Special Health Services
United States Public Health Service
Department of Health, Education and
  Welfare
Washington, DC 20025
(heart diseases and education)

Heart Information Center
National Heart Institute
United States Public Health Service
Bethesda, MD 20014
(heart diseases and heart research)

Information Center on Children's Cultures
United States Committee for UNICEF
866 United Nations Plaza
New York, NY 10017

Johnson and Johnson Health Care
   Division
New Brunswick, NJ 08903
(first aid and dental health)

Kellogg Company
Department of Consumer Education
Battle Creek, MI 49016

Joseph P. Kennedy Jr. Foundation
Suite 205
1701 K Street, NW
Washington, DC 20006
(mental retardation)

Lever Brothers Company
390 Park Avenue
New York, NY 10022
(dental health)

March of Dimes Birth Defects
   Foundation
1275 Mamaroneck Avenue
White Plains, NY 10605

Metropolitan Life Insurance Co.
School Health Bureau
Health and Welfare Division
1 Madison Avenue
New York, NY 10010
(health, safety and first aid)

Muscular Dystrophy Association of
   America, Inc.
Public Information Department
1790 Broadway
New York, NY 10019

National Academy of Sciences
National Research Council
2101 Constitution Avenue, NW
Washington, DC 20418
(food and nutrition)

National Aid to the Visually Handicapped
3201 Balboa Street
San Francisco, CA 94121

National Association for Mental
   Health, Inc.
10 Columbus Circle
New York, NY 10019
(mental health)

National Association for Retarded
   Children
2709 Avenue E, East
Arlington, TX 76011

National Association for the Education of
   Young Children
1834 Connecticut Avenue, NW
Washington, DC 20009

National Association of Hearing and
   Speech Agencies
919 18th Street, NW
Washington, DC 20006

National Board of Fire Underwriters
American Insurance Company
85 John Street
New York, NY 10038
(fire prevention education)

National Commission on Safety
   Education
National Education Association
1201 16th Street, NW
Washington, DC 20036
(safety education)

National Congress of Parents and
   Teachers
700 North Rush Street
Chicago, IL 60611
(child health and safety)

National Council for Homemaker-Home
   Health Aide Services, Inc.
1740 Broadway
New York, NY 10019

National Council on Family Relations
1219 University Avenue, SE
Minneapolis, MN 55414
(teacher's kit on family living, $2.50)

National Cystic Fibrosis Foundation
3379 Peachtree Road, NE
Atlanta, GA 30326

National Dairy Council
6300 North River Road
Rosemont, IL 60018–4233
(nutrition and health education)

National Easter Seal Foundation for
   Crippled Children and Adults
2023 West Ogden Avenue
Chicago, IL 60612

National Epilepsy League
203 North Wabash Avenue
Chicago, IL 60610
(epilepsy)

National Fire Protection Association
Public Relations Department
60 Batterymarch Street
Boston, MA 02110
(fire prevention and education)

National Foundation
Division of Scientific and Health
   Information
800 Second Avenue
New York, NY 10017
(poliomyelitis, arthritis, birth defects and
   disorders of the central nervous
   system)

National Health Council
1790 Broadway
New York, NY 10019
(health education)

National Hemophilia Foundation
25 West 39th Street
New York, NY 10018

National Institute of Health
U.S. Public Health Service
Bethesda, MD 20014
   1. Allergy and Infectious Diseases
   2. Arthritis and Metabolic Diseases
   3. Cancer
   4. Child Health and Human
      Development
   5. Dental Research
   6. General Medical Sciences
   7. Heart
   8. Mental Health
   9. Neurological Diseases and
      Blindness
      (arthritis, metabolic diseases,
      dental, mental health, blindness,
      child health, medical, microbiologic
      data)

National Kidney Foundation
342 Madison Avenue
New York, NY 10017
(kidney diseases)

National Live Stock and Meat Board
36 South Wabash Avenue
Nutritional Department
Chicago, IL 60603
(nutrition)

National Multiple Sclerosis Society
257 Fourth Avenue
New York, NY 10010

National Nephrosis Foundation, Inc.
143 East 35th Street
New York, NY 10016
(kidney disease)

National Paraplegia Foundation
333 North Michigan Avenue
Chicago, IL 60601

National Safety Council
444 North Michigan Avenue
Chicago, IL 60611
(safety materials, films, posters)

National Society for the Prevention of
   Blindness
16 East 40th Street
New York, NY 10016
(eye health and safety)

National Tuberculosis and Respiratory
   Disease Association
1790 Broadway
New York, NY 10019
(tuberculosis, respiratory diseases)

National Wildlife Federation
Educational Services Section
1412 Sixteenth Street, NW
Washington, DC 20036
(air/water pollution, energy)

Nationwide Insurance
Safety Department
246 North High Street
Columbus, OH 43216
(traffic and child safety)

Nutrition Foundation, Inc.
888 Seventeenth Street, NW
Washington, DC 20036
(nutrition education)

Office of Child Development
U.S. Department of Health and Human
   Services
P.O. Box 1182
Washington, DC 20013

Office of Civil Defense/Emergency
   Preparedness
Public Information
The Pentagon
Washington, DC 20310

Personal Products Corporation
Education Department
Milltown, NJ 08850
(cleanliness)

Pet Milk Company
Director of Home Economics
400 South Fourth Street
St. Louis, MO 63101

Pied Piper Shoe Company
Box 118
Wausau, WI 54402
(foot health)

The Pillsbury Company
1177 Pillsbury Building
608 Second Avenue, South
Minneapolis, MN 55402
(nutrition education)

Prudential Insurance Company of
    America
Education Department
P.O. Box 36
Newark, NJ 07101

Public Affairs Pamphlets
22 East 38th Street
New York, NY 10016
(family relations, health and science)

Public Health Service
Public Inquiries Branch
United States Department of Health,
    Education and Welfare
Washington, DC 20201
(health and poison prevention)

Ross Laboratories
Director of Professional Services
625 Cleveland Avenue
Columbus, OH 43216

School Health Education Study
1507 M Street, NW, Room 800
Washington, DC 20005
(health education)

Science Research Association, Inc.
259 East Erie Street
Chicago, IL 60611
(health)

Sex Information and Education Council
    of the United States
1855 Broadway
New York, NY 10023
(sex education)

Society for Nutrition Education
1736 Franklin Street
Oakland, CA 94612

State Farm Insurance Companies
Public Relations Department
One State Farm Plaza
Bloomington, IL 61701
(first aid, safety)

The Toni Company
Merchandise Mart Plaza
Chicago, IL 60654
(grooming)

John Tracy Clinic
807 West Adams Boulevard
Los Angeles, CA 90007
(education of deaf children)

Travelers Insurance Companies
Public Information and Advertising
    Department
700 Main Street
Hartford, CT 06115
(traffic safety)

United Cerebral Palsy
369 Lexington Avenue
New York, NY 10017
(cerebral palsy)

United Cerebral Palsy Associations
66 East 34th Street
New York, NY 10016

United States Department of Agriculture
Agricultural Research Administration
Bureau of Human Nutrition and Home
    Economics
Washington, DC 20250
(nutrition)

U.S. Government Printing Office
Superintendent of Documents
Washington, DC 20402

United States Office of Education
Department of Health and Human
    Services
P.O. Box 1182
Washington, DC 20013

The Upjohn Company
Trade and Guest Relations Department
Kalamazoo, MI 49003

Wheat Flour Institute
309 West Jackson Boulevard
Chicago, IL 60606
(nutrition)

World Health Organization
Office of Public Information
525 23rd Street, NW
Washington, DC 20037
(international health)

Yankee Shoemakers
Newmarket, NH 03857
(foot health)

APPENDIX F   SOURCES AND TITLES OF NUTRITION-RELATED SONGS AND POEMS

Source	Song Titles
Bertail, I. *Complete Nursery Song Book.* New York: Lothrop, Lee, and Shepard, 1967.	*Cherries Ripe* *King Arthur* *Thanksgiving Day* *Oats, Peas, Beans* *Can You Show Me How The Farmer?* *Jolly Is The Miller*
Kapp, P. *Cock-a-Doodle-Doo! Cock-a-Doodle-Dandy!* New York: Harper and Row, 1966.	*Beautiful Soup*
Glazer, T. *On Top of Spaghetti.* Garden City, NY: Doubleday and Co., 1963.	*On Top of Spaghetti*
Larrick, N. *The Wheels of the Bus Go Round and Round.* San Carlos, CA: Golden Gate Junior Books, 1972.	*Who Stole The Cookies From The Cookie Jar?*
Boy Scouts of America	*Tarzan Of The Apes*

Source	Poem Titles
Christopher Morley	*Animal Crackers*
Katherine Edelman	*Saturday Shopping*
Aileen Fisher	*Shelling Peas*
Christina Rosetti	*Mix A Pancake*
Christina Rosetti	*Bread and Milk For Breakfast*
Christina Rosetti	*Hot Cross Buns*

GLOSSARY*

abdomen – the portion of the body located between the diaphragm (located at the base of the lungs) and the pelvic or hip bones.

absorption – the process by which the products of digestion are transferred from the intestinal tract into the blood or lymph or by which substances are taken up by the cells.

abuse – to mistreat, attack or cause harm to another individual.

accident – an unexpected or unplanned event that may result in physical harm or injury.

accreditation – the process of certifying an individual or program as having met certain specified requirements.

acuity – sharpness or clearness, as in vision.

acute – the stage of an illness or disease during which an individual is definitely sick and exhibits symptoms characteristic of the particular illness or disease involved.

alignment –the process of assuming correct posture or of placing various body parts in proper line with each other.

alkali – a group of bases or caustic substances which are capable of neutralizing acids to form salts.

allowed foods – foods which are eligible for reimbursement under School Lunch or Child Care Food Program Guidelines.

amblyopia – a condition of the eye commonly referred to as ''lazy eye''; vision gradually becomes blurred or distorted due to unequal balance of the eye muscles. The eyes do not present any physical clues when a child has amblyopia.

amino acids – the organic building blocks from which proteins are made.

anecdotal – a brief note or description that contains useful and important information.

anemia – a disorder of the blood commonly caused by a lack of iron in the diet, resulting in the formation of fewer red blood cells and lessened ability of the cells to carry oxygen. Symptoms include fatigue, shortness of breath and pallor.

anthropometric – pertains to measurement of the body or its parts.

antibodies – special substances produced by the body that help protect against disease.

appraisal – the process of judging or evaluating; to determine the quality of one's state of health.

assessment – appraisal or evaluation.

attitude – a belief or feeling one has toward certain facts or situations.

atypical – unusual; different from what might commonly be expected.

autonomy – a state of personal or self-identity.

basal metabolic rate – minimum amount of energy needed to carry on the body processes vital to life.

biochemical – pertains to chemical evaluation of body substances such as blood, urine, etc.

bonding – the process of establishing a positive and strong emotional relationship between an infant and its parent; sometimes referred to as attachment.

---

*Definitions are based on usage within the text.

bottle-mouth syndrome – a pattern of tooth decay, predominantly of the upper teeth, that develops as the result of permitting a child to go to sleep with a bottle containing juice, milk, or any other caloric liquid which may pool in the mouth.

calories – units used to measure the energy value of foods.

catalyst – a substance that speeds up the rate of a chemical reaction but is not itself used up in the reaction.

catalyze – to accelerate a chemical reaction.

characteristics – qualities or traits that distinguish one person from another.

chronic – frequent or repeated incidences of illness; can also be a lengthy or permanent status, as in chronic disease or dysfunction.

clinical – pertains to evaluation of health by means of observation.

cognitive – the aspect of learning that refers to the development of skills and abilities based on knowledge and thought processes.

collagen – a protein that forms the major constituent of connective tissue, cartilage, bone, and skin.

communicable – a condition that can be spread or transmitted from one individual to another.

complementary proteins – proteins with offsetting missing amino acids; complementary proteins can be combined to provide complete protein.

complete proteins – proteins which contain all essential amino acids in amounts relative to the amounts needed.

compliance – the act of obeying or cooperating with specific requests or requirements.

concept – a combination of basic and related factual information that represents a more generalized statement or idea.

contagious – capable of being transmitted or passed from one person to another.

contrasting sensory qualities – differing qualities pertaining to taste, color, texture, temperature, and shape.

convalescent – the stage of recovery from an illness or disease.

cost control – reduction of expenses through portion control inventory and reduction of waste.

criteria – predetermined standards used to evaluate the worth or effectiveness of a learning experience.

cycle menus – menus which are written to repeat after a set interval, such as every 3–4 weeks.

deciduous teeth – a child's initial set of teeth; this set is temporary and gradually begins to fall out around five years of age.

dehydration – a state in which there is an excessive loss of body fluids or extremely limited fluid intake. Symptoms may include loss of skin tone, sunken eyes and mental confusion.

development – commonly refers to the process of intellectual growth and change.

developmental norms – the mean or average age at which children demonstrate certain behaviors and abilities.

diagnosis – the process of identifying a disease, illness or injury from its symptoms.

digestion – the process by which complex nutrients in foods are changed into smaller units which can be absorbed or used by the body.

digestive tract – pertains to, and includes the mouth, throat, stomach and intestines.

direct contact – the passage of infectious organisms from an infected individual directly to a susceptible host through methods such as coughing, sneezing or touching.

discipline – training or enforced obedience that corrects, shapes or develops acceptable patterns of behavior.

disorientation – lack of awareness or ability to recognize familiar persons or objects.

DNA – deoxyribonucleic acid; the substance in the cell nucleus that codes for genetically transmitted traits.

elevate – to raise to a higher position.

endocrine – refers to glands within the body that produce and secrete substances called hormones directly into the blood stream.

energy – power to perform work.

enriched – adding nutrients to grain products to replace those lost during refinement; thiamin, niacin, riboflavin, and iron are nutrients most commonly added.

environment – the sum total of physical, cultural and behavioral features that surround and affect an individual.

enzymes – proteins which catalyze body functions.

essential nutrient – nutrient which must be provided in food because it cannot be synthesized by the body at a rate sufficient to meet the body's needs.

ethnic – pertaining to races or groups of people who share common traits or customs.

evaluation – a measurement of effectiveness for determining whether or not educational objectives have been achieved.

expectations – behaviors or actions that are anticipated.

failure to thrive – a term used to describe an infant whose growth and mental development is severely slowed due to lack of mothering or mental stimulation.

family nutrition programs – nutrition programs which focus on the family unit. Examples are Food Stamps, WIC, and the Food Distribution Program.

fever – an elevation of body temperature above normal; a temperature over 99.4°F or 37.4°C orally is usually considered a fever.

food-borne illnesses – food infections due to ingestion of food contaminated with bacteria, viruses, some molds, or parasites.

fruit drink – a product which contains 10 percent fruit juice, added water, and sugar.

full-strength juice – undiluted fruit or vegetable juice.

giardiasis – a parasitic infection of the intestinal tract that causes diarrhea, loss of appetite, abdominal bloating and gas, weight loss and fatigue.

gram – a metric unit of weight; approximately 1/28 of an ounce.

growth – increase in size of any body part or of the entire body.

habit – the unconscious repetition of a particular behavior.

hands-on – active involvement in a project; actually doing something.

harvesting – picking or gathering fruit or grains.

head circumference – the distance around the head obtained by measuring over the forehead and bony protuberance on the back of the head; it is an indication of normal or abnormal growth and development of the brain and central nervous system.

health – a state of wellness. Complete physical, mental, social and emotional well-being; the quality of one element affects the state of the others.

hemoglobin – the iron-containing, oxygen-carrying pigment in red blood cells.

hepatitis – an inflammation of the liver.

heredity – the transmission of certain genetic material and characteristics from parent to child at the time of conception.

hormones – special chemical substances produced by endocrine glands that influence and regulate certain body functions.

hyperactivity – a condition characterized by attention and behavior disturbances, including restlessness, impulsive and disruptive behaviors. True cases of hyperactivity respond to the administration of stimulant-type medication.

hyperopia – farsightedness; a condition of the eyes in which an individual can see objects clearly in the distant but has poor close vision.

hyperventilation – rapid breathing often with forced inhalation; can lead t sensations of dizziness, lightheadedness and weakness.

immunized – a state of becoming resistant to a specific disease through the introduction of living or dead microorganisms into the body which then stimulates the production of antibodies.

impairment – a condition or malfunction of a body part that interferes with optimal functioning.

incidental learning – learning that occurs in addition to the primary intent or goals of instruction.

incomplete proteins – proteins which lack one or more essential amino acids.

incubation – the interval of time between exposure to infection and the appearance of the first signs or symptoms of illness.

indirect contact – transfer of infectious organisms from an infected individual to a susceptible host via an intermediate source such as contaminated water, milk, toys, utensils or soiled towels.

infection – a condition that results when a pathogen invades and establishes itself within a susceptible host.

ingested – the process of taking food or other substances into the body through the mouth.

INQ – Index of Nutrient Quality, a system of expressing nutrient density; the amount of nutrients present in relation to calories.

inservice – educational training provided by an employer.

intentional – a plan of action that is carried out in a purposeful manner.

intervention – practices or procedures that are implemented to modify or change a specific behavior or condition.

intestinal – pertaining to the intestinal tract or bowel.

iron deficiency anemia – a failure in the oxygen transport system caused by too little iron.

judicious – wise; directed by sound judgment.

lactating – producing and secreting milk.

language – form of communication that allows individuals to share feelings, ideas and experiences with one another.

lethargy – a state of inaction or indifference.

liability – legal responsibility or obligation for one's actions owed to another individual.

licensing – the act of granting formal permission to conduct a business or profession.

linoleic acid – a polyunsaturated fatty acid which is essential (must be provided in food) for humans.

listlessness – a state characterized by a lack of energy and/or interest in one's affairs.

lymph glands – specialized groupings of tissue that produce and store white blood cells for protection against infection and illness.

macrocytic anemia – a failure in the oxygen transport system characterized by abnormally large immature red blood cells.

malnutrition – prolonged lack or inadequate intake of nutrients and/or calories required by the body.

mandatory – something that is required; no choices or alternatives available.

megadose – an amount of a vitamin or mineral at least ten times that of RDA.

metabolism – all chemical changes that occur from the time nutrients are absorbed until they are built into body tissue or are excreted.

microcytic anemia – a failure in the oxygen transport system characterized by abnormally small red blood cells.

microgram – a metric unit of measurement; one-millionth of a gram.

milligram – a metric unit of measurement; one-thousandth of a gram.

minerals – inorganic chemical elements that are required in the diet to support growth and repair tissue and to regulate body functions.

misarticulation – improper pronunciation of words and word sounds.

mold – a fuzzy growth produced by fungi.

mottling – marked with spots of dense white or brown coloring.

myopia – nearsightedness; an individual has good near vision, but poor distant vision.

neglect – failure of a parent or legal guardian to properly care for and meet the basic needs of a child under eighteen years of age.

negligence – failure to practice or perform one's duties according to certain standards; carelessness.

neurological – pertaining to the nervous system which consists of the nerves, brain and spinal column.

neuromuscular – pertaining to control of muscular function by the nervous system.

normal – average; a characteristic or quality that is common to most individuals in a defined group.

notarized – official acknowledgement of the authenticity of a signature or document by a notary public.

nutrient – the components or substances that are found in food.

nutrient strengths – nutrients which occur in relatively large amounts in a food or food group.

nutrient weaknesses – nutrients which are absent or occur in very small amounts in a food or food group.

nutrition education – activities which impart information about food and its use in the body.

obese – a term used to describe an individual who has an excessive accumulation of fat.

obesity – excessive body fat, usually 15–20 percent above the individual's ideal weight based on height, age and sex.

objective – a clear and meaningful description of what an individual is expected to learn as a result of learning activities and experiences.

observations – to inspect and take note of the appearance and behavior of other individuals.

odd-day cycle menus – menus planned for a period of days other than a week that repeat after the planned period; cycles of any number of days may be used. These menus are a means of avoiding repetition of the same foods on the same day of the week.

overnutrition – the result of eating too much food, especially excess calories and excess fat. Overnutrition may or may not be accompanied by deficiencies of essential nutrients.

pallor – paleness.

parallel play – a common form of play among young children in which two or more children, sitting side by side, are engaged in an activity but do not interact or work together to accomplish a task.

paralysis – temporary or permanent loss of sensation, function or voluntary movement of a body part.

pathogen – a microorganism capable of producing illness or infection.

peers – one of the same rank; equals.

personal sanitation – personal habits, such as hand washing, care of illness, cleanliness of clothing.

poverty guidelines – family-size and income standards for determining eligibility for free or reduced-price meals under the National School Lunch Program.

precipitating – factors that trigger or initiate a reaction or response.

pre-planning – outlining a method of action prior to carrying it out.

prevention – measures taken to avoid an event such as an accident or illness from occurring; implies the ability to anticipate circumstances and behaviors.

preventive – the act of taking certain steps and measures so as to avoid or delay unfavorable outcomes, as in preventive health care.

primary goal – the aim which assumes first importance.

prodromal – the appearance of the first nonspecific signs of infection; this stage ends when the symptoms characteristic of a particular communicable illness begin to appear.

PUFA – polyunsaturated fatty acids; fatty acids which contain more than one bond that is not fully saturated with hydrogen.

punishment – a negative response to what the observer considers to be wrong or inappropriate behavior; may involve physical or harsh treatment.

RDA – Recommended Daily Dietary Allowances; suggested amounts of nutrients for use in planning diets. RDAs are designed to maintain good nutrition in healthy persons. Allowances are higher than requirements in order to afford a margin of safety.

reduced-price meals – a meal served under the Child Care Food Program to a child from a family which meets income standards for reduced-price school meals.

referral – directing an individual to another source, usually for additional evaluation or treatment.

regulation – a standard or requirement that is set to insure uniform and safe practice.

reimplant – to replace a part from where it was removed, such as a tooth.

reprimand – to scold or discipline for unacceptable behavior.

resistance – the ability to avoid infection or illness.

respiratory diseases – diseases of the respiratory tract, such as colds, sore throats, flu.

respiratory tract – pertains to, and includes the nose, throat, trachea and lungs.

resuscitation – to revive from unconsciousness or death; to restore breathing and heartbeat.

retention – the ability to remember or recall previously learned material.

Reye's syndrome – an acute illness of young children that severely affects the central nervous system; symptoms include vomiting, coma and seizures.

RNA – ribonucleic acid; the nucleic acid which serves as messenger between the nucleus and the ribosomes where proteins are synthesized.

Salmonella – a bacteria which can cause serious food-borne illness.

salmonellosis – a bacterial infection that is spread through contaminated drinking water, food or milk or contact with other infected persons. Symptoms include diarrhea, fever, nausea and vomiting.

sanitizing solution – a solution of dilute chlorine bleach (¼ cup chlorine to 1 gallon of water), used to sanitize utensils and work surfaces.

scald – to rinse with boiling water.

sedentary – unusually slow or sluggish; a life-style that implies a general lack of physical activity.

seizures – a temporary interruption of consciousness sometimes accompanied by convulsive movements.

sensorimotor – Piaget's first stage of cognitive development, during which children learn and relate to their world primarily through motor and sensory activities.

serrated – saw-toothed or notched.

skeletal – pertaining to the bony framework that supports the body.

skinfold – a measurement of the amount of fat under the skin; also referred to as fat-fold measurements.

speech – the process of using words to express one's thoughts and ideas.

spina bifida – a birth defect in which incomplete formation of the body vertebrae allows a portion of the spinal cord to be exposed to the outside. Varying degrees of paralysis and lack of function are common in the portion of the body below the defect.

standardized recipe – a recipe that has been tested to produce consistent results.

Staphylococcus – a bacteria that can cause serious food-borne illnesses.

sterile –free from living microorganisms.

strabismus – a condition of the eyes in which one or both eyes appear to be turned inward (crossed) or outward (walleye).

submerge – to place in water.

supervision – watching carefully over the behaviors and actions of children and others.

susceptible host – an individual who is capable of being infected by a pathogen.

symptom – changes in the body or its functions that are experienced by the affected individual.

syndrome – a grouping of symptoms and signs that commonly occur together and are characteristic of a specific disease or illness.

synthesis – the process of making a compound by the union of simpler compounds or elements.

tax exempt – excused from taxation, often on the basis of nonprofit status.

temperature – a measurement of body heat; varies with the time of day, activity and method of measurement.

toxicity – a state of being poisonous.

tuberculosis – an infectious disease caused by the tubercle bacillus, characterized by the production of lesions.

undernutrition – an inadequate intake of one or more required or essential nutrients.

urinate – the act of emptying the bladder of urine.

values – the beliefs, traditions and customs an individual incorporates and utilizes to guide behavior and judgements.

verbal assault – to attack another individual with words.

viruses – any of a group of submicroscopic infective agents, many of which cause a number of diseases in animals and plants.

weekly menus – menus that are written to be served on a weekly basis.

whole grains – grain products which have not been refined; they contain all parts of the kernel of grain.

Index